Dr. Randine Lewis's patients and readers of *The Infertility Cure* express their gratitude and joy

"It's a healthy BOY! We are thrilled! And relieved, as everything looked good on the ultrasound. I feel like I can relax a little now and enjoy the rest of this pregnancy. It amazes me every day that I was able to conceive this baby, especially after what I was told by doctors. I thank you so much for your guidance and wisdom because if I hadn't picked up your book seven months ago, I know I probably wouldn't be carrying this life inside me now."

— L. K., Washington, DC

"Dr. Lewis was a true gift from God during my journey with infertility. I believe that the traditional Chinese medicine she administered during my IVF cycle contributed to my success of giving birth to a precious little boy. It provided the support my body needed and allowed me to relax during the procedure. I don't fully understand the magic of the medicine, but I would not consider another IVF cycle without supplementing it with acupuncture."

— Kim C., Houston, Texas

"Starting out as the biggest skeptic on TCM, I have been having treatments for nine months and am currently eleven weeks pregnant with my second IVF cycle. Dr. Lewis's knowledge of Eastern and Western medicine and her ability to understand and leverage both, as appropriate, obviously helps her success rates with her patients."

— Renee B., Seattle, Washington

"My body, mind, and soul have been greatly enhanced as a result of experiencing Dr. Lewis's program. Through her truly caring spirit she not only provided me hope (I now know that there's no such thing as 'old eggs'!), she also gave me the greatest blessing of all — the tools to attain outstanding health on every level. For this, and so much more, I am forever grateful."

— Denise N., Jupiter, Florida

"I combined Western and Eastern treatments for infertility. I know the traditional Chinese medicine treatment made the difference in the success of my IVF cycle. . . . We now have a beautiful two-week-old boy!!"

— Lisa S., Houston, Texas

"Dr. Lewis, I am not sure if you will remember me but I am an acupuncturist near Charlotte, North Carolina, and we spoke on the phone in the spring of last year. Well, long story short . . . I continued with your nutritional supplementation advice and with my TCM doc over the summer of '03 and then we decided to start the adoption process. . . . Four days later I found out that I was pregnant. Currently we are eighteen weeks and everything looks good. THANK YOU SO MUCH!"

— Marcia H., Charlotte, North Carolina

"Although my husband had low sperm count and motility, we both went to see Dr. Lewis. We were about to begin the process of our second IVF cycle with ICSI (intracytoplasmic sperm injection). We were becoming more desperate and less hopeful. The treatments were to prepare me to respond better to the medications and the entire stressful medical procedure. I felt better immediately; the most miraculous result, however, was that when my husband had his next sperm analysis, his sperm count was normal! We decided to try naturally, and realized we didn't even know when the timing was right. Dr. Lewis became our fertility counselor. I am so proud and elated to report that we are now pregnant with our first child. We have so much hope now that we will be able to have the family we had always dreamed of."

— Kei H., Houston, Texas

"I went through IVF last month and just found out that I am pregnant! We had two embryos implanted; I've had two blood tests to date — the first beta was 125 and the second was 334, so everything looks good so far. I wanted to thank you, Dr. Lewis, for giving me your treatments and recommendations, which led to my miracle. On a more personal note, you were the one who gave me the hope and belief to try one last time. We still can't believe it is true and probably won't believe it until I'm delivering. I had continued my acupuncture throughout the rest of the year and up until my transfer. I also went through the pre- and post-transfer acupuncture and I believe all of it made my pregnancy come true. I will always be grateful."

— Maria H., Houston, Texas

"After many months of medical intervention (injections and IUI's) for unexplained infertility, I began treatments with Randine Lewis. The weekly sessions were very relaxing, and within a month I had more energy and generally felt better. My reproductive endocrinologist began noticing physical and physiological changes after just two months of acupuncture and herbal treatments. Four months after I met Dr. Lewis, I became pregnant. My precious daughter will go through life hearing the story of how she would not be here if it were not for the caring hands of Dr. Lewis. It saddens me to think that there are women who are not informed, or who hesitate to seek Dr. Lewis's help, and continue to struggle needlessly with infertility."

— Sharon L., Houston, Texas

"I read this book cover to cover, then went back to page one and read it again. The wisdom, information, and hope it provided gave me the power to help myself and, ultimately, find my fertile soul."

— Suzanne R., Los Angeles, California

"My reproductive endocrinologist is very excited about my FSH level and gave me instructions to begin Fallistim injections. I am taking two vials per day. I just wanted to tell you how grateful I am for Dr. Lewis's help and how amazed I am at how quickly these changes have taken place in my cycle! I can't thank you enough!"

— D.C., Wilmington, Delaware

"When I first came to see Dr. Lewis, I had many medical problems other than infertility. I had severe depression, and an autoimmune condition, which I believed was part of my inability to get pregnant. Dr. Lewis assured me that as we worked on my mood disorder and autoimmunity, my reproductive system would become healthier in the process. With her help, I was able to wean myself off my antidepressants (with my psychiatrist's consent). We were successful in having a baby, and my autoimmune condition is now in remission. I trust Dr. Lewis completely and always knew that my overall well-being was more important to her than anything else. She steered me in the right direction at every step of the way."

— Michelle H., Houston, Texas

"I am sitting here nursing our two-day-old son. . . . I am eternally grateful for your guidance and expertise."

— Diana K., Houston, Texas

"I was very skeptical about going to an acupuncturist. I was from a traditional medical family, but during my first appointment I was so relaxed that I fell asleep! After going to Dr. Lewis for a couple of weeks, I had much more energy and felt a lot more relaxed in general. She predicted that I would get pregnant within six weeks to six months of seeing her, and at the six-week mark I was pregnant! We are expecting our baby at the end of October."

— Laura W., Houston, Texas

"I am now almost nineteen weeks. My morning sickness is gone and I'm well into the second trimester. The amnio results came back Wednesday with the great news of us growing a normal boy. I hope/think we are finally now at a point where we can truly enjoy every kick and doctor's visit. I credit you and your herbs and needles for giving us this normal little bean to grow. Saying thank you doesn't seem to be enough. But thank you for the miracle you have performed."

— Shaye H., Galveston, Texas

THE INFERTILITY CURE

The Ancient Chinese Wellness
Program for Getting Pregnant
and Having Healthy Babies

Randine Lewis, Ph.D.

Master of Science in Oriental Medicine

LITTLE, BROWN AND COMPANY
New York Boston London

Dedicated to all women whose yearning to express life
will bring forth the children of tomorrow.
To the children born of these dedicated women:
may you always know how much you were cherished —
even before you were born.
    For Theresa
    For Kyra
    For Lars
    Thank you for expressing yourselves in my life.

Little, Brown and Company
Hachette Book Group
237 Park Avenue, New York, NY 10017

www.hachettebookgroup.com

Little, Brown and Company is a division of Hachette Book Group, Inc.
The Little, Brown logo is a trademark of Hachette Book Group, Inc.

Originally published in hardcover by Little, Brown and Company, January 2004
First paperback edition, March 2005

Acknowledgment of permission to reprint previously copyrighted material appear on page 302.

Library of Congress Cataloging-in-Publication Data
Lewis, Randine A.
    The infertility cure : the ancient Chinese wellness program for getting pregnant and having healthy babies/Randine Lewis.
        p.   cm.
    Includes index.
    ISBN 978-0-316-17229-5 (hc) / 978-0-316-15921-0 (pb)
        1. Infertility, Female — Alternative treatment. 2. Medicine, Chinese. I. Title.
RG201.L49 2004
    618.1'7806 — dc22   2003054642

10 9 8 7

RRD-C

Designed by Meryl Sussman Levavi/Digitext

Printed in the United States of America

Contents

How to Use This Book

If you have been diagnosed with specific conditions that affect your fertility, your natural inclination may be to turn directly to the chapters in part 3 that deal with your particular problem. But to benefit most from this book, you need to know the basics of traditional Chinese medicine (TCM) so you may correctly apply the suggestions contained in the book's later chapters. With a little background in the principles of TCM, you will be able to understand of the causes of your own particular fertility challenges and then discover how to treat them using this ancient form of healing.

At a minimum I suggest that you do the following:

◆ Read chapter 3. It will give you a foundation in the principles of TCM.
◆ Read chapter 4 and take the diagnostic test. This is essential if you wish to discover and understand the causes of your infertility according to TCM. In chapter 4 you'll also learn a series of abbreviations that are used throughout the book to refer to specific imbalances in the different Organ systems of the body. Once you know which imbalances are affecting you, you can look for the symbol for your particular imbalances in the chapters on diet, lifestyle, acupuncture, and herbs, as well as in any chapters dealing with Western-diagnosed conditions.
◆ I also recommend that you read all of part 2, "The Ancient Chinese Program for Reproductive Wellness." This section describes the various treatments of TCM, that you can apply to your diagnosis later in the book.

While I have done my best to make the material in this book easy to read and comprehend, keep in mind that there may be new and unfamiliar material in these pages. However, as a Chinese proverb tells us, "With time and patience the mulberry becomes a silk gown." With a little persistence you will understand how TCM can help enhance or restore your fertility.

NOTE: This book is intended as complementary in nature. It is not designed to take the place of medical care, Eastern or Western. It is an attempt to put into plain English how natural forms of treatment, based upon an Eastern paradigm, can assist in improving your fecundity. You should consult a physician before embarking on any treatment plan.

Contained within this book are exercises you can perform to help your body put maximum emphasis on your reproductive capacity. These exercises, based upon individual patterns, will give you the benefit of traditional Chinese medicine. More sophisticated treatments will require consultation with a licensed acupuncturist or doctor of Oriental medicine.

Many of the articles referenced in this book come from European or Asian medical sources. The international medical community has been supporting natural alternatives for many years. The American medical community is just beginning to support scientific studies to investigate natural, complementary care. Gratefully, this trend is improving, thanks to public demand.

Also, please note that all patients' names used in this book have been changed to protect their privacy.

Introduction

From Infertility to Motherhood

I was born to Scandinavian parents and grew up in northern Minnesota. My family included two older twin sisters and a younger brother. For as long as I can remember, I wanted a family of my own. Having children just seemed a part of my destiny. Although I was a tomboy and didn't play house or typical girls' games, I knew I would be a mom someday.

My parents couldn't afford to pay for my education, so at eighteen I joined the air force. I moved to Italy and married at age twenty; six months later, through no effort or concentrated planning, I was with child. My pregnancy transformed me. My life had never had such meaning. The miracle of this child growing in me was beyond words. I gave birth to a beautiful daughter, Theresa. My marriage, however, was another story. My husband and I had lost our passion for each other, and the partnership ended.

With my marriage over, I turned my sights toward a professional goal. The zeal I felt for the miracle of pregnancy never left me, and I decided on a career in medicine — maybe obstetrics gynecology (OB-GYN). Theresa was in third grade when I was accepted into medical school. My studies were intense and required maternal sacrifice, but I had found my life's work.

Upon completion of the academic portion of medical school, I met Ed, a physician from Texas, and we got married. I began work in Houston as a medical consultant. We decided that before I went into a fast-paced medical practice, we were going to start a family of our own. Okay, *I* wanted to increase the size of our family; Ed was content with our life as it was. Yet my yearning to bear another child grew into an obsession.

At the same time, I was experiencing hormonal problems. My joints ached, I had lower back and knee pain, I had to urinate frequently, I had night sweats, I was experiencing hair loss, and my periods were extremely irregular and sometimes nonexistent. A medical work-up revealed my estrogen and progesterone levels were alarmingly low, resulting in an inability to conceive. The doctor recommended Clomid, a drug designed to hyperstimulate a woman's ovaries to produce more eggs, thus increasing the chances of pregnancy. This advice seemed wrong to me; why hyperstimulate my ovaries when the problem obviously resided in my whole hormonal system? Ed was also against this prospect. During his medical training he had seen firsthand the unfortunate outcomes of multiple births: fetal distress and death; two-pound babies barely kept alive on life support, only to be irreparably harmed for life.

But in my desperation I would have subjected myself to *any* medical procedure to get pregnant. I eventually became convinced that I had to solve my own hormonal problem. But I could recall very little practical information from my medical training — for the very good reason that it was never provided! We learned about gynecological diseases but not about gynecological *health*, and even less about reproductive well-being. So I started reading everything I could find in the library, at bookstores, and on medical search engines. I began to eat healthfully and exercise, while devouring every book ever written on how to conceive naturally. Gradually, I stopped drinking alcohol, gave up smoking, quit drinking coffee and diet soda, and stopped eating sugar, milk, and meat. I shopped only at an upscale health-food supermarket specializing in organic foods. I ate a strictly vegan diet; I drank a shot of wheatgrass every day and took a plethora of nutritional supplements. In one book, I read that acupuncture could treat infertility. While this seemed a little far-fetched, I was intrigued. I found one acupuncture general practitioner, another who practiced acupuncture and prescribed Chinese herbs, and one who specialized in herbal medicine for gynecology. And I went to all three! I also began to research herbal fertility remedies. I began taking herbs like wild yam, Vitex, and other reproductive herbal tonics. I made teas, tinctures, and other concoctions, each one smelling and tasting worse than the other. I brewed mixtures of raw Chinese herbs on the stove, plug my nose, and choke down my special herbal potions every day.

But still I couldn't get pregnant. Desperately, I started reaching for anything. I stood on my head, put pillows under my hips during sex, waited and prayed a lot. Each month was a cycle of anticipation and despair. I almost developed an addiction to home pregnancy tests. At the first notion of a potential symptom of pregnancy (a twinge in the uterus, tender breasts, nausea), I would buy *just one* early pregnancy test and promise myself if it was negative I wouldn't buy another one. But each time I was let down. I began to detest the appearance of the single pink line, only to try again the next morning.

When you're trying to get pregnant, it seems as if every woman around you gets pregnant by accident. I began to resent the drivers of the minivans that occupied the "Stork Club" parking spaces at the supermarket. It felt as if I was the only one who wasn't allowed to join this club. I noticed homeless women living under the bridge with swollen bellies, a cigarette in one hand and a beer in the other. Couldn't I provide a better home for a child? Every aspect of my being was challenged: my self-worth, my femininity, my profession, my marriage, my faith.

In the meantime, however, I noticed changes occurring within my body. My hair no longer fell out. My joints stopped hurting. I had more energy and generally just felt better. Three months later, I became pregnant with Kyra. I was beyond delighted. My fascination with Oriental medicine intensified. I felt that I needed to understand this noninvasive, healthy way of thinking. I matriculated at Chinese medical school at night and finished the four-year program in two and a half years. My friends and family stood by, amazed. Give up a career in "real" medicine to pursue this gibberish? But I had experienced the efficacy of this novel form of medicine firsthand, and I wanted to know how and why it worked. More important, I wanted to help other women who were challenged with infertility.

When I finished my training, however, I still didn't feel as though I knew enough about Chinese medicine to apply it effectively to others. So I took my family to a city on the eastern coast of China, where I worked in a hospital of traditional Chinese medicine. This particular hospital had departments much like any American hospital — neurology, cardiology, dermatology, emergency medicine. The diagnostic equipment was similar; the difference was that every patient was treated only with acupuncture or herbs. Although I'd like to paint a picture of this experience as being beautiful and exotic, in truth the hospital lacked central heating and wasn't as clean as I would have wished. But all the doctors, including me, worked exceptionally hard, and the system was extremely efficient and friendly.

My internship focused on patients with gynecological problems, especially infertility. (Chinese women are usually alerted to any conception difficulties by their thirties at the latest. This health impairment is taken very seriously and addressed straightaway.) I saw up to forty patients a day; I assessed their patterns, evaluated their pulse, and viewed the appearance of their tongue. As different as this routine was from the American hospital system, it worked. I treated patients until Chinese medical philosophy became second nature.

Most patients came for diagnosis and herbal prescriptions; others came for acupuncture. Some treatment rooms held eight to ten beds to accommodate the mass of patients, yet each individual received complete attention from her physician. The patients would converse among themselves and with the doctors during their treatments, and it seemed they truly enjoyed their weekly outings to the hospital. I learned a very different approach to health care: here, the doctors and patients were a team.

Upon returning from China, I opened up a clinic in Houston specializing in gynecology. I did my own research and earned a Ph.D., completing my dissertation on addressing and treating fertility issues with traditional Chinese medicine. Helping women conceive continued to be my real passion.

After Kyra's birth, I never used any type of birth control, although I did resume my normal unhealthy American lifestyle. A couple years later, the idea of having another baby emerged. I began eating healthfully, changing my exercise routine, taking my basal body temperature, and consuming vitamins and herbs. This time I became pregnant rather quickly. Nine weeks later, however, I woke up one morning and knew that I had lost the baby. My breasts were no longer tender, and I just didn't *feel* pregnant anymore. I called my obstetrician, who reassured me that everything was fine. My subjective signs were not clinically significant, he said, but I could come in for reassurance. My instincts had been right: the blood test showed my hCG dropping, and the ultrasound revealed no heartbeat. I miscarried at ten weeks.

I was devastated. My whole life had become focused on fertility, but I couldn't handle the loss of my own child. I went through four of the five stages of grief — denial, anger, bargaining, and depression — but never made it to acceptance. Nobody, not even my husband, understood. My friends and family urged me to "get on with my life." But this was more than a material loss — a part of my soul had died. I couldn't deal with the all-encompassing despair. I went in for a D & C (dilation and curettage) on Christmas Eve. My doctor gave me pain pills for the recovery period. Although the physical pain was nominal, the emotional pain was intolerable. I took enough pills to make me completely numb. For the next month, I continued to take herbs and had a few acupuncture treatments, but in truth I felt shut down physically and emotionally. Thankfully, I got pregnant again in February.

But when my hCG tests started dropping again, I feared the worst. On the way to my scheduled ultrasound I was petrified that my baby would be gone. I couldn't comprehend why I was being put through these trials. My greatest fear was that perhaps I wasn't meant to have another child. I changed my prayers and pleaded for the strength to get through this, rather than to make it turn out the way I wanted it. The thought that maybe my losses could help someone else gave me some peace. All of a sudden I knew that everything would be all right no matter what the outcome. A stoic composure overtook me, and I went to my appointment with a new sense of strength. My eyes were glued to the ultrasound screen as my doctor repositioned the wand to look for the fetus, and there it was — a heartbeat! Life was worth living again. Six weeks later my amniocentesis was normal. And I was going to have a boy!

However, five months into my pregnancy I started bleeding heavily. I was diagnosed with placenta and vasa previa, meaning that the placement of the placenta was too low, over the cervical opening. When the uterus expanded to accommodate the growing baby, a large vessel had started to hemorrhage. I was ordered on bed rest for the remainder of my pregnancy. I lay flat on my back for almost three months, doing nothing but watching TV.

At thirty-two weeks, the bleeding wouldn't stop. Lars was born via emergency cesarean section eight weeks prematurely; his cord was knotted and wrapped around his neck three times. The little guy overcame some big obstacles to get here! He spent two weeks in the neonatal intensive care unit. Today Lars and my other children are perfectly healthy. But my combined experiences taught me that I had to take charge of my own reproductive health.

Western medicine had once misled me into thinking I was infertile or somehow "broken." But I wasn't infertile: I was imbalanced. To heal myself, I had to open my mind to other ways of thinking based on a concept of wellness rather than disease. I had to look at my body as an ally rather than an enemy, as something that needed nurturing and healing in order to support the growth of a child inside it.

From my own fertility struggles arose a compassion and determination to do everything I could to make sure other women would not have to go through such events without the availability of *everything* that medicine — Western or Eastern — has to offer.

Today I can give my rocky path toward motherhood its proper meaning. My fertility struggle was not a medical condition: it was a lack of reproductive and hormonal balance. I don't accept that I was being spiritually punished or rewarded. I believe I was being challenged, sometimes beyond my capacity to bear it. But I know that the experiences I went through give me strength. I am a better parent and a better practitioner because of the obstacles I overcame. My hope is that this book will help you conquer your fertility impairments as well. I hope it will be a valued guide; that it will provide ideas, treatments, and solutions that are outside what you may have heard from your Western medical doctor; and that it will open you up to a more natural and supportive way of bringing a baby into your womb. We in the West may not be familiar with TCM techniques, but they have worked for millions of women for thousands of years. They are designed to promote greater health and well-being, to work with nature and make us fruitful.

I can't know the pain you may have experienced in your quest for conception — the disappointment, the frustration, the hope and the hopelessness of each negative pregnancy test. Perhaps you, like me, have felt the heartbreak of conceiving and losing a child. Perhaps, like me, you have given the power over your own body to doctors in the hope that somehow they will make everything better. I don't know why we have been chosen to undertake such a painful journey, why we must go through such struggles to bring our children into the world. But I do know that when we look into our babies' faces, they will *never* have to wonder if they were really wanted. Ours are the children who, no matter how they came to us, will look at their parents and *know,* from the deepest place in their heart, how much we cherish them, and how we labored to give them life. And in that there is no greater security and no greater gift.

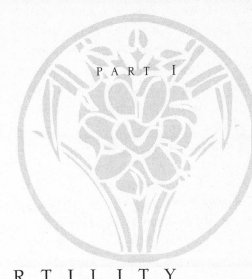

PART I

CHANGING YOUR MIND ABOUT INFERTILITY

The superior physician does not just treat disease but teaches society and helps form the intentions of humanity.

— SUN SI MIAO

When I first began studying TCM it was difficult to believe what was presented to me. I found myself arguing with my TCM professors, until one of them told me to forget all the ideas of Western medicine that I had come to accept as the only truth. What a challenge — to put aside my scientific background and allow for new ideas and a new paradigm!

But I thought that since TCM has worked for millions of people for thousands of years, and since its practices had helped me get pregnant naturally when my Western doctor's only solution was to use drugs like

Clomid, I would grasp everything that I could about TCM, especially as it related to infertility. So I learned how to use the principles of Chinese medicine and watched my patients' astonishment as they became pregnant after Western medicine had given them no hope.

I am grateful for both my Western and Eastern training because it allows me to serve as a bridge between the two medical worldviews. I value the ability of Western medicine to quantify every moment of a woman's reproductive cycle, allowing me to pinpoint exactly where the potential lack of harmony might be. I also respect enormously the technological wizardry of Western science that allows us to see inside the body with great accuracy, the microsurgery that can repair the smallest tears and blockages, and, above all, the assisted reproductive technology (ART) that permits women with no hope of conceiving to bear children.

However, my Eastern medical training has given me a different perspective. Eastern medicine sees the body as a microcosm of nature. Disease or malfunction is a disturbance in the "ecosystem" of the body, and health is restored by treating the entire system rather than fixing one part of it. As the sixteenth-century physician Paracelsus put it, "The physician is only the servant of nature, not her master. Therefore, it behooves medicine to follow the will of nature."

Our reproductive systems are not made up of isolated organs and batches of separate hormones. Each element of the system must work together seamlessly so conditions will be right for pregnancy to occur. When you restore the health of the body, a woman's reproductive system will do what it was designed to do naturally: conceive and carry to term a healthy child.

The first step to fertility isn't another drug or procedure, or even an acupuncture treatment: it's discovering a new way of thinking about yourself, your body, and your health. The first few chapters of this book will introduce you to the different approaches taken by Western and Eastern medicine for the treatment of infertility. Both of these medical disciplines have a coherent worldview. But I believe that in many cases the Eastern method offers alternatives for women who have been walking the painful road of infertility and would like to try another path — or, at the very least, would like to see if Eastern methods can help make their Western treatments more effective.

There is a Chinese saying: "We never wander so far as when we think we know the way." I'm not asking you to leave your critical faculties behind and accept any of these ideas on faith alone. I only ask of you what was required of me: that you keep an open mind. Approach this material with a sense of interest and possibility, and I believe you may find the help you need.

1

There's No Such Thing as Infertility

It can be frightening, this yearning for a child — it's hard to fathom the desperate urgency.

— WENDY WASSERSTEIN, AWARD-WINNING PLAYWRIGHT AND FIRST-TIME MOTHER AT AGE FORTY-SIX, FROM *CREATING A LIFE* BY SYLVIA HEWETT

While the question "When does life begin?" has been debated throughout the ages, one issue that is virtually undebatable is the intense desire of most women to bear children. Young girls jump rope singing, "First comes love, then comes marriage, then comes Mary with a baby carriage!" Maternal conditioning prepares us to become mothers. Even girls who show no interest in babies or dolls while growing up still assume they possess the capacity, if not the desire, to have children.

However, when children become teenagers the focus shifts to *not* having babies too soon. Most adolescents in the United States are well schooled in preventing pregnancy through condoms, birth control pills, abstinence, and so on. Certainly, this is an important message for teenagers, but what happens to women who, when they are ready to have babies, find that it's not as easy to conceive as they were led to believe it would be? This is neither a small nor an isolated problem. *Fertility issues affect at least one in six couples in the United States. This statistic means that every month more than 7 million U.S. couples experi-*

ence the pain and disappointment of failing to conceive. (The American Fertility Society states that a couple is considered infertile when pregnancy has not occurred after one year of coitus without contraception.)

The causes of infertility are wide-ranging — unfortunately, partners usually don't know there's a problem until they want to conceive and are then thrown into an endless spiral of diagnosis, treatment, trying to get pregnant and failing, more diagnosis, more treatment, and more failure. As a med-ical practitioner involved in fertility issues, I know firsthand the desperate hunger of couples who want to have children. And as a woman, I know personally the pain of wanting to conceive and failing. I, too, have suffered through miscarriage and unexplained infertility. I traveled around the world to make my dream of having more children come true. I know your journey and your pain, and your desire to create new life. If you will walk with me, I will show you a path that may lead you to both healing and hope.

❧ MOTHERHOOD AT ANY COST

Oh, what a power is motherhood, possessing
A potent spell. All women alike
Fight fiercely for a child.

EURIPIDES, *IPHIGENIA IN AULIS*, C. 405 B.C.

For a couple, the diagnosis of infertility can be difficult, but for a woman it can be devastating. Being told you are infertile is like being told your body has failed its very reason for existence. Throughout the ages, a woman who was "barren" was considered extremely ill fated. The Old Testament includes several stories of women who prayed ceaselessly for a child. Rachel, Jacob's wife, went so far as to ask Jacob to impregnate her servant so she could then claim the child as her own. Fairy tale after fairy tale (*Rumpelstiltskin, Thumbelina, Sleeping Beauty*) describes the hunger for children experienced by queen and peasant alike. Women have resorted to everything — from prayer to magic potions to strange sexual positions to drugs to surrogacy — to enhance their fertility.

Today fertility is complicated by the fact that women are waiting longer to become mothers. The average age at marriage for both women and men has been rising steadily since the 1950s. We are not marrying until we're in our late twenties or thirties, and we're postponing having our children until even later. We believe that we can have children any time between menarche and menopause, and ask ourselves, why not wait until everything is just right?

I wish it were that easy. Far too many of us are discovering that when we're ready for children, our bodies are not. According to some statistics, a woman's fertility peaks in her early twenties and starts to decline as early as age twenty-seven. By the time a woman is thirty-five, her chances of conceiving are decreased by 50 percent, and they shrink to 20 percent by the time she hits forty. (While these statistics may be valid, there are ways a woman of almost *any* age can increase her fertility.) Age, the effects of which are often exacerbated by years of poor diet and stress, depletes the reproductive system of both men and women. Women's bodies become ill prepared to accept the burden of conceiving and carrying a healthy child to term. Month after month their hopes rise, only to fall again with the onset of menstruation.

But women are tenacious. We don't give up our dream of children that easily — especially since Western reproductive medicine has provided some of the best-publicized miracles of modern science. The "infertility epidemic" has spawned a huge biomedical industry treating those who want children but can't have them. And indeed, assisted reproductive technology (ART) has given hope to many women who could never bear children otherwise. But the physical, emotional, and financial costs of these treatments are high. Women spend every penny they have and borrow more for in vitro fertilization (IVF) cycles. They take drugs that

hyperstimulate their ovaries, turning them into egg-producing, hormone-raging madwomen. Women have sex, don't have sex, have sex on schedule, have sex all the time — whatever they're told will work. They allow their eggs to be harvested, fertilized outside their bodies, and inserted back into the uterus, hoping that at least one egg will "take." They resort to surrogate mothers, or use someone else's eggs. We women will literally undergo almost any kind of procedure, no matter how dangerous or humiliating, in our craving for motherhood. Yet all too often we end up broke and heartbroken, our arms empty and our bodies exhausted.

Unfortunately, while we hear a great deal about how Western reproductive medicine has helped women conceive, we hear a great deal *less* about the pain, expense, and statistically low success rates of such procedures. Research shows that even young women using IVF techniques have between a 20 and 30 percent chance of conceiving (at a cost of at least ten thousand dollars per attempt). The chances fall to less than 10 percent for women at age thirty-nine, and only 3 percent for women at age forty-four. On average, women go through seven cycles of ART before they either conceive or quit, spending tens to hundreds of thousands of dollars in their attempts to have children.

Fortunately, the failures of Western reproductive medicine have galvanized women to seek out healthier, more holistic methods of fertility enhancement. For these women, my practice at the Eastern Harmony Clinic and at Fertility Retreats —

where I use traditional Chinese medical techniques to enhance both women's and men's fertility and improve their health — offers an alternative. Traditional Chinese medicine can be used in conjunction with cutting-edge Western reproductive medicine to increase the chances for conception. It also can help a woman move gently and naturally to a state of health and well-being that will allow her body to conceive and carry to term a healthy child.

This book outlines the basics of the fertility and wellness program used by women at my clinic. Let us begin with the story of one such woman, who represents the many hundreds who bring me their fertility issues, along with their despair and hope.

THE THIRD WAY TO CONCEPTION: SUSIE'S STORY

Susie had been diagnosed with "unexplained infertility." This meant that her doctors could find no specific hormonal or physical reason for her inability to conceive. Her reproductive endocrinologist had put her on courses of hormone injections to stimulate her ovaries to produce more eggs, as well as intrauterine inseminations to bypass any potential cervical or sperm factors. But nothing had worked. A friend had told her about my program, and Susie decided to try it. "What did I have to lose?" she told me later.

When Susie first made the appointment at our clinic, she downloaded a set of forms, which we asked her to complete in advance and bring with her. These forms asked about her general health, diet, emotions, and specific menstrual and hormonal symptoms. Susie thought some questions were irrelevant to her fertility problem, but she filled in her answers and brought the forms with her on the appointment day.

When Susie walked in for her first appointment, she was frustrated, fearful, and skeptical. She knew a lot about what Western medicine had to offer in her quest for a child but was unfamiliar with more natural approaches to fertility enhancement. When she passed through the doors of Eastern Harmony, however, she knew she was in for a far different experience from her other doctor's sterile clinic. When a patient comes into our clinic, she is surrounded by an atmosphere of tranquillity created by music, water fountains, plants, scented candles, and incense.

My consulting room is also warm and inviting, a place of comfort and hope. I could see Susie start to relax as soon as she walked in the door. We chatted about her general health and the problems she had had conceiving, and I looked at her questionnaire to familiarize myself with her symptoms. Then I took Susie's wrist and listened to her pulse — one of the primary methods of diagnosis used in TCM. (Practitioners of TCM are taught to read nine different positions of a patient's pulse.) I looked at her eyes and her tongue for outward manifestations of internal energies. I wanted to see where the flow of Susie's life force energy, or Qi (pronounced *chee*), was blocked or out of balance.

After I had assessed Susie's condition, I told her, "I believe you have an energy imbalance in the meridians running to your reproductive organs. In traditional Chinese medicine, for the ovaries and uterus to be in balance the Kidneys, Liver, and Spleen must be also, as these energy systems are intricately linked to reproduction. The imbalance of energy is affecting your hormones as well as your overall health."

"But my reproductive endocrinologist didn't find anything wrong with my hormones," Susie replied.

"Many hormonal problems occur because of slight imbalances in the endocrine system, altering the way the body produces hormones," I told her. "Modern Western diagnostic techniques may not detect any abnormality, but even a slight aberration can throw the entire system off so it no longer functions smoothly. We need to get your hormones and the other systems in your body back into balance."

"I've had my hormones stimulated, and it didn't work," Susie objected.

"I'm not talking about stimulating your hormones but rather restoring your body's natural balance," I reassured her. "Think of your body like a river. The health of the river depends upon the natural flow of water. When nature is doing its job, rain falls in the hills, runs downhill in rivulets into streams, then into bigger streams, then into the river.

But if the river isn't getting enough water — if there's a drought, for example — the system won't flow the way it's supposed to. The Western solution to a drought is to open the floodgates of a dam upstream and release an enormous amount of water all at once. That will cause water to flow into the river, but it also may cause enormous problems because the river's ecosystem isn't equipped to handle that much water all at once. Hormonal stimulation can have the same effect on a woman's body: it floods the system with a huge amount of stimulation that the body simply isn't equipped to handle.

"The Eastern method is different. Instead of flooding the river with water from a dam, the natural approach is to seed the clouds and release just enough rain to restore the proper level of water in the river. Traditional Chinese medical treatments are designed to stimulate the body's own natural production of hormones while restoring the health and harmony of the entire system. Once the body is in balance and its hormones are restored, conception can occur."

"You're sure it's effective?" Susie asked.

"The first records of fertility treatments using traditional Chinese medicine date back to well before the Christian era," I answered.

"I advocate a simple four-step program that can help you balance your energies and prepare your body to nurture a child. Each program is designed specifically for the individual patient. The first step is to diagnose what's going on with your system and how your reproductive energies need to be harmonized. The second step is to change your diet. In the Chinese medical system, certain foods have specific properties — generating heat or dampness, for example. Depending on your Chinese medical diagnosis, you may need to choose foods that will help purify your Blood, or increase energy flow to your Kidneys, or eliminate stagnation in your Liver. And we'll explore adding certain vitamin and mineral supplements to your diet, too.

"The next step is to clear your energy meridians. In your case, I believe a series of acupuncture treatments would be helpful. I may also prescribe specific exercises."

"My friend swore that your acupuncture treatments helped her get pregnant," Susie said. "But after all the injections I've been getting for the last few months, I hate the idea of needles."

I shook my head. "Acupuncture is nothing like an injection. Most of my patients say they can't even feel the needles, and many tell me that they are more relaxed after a treatment. I suggest you try one treatment and see how you feel. If it's not for you, we can pursue other options, like acupressure. The goal is to balance your energy meridians and get the Qi flowing smoothly again.

"The final step is to increase your chances of conception through the use of herbs, natural energetic substances that gently correct underlying deficiencies or clear obstructions. Herbal preparations and tonics have been used for thousands of years in China to help increase fertility. We'll individualize each herbal formula based upon your diagnostic pattern. There will be different herbs for various segments of your cycle. I'll also give you an herbal mix designed to enhance your overall health and well-being.

"We'll keep assessing our progress and make changes as needed. Simply by following these steps — diet, acupuncture, and herbs — and using relaxation and stress-reduction techniques, many women in our clinic are able to conceive within a period of months."

Susie looked at me expectantly. "Do you really think I can have a child?"

I knew what she was feeling because I've seen it in hundreds of patients and have felt the same need for hope myself. "Susie, we're not talking about a quick fix here. Chinese medical treatments are designed to work *with* nature rather than against it, to allow conception to occur rather than force it. Most of my patients need to be on this program for at least three cycles before they can expect noticeable hormonal changes. But many of them report almost instantaneous improvement in their level of health and well-being, as well as greater energy, more emotional calm, and a sense that they are working with their bodies to prepare themselves to become pregnant. My patients will attest that these techniques work. Yes, I truly believe they can help you have a child."

Susie left my office that day with a renewed sense of hope and possibility. She came in weekly for acupuncture sessions (which, she told me, didn't hurt at all), changed her diet, and began taking the herbal mixtures I prescribed. Within a month her energy and overall health were much better. Four months after her first visit to my office, Susie became pregnant naturally. She had a beautiful daughter and is currently expecting her second "acupuncture baby."

THE MYTH OF INFERTILITY

Susie's story is similar to that of many women who find their way to my clinic. They arrive discouraged, disheartened, hoping against hope there might be an alternative that will allow them to have a child. It is my blessing and responsibility to offer these women a source of hope that they, too, can feel a child quickening within them and hold that child in their arms.

My work with fertility issues began as a result of my personal struggles. Now I only treat women who are trying to get pregnant. Though I suffer through their heartache, I also get to experience their joy when, as a result of my treatment, they become pregnant after being told they were infertile.

If you too have been told you are infertile, I have one message for you: *There is no such thing as infertility; it is a myth!* Rarely have I met a woman of childbearing age with all her reproductive organs intact who isn't capable of bearing children. As long as the anatomical structures are present, a medical diagnosis of "infertility" is often a fallacy. Many factors can cause a woman to have difficulty conceiving, but once these factors are overcome and a woman's body is restored to health, conception can occur naturally.

The focus of my program is to remove obstructions to conception. The stories of the patients I have treated are not unusual. Women around the world are finding more natural means to overcome their fertility barriers. Restoring optimal health permits the expression of our natural fertile state. Our job is simply to be ready for the occasion when the universe says, "It's time."

I advise you to devour all the knowledge you can about fertility. Take control of your own health, and trust yourself. No one is in tune with your body like you are. You have to learn to trust your instincts until your individual solution emerges. Above all, know that you are *not* broken; you are *not* deficient. No matter what the outcome of your own personal journey, you are whole.

You can conceive. It may take more motivation and perseverance than you ever thought possible. But Nature is on your side. With her gentle help and support, *your child will come.*

2

Correcting the "Conception Misconceptions" of Western Medicine

To create health, you need a new kind of knowledge, based on a deeper concept of life.

— DEEPAK CHOPRA, M.D., *QUANTUM HEALING*

Let's take a look at a typical course of Western medical treatments for a woman with fertility problems. Joanne was an attractive, slender woman of thirty-seven. Two years ago she married Bill, an oil executive. After trying for a year, they were still unable to conceive, so her gynecologist referred her to a reproductive endocrinologist for an endocrine workup. Joanne's doctor found that she had antithyroid antibodies and low levels of circulating thyroid hormone in her blood. The diagnosis was Hashimoto's thyroiditis, meaning that her immune system was attacking her thyroid gland, causing her thyroid to function below optimum. (Low levels of thyroid hormone have been associated with infertility and recurrent pregnancy loss.) Her reproductive endocrinologist prescribed Synthroid, a synthetic thyroid supplement. Joanne was hopeful that with this treatment she might become pregnant.

However, months went by and she still hadn't conceived. With her thyroid imbalance "corrected," she entered a new diagnostic category: unexplained infertility. Joanne's doctor suggested she take Clomid to help stimulate her ovaries to produce more eggs. This drug made her feel crazy, but it offered her hope.

Joanne was not aware that if Clomid (an anti-estrogenic drug) is administered to the wrong subset of women it can actually produce more problems: ovulatory dysfunction, decreased cervical mucus, and thinning of the uterine lining. But for most patients, Clomid is the first drug prescribed by both gynecologists and reproductive endocrinologists, unless its use is specifically contraindicated. In Joanne's case, her doctor assured her that she would be able to get pregnant with the Clomid — but all she got was cysts.

After three months on Clomid, Joanne still hadn't become pregnant, and her doctor recommended that she proceed to gonadotropic hormones. Joanne had to give herself a series of injections to stimulate her ovaries to produce more follicles. When the time was right and her eggs had been released with another hormone shot, Joanne reported to the clinic. Bill previously had provided a sample of seminal fluid, which had been "washed" to make sure it contained only the most motile sperm. The sperm was placed into a syringe, and a nurse threaded a catheter through Joanne's cervix and released the sperm directly into her uterus (an intrauterine insemination, or IUI).

The drugs had cost Joanne and Bill upwards of two thousand dollars per month, and none of the expenses were covered by health insurance. But after five stimulated inseminations, Joanne was still not pregnant. The doctor now urged the couple to consider IVF. This ten-thousand-dollar procedure

would not be covered by their insurance either, but Joanne and Bill decided to go for it.

Joanne quickly discovered that the drugs she had to take to prepare for IVF stimulation were infinitely worse than anything she had taken thus far. Before a course of IVF, a woman's endocrine system has to be suppressed by a drug that simulates menopause, so for three weeks Joanne took Lupron, which shut off her own hormones and gave her horrible headaches. She developed hot flashes and night sweats; the physical and mental stress were horrendous. Once Joanne's hormones had been adequately curtailed, she was injected with follicle-stimulating hormone (FSH), which hyperstimulated her ovaries to produce several mature eggs. She went in for blood work and an ultrasound every few days and was pleased when the technicians told her she was responding fairly well to the drugs. Two weeks later they informed her she had six follicles, whose eggs would be retrieved through the vagina via needle aspiration when the time came.

Once Joanne's follicles were ready, she took a shot to further mature the eggs, which were then surgically extracted and placed with another sample of Bill's washed sperm in a petri dish in the laboratory, where the mixture was allowed to cultivate for eighteen hours. Joanne was delighted when the nurse called to tell her that most of her eggs were fertilized. She told Joanne to relax and come back for the embryo transfer in two days. But how could Joanne relax? She had put all her hopes on this procedure.

When Joanne returned (not relaxed) the nurse told her that two of the embryos were of high enough quality to implant in her uterus. Joanne resumed the standard "Pap smear" position — on her back, her feet held apart in cold metal stirrups, her most intimate organs exposed — and the doctor transferred the embryos into her uterus. He put Joanne on daily progesterone injections to improve the chances of the embryos implanting successfully and told her to resume normal activity and return in two weeks for a pregnancy test. Joanne couldn't sleep and could barely eat, yet the hormones were making her gain weight. She was so anxious that she didn't want to socialize with her friends. Only her closest family members knew what was going on. She felt depressed, alone, scared to death that the procedure wouldn't work, and guilty for being so pessimistic. She cried all the time, and even her husband couldn't console her.

Two weeks later, the pregnancy test came back negative, just as she feared. The doctor told them both that they could try another IVF or they could explore using donor eggs. Joanne wasn't pregnant; she and her husband were tens of thousands of dollars in debt; she was fat and depressed and still didn't have a child. Joanne and Bill gave up. Every time someone asks them why they don't have children, she slowly dies inside.

❧ THE BASIS — AND BIAS — OF WESTERN MEDICINE

The more doctors have to intervene with drugs, needles and surgery to get sperm to meet egg, the greater the chance that something will go wrong.

— CHRISTINE GORMAN, *TIME*, APRIL 15, 2002

Joanne's case is typical of the medical treatment received by most women with fertility issues. When all the mechanical functions of the uterus and ovaries are assessed as normal, Western reproductive medical protocols do not vary much in approach, and each step adds more medical control over a woman's cycle. Yet we women still do this willingly in our desperate quest for children.

The number of Western medical procedures to correct infertility rose 40 percent between 1995 and 1999. The "fertility industry" in the United States brings in over *$2 billion* a year. The problem arises when Western medicine fails us, as it did in Joanne's case and as it does thousands of women every month.

Conception is a fragile miracle that can

be affected by any one of a thousand factors. If there are physical obstructions in the ovaries, fallopian tubes, or uterus, if any of her hormones are slightly off, if her menstrual cycle is out of phase, if her egg doesn't release at the proper time, if she doesn't produce enough estrogen to thin her cervical mucus to allow sperm to enter her uterus, if her uterine lining is too thin or too thick by even a millimeter, if cellular adhesion molecules aren't present, if the endometrial glands don't respond to the progesterone — if any one of these problems is present, she has a minuscule chance of conceiving that month, if at all. And all of these factors are affected not just by a woman's reproductive organs and hormones but also by her general health, levels of stress, exercise, and dietary habits.

Western medicine shines in pinpointing the minutiae of physical ailments and disease. The diagnostic tests, measurements of hormone levels, ultrasounds, genetic testing, and so on, are often excellent in telling us what is wrong with our organs, hormones, or genes. However, such tests can sometimes miss the forest because they're so busy looking at the veins in the leaf of a single tree. And conventional medicine isn't capable of correcting some of the subtle underlying imbalances that might make a couple infertile in the first place, especially if those imbalances have to do with overall well-being.

Joanne's case is a perfect example. Her problem seemed to be low levels of thyroid hormone. Correcting the thyroid imbalance was definitely proper treatment, and her Western medical doctor's prescription of Synthroid was designed to do just that. But wouldn't it be better if Joanne's body produced more thyroid hormone itself? Shouldn't the goal be to help the patient's body function at the highest possible level, with all systems, including reproduction, working as designed? Shouldn't the best kind of treatment focus not on curing individual symptoms but rather on restoring balance to entire systems that are out of whack? I believe that the "conception misconceptions" of Western medicine arise from this tendency to focus completely on individual components of a system — a disease or an organ — and then treat the mere manifestation.

As every patient will tell you, there is no symptom or disease whose effects are confined to one part of the body. If you break your leg, your entire body will be affected by your leg's altered condition. Your balance will be off; your gait will shift; even the way you sleep at night will be upset. And that's not even taking into account the thousands of changes occurring within the biochemistry of your blood, bone, lymph, muscles, and nerves as your body goes about the process of healing the fracture.

The same is true when it comes to modern reproductive medicine's isolated treatment of infertility. Certainly, there are some causes of impaired fertility that benefit from the approach of treating the diseased parts. If the fallopian tubes are blocked or scarred, for example, or if the uterus or cervix is compromised, eliminating such physical blockages can allow conception and/or implantation to occur. But there are far more complex factors at work when it comes to many other conditions that impair fertility. If a patient receives a diagnosis of luteal phase defect (LPD), for instance, she may produce follicles and eggs correctly every month, and those eggs may even become fertilized. But because her corpus luteum is not producing enough progesterone to allow the fertilized egg to be implanted in the uterus, she appears to be infertile. What's her real problem? Not enough progesterone, or the fact that the corpus luteum isn't doing its job? How do you address a problem whose cause is unknown?

The Western medical approach often is to flood the system with a synthetic version of the hormones the body should be producing in small amounts on its own. However, Chinese medicine strives to return the body to balance so it can not only produce but also respond to its own hormones. To use a metaphor from nature, it's the difference between dumping chemical fertilizer on a plant versus nurturing the soil with compost and other natural materials, thus bringing the plant into balance and producing healthy fruit organically. I would argue that the natural approach is better, especially since the "chemical fertilizer" (i.e., synthetic hormone) of Western medicine may bring with it unhealthy side effects while still not producing the "fruit" a woman desires.

Let me state clearly that I believe there is much to admire in Western medicine.

When my son, Lars, was born eight weeks prematurely, I thanked God for the neonatal unit at the hospital that kept him alive and helped him grow to be a healthy, happy baby. I believe in the principles of medicine. I admire its emphasis on scientifically based testing and its demands for proof based on measurable data. I subscribe to reproductive medical journals and keep up to date on the latest infertility research and information. I have very cordial relationships with many respected reproductive endocrinologists throughout the United States. That said, I believe that some fertility treatments are like using a sledgehammer to drive a tack. Women who choose IVF can be taking upwards of fifteen different medications during just one cycle, and their hormone levels can be hugely elevated. These hormone levels can remain artificially high for weeks or even months. Drugs like Clomid and Gonal-F (FSH) are designed to mimic the body's own hormones in stimulating the growth of follicles and eggs in the ovaries and the release of mature eggs into the fallopian tubes for fertilization. Yet the effects of these drugs — multiple egg development, possible ovarian cysts, and side effects such as mood swings, headaches, insomnia, abdominal pain, breast tenderness, nausea, rashes, and so on — indicate that they are a less-than-perfect substitute for the hormones produced by a healthy woman's body in the course of a normal monthly cycle. And since the science of fertility enhancement is still in its infancy, we have yet to see the long-term effects of such elevated hormone levels on women in their later years.

The drugs and ART certainly have their place. But what if there was a way to stimulate a woman's body to *naturally* produce, at the right levels and at the right time, the hormones needed for conception? Wouldn't it make sense for women to use these methods first, to use a thumb instead of a sledgehammer to put the "tack" of their hormones back into balance? Doesn't it also make sense to restore health to the whole person rather than zero in on the few hormones and organs involved specifically in reproduction?

Traditional Chinese medicine holds that a woman's body must be gently nourished and encouraged to bear fruit. It works to rebalance the delicate interplay of energies that occur each month, causing a woman to produce a healthy egg capable of fertilization and to prepare her uterine lining to receive that egg. In my many years of practicing TCM and applying its tenets to infertility, I have found that most hormonal imbalances (which contribute to 40 percent of documented cases of infertility, yet are considered untreatable by conventional Western medicine) respond to Eastern methods of treatment. Many patients come to me having been diagnosed with high FSH levels, luteal phase defect, polycystic ovarian syndrome (PCOS), endometriosis, and so on, or having gone through months or years of trying to get pregnant using ART. And many of them are delighted to discover that after three to six months of the dietary

changes, herbs, and acupuncture treatments that I prescribe, they become pregnant with no further effort.

Let me tell you how I would treat a patient with a condition similar to Joanne's. Carla, age forty, came to see me with a history of being unable to conceive. She had been diagnosed with low circulating levels of thyroid hormone, but she hadn't yet agreed to go on any medication. When I interviewed Carla, I noticed her complexion was pale and yellowish, her hair was thin and dry, her fingernails were brittle, and her eyebrows were missing over the outer half of her eyes (all symptoms of low-functioning thyroid). I asked her, "What are your sleep patterns? What is your diet? What happens premenstrually? What emotions are you experiencing?" The interview revealed that Carla had a history of dietary allergies, hair loss, extreme fatigue, and migraine headaches. Her vaginal discharge seemed abnormal, and every month her urinary and bowel patterns changed premenstrually. She got a "fever" each month before her period came, her period was heavy and crampy, and her menstruate contained clotty tissue.

Using the principles of TCM, I diagnosed Carla with a pattern of imbalance that affected her hormones. I suggested some dietary changes, including staying away from sugar and refined carbohydrates, avoiding unfermented soy products like soy protein powders, and cooking greens like Brussels sprouts, cabbage, and broccoli rather than consuming them raw. I asked her to include kelp and seaweed in her diet (both good sources of iodine, which the thyroid needs to function properly). I told her to avoid fluoride, which interferes with proper thyroid functioning, and advised her to take 500 milligrams of tyrosine (a thyroid hormone precursor) before breakfast, and supplement with magnesium and B vitamins.

Once a week I gave Carla acupuncture treatments to strengthen her weaker energies. I put her on an herbal formula, which I modified as her symptoms changed. Although I knew her primary purpose was to become pregnant, we never discussed the "I" word. (I believe that even the word *infertility* sets up a negative internal stressor that works against any woman who is trying to conceive.)

After two months, Carla reported that her fatigue and allergic symptoms were gone. After three months, she no longer had any premenstrual symptoms, and her periods became more regular and weren't so heavy. The next month, she became pregnant naturally. Her obstetrician repeated the thyroid studies and discovered her thyroid levels were within normal limits. Carla carried the baby to term and went on to have more children.

Western medicine relies on scientific measurements to determine the problem, and then it provides remedies that are supposed to overcome that particular effect. Chinese medicine, on the other hand, looks at the whole patient, seeking imbalances in the system rather than focusing on disease. In Carla's case, an underlying imbalance made her body inhospitable for conception. The treatments I prescribed restored her body's normal function, allowing her to conceive.

WORKING WITH YOUR DOCTOR(S) IN YOUR JOURNEY TO CONCEPTION

As someone who is trained in both Eastern and Western medicine, I am supportive of whatever treatments a woman chooses for her fertility problems. For women who choose to use TCM exclusively, I am happy to be their primary source of infertility treatment. Others want to avail themselves of Western medicine, and in those circumstances, I step back and become a support system for their Western treatment. But I encourage every woman to take charge of her own fertility treatments. Far too many of us view our doctors as omniscient beings who must know exactly what we need to do in order to get pregnant, when in truth, doctors (including me) are merely human.

You need to be willing to learn as much as you can about every aspect of your treatment. Get clear on the drugs you're prescribed, their effects and possible side effects. Make sure you understand every procedure, what the doctors believe will happen, and the conditions necessary for the best possible result. Read. Research medical articles on the Internet. Converse with other patients. Your body and its hormones and cycles are unlike anyone else's, and no one is going to care about your fertility as much as you will. You have to stand up for what you want the most: a healthy child conceived and carried to term in a healthy body.

If you choose complementary treatments, great! Because most alternative medical treatments (like TCM) focus on restoring health and balance to the body, they can help Western medical treatments work better. But your Western medical doctor needs to know what you are doing. *Tell your doctor if you're taking herbs, vitamins, or any kind of supplements, or if you're doing meditation, yoga, or acupuncture — anything that might affect your fertility.*

I personally think it's foolhardy for people to advocate vehemently for using one kind of medicine or another. The best way for you to get pregnant may be medicine, Eastern medicine, or a combina-tion of the two. Be willing to keep an open mind. Do your research. Find something that makes sense to you, try it, and see how your body responds. If you're getting good results, keep on that path; if not, explore other options.

Ultimately, no matter what path or paths we choose in our pursuit of fertility, *we* must be willing to take command of our medical care. We must not rely on the word of any one medical tradition or practitioner. Above all, we must learn to listen to our own body, mind, soul, and heart. In *Inconceivable*, by Julia Indichova, Christiane Northrup, M.D., the author of *Women's Bodies, Women's Wisdom*, writes: "When we're willing to listen to our bodies and begin trusting ourselves as much as we trust outer authorities, all the rules change. And so does our biology. Statistics no longer apply to us. We enter the realm of miracles and undreamed-of possibilities."

3

The Eastern View
of Your Body and Its Needs

Just imagine what would happen if the practicing physicians, the ones who come into contact directly with suffering humanity, had some acquaintance with Eastern systems of healing! The spirit of the East surges in through every pore, as balm for all the afflictions.

— C. G. Jung

Human beings are not machines; we act in accordance with the laws of nature. Our bodies and psyches are attuned to the time and tides of nature — the rhythm of day and night, the lunar cycle, the four seasons. The health of humanity is directly tied to conditions in the environment. If the climate is too hot or too cold, we suffer. If our water is tainted, we get sick. If our air is fouled, we can't breathe. It's as if we are linked to nature with an invisible web of cause and effect, substance with substance, energy with energy. As philosopher Chuang Tzu wrote in the second century B.C.E., "Heaven, Earth, and I are living together, and all things and I form an inseparable unity."

Traditional Chinese medicine draws its philosophy and treatments from the recognition of this connection between humanity and nature. Chinese medicine regards the human body as an ecosystem. In the same way ecosystems in nature consist of rivers, land, mountains, clouds, and so on, the ecosystem of the human body consists of organs, fluids, and energy. Just as there are complex relationships in nature — clouds delivering water to the mountains in the form of rain, rain flowing down the mountains and washing soil toward the plains, land being refreshed and replenished by this soil while rivers fill with water from the rain — there are equally complex yet traceable relationships between the different systems of the body. And just as the health of the external ecosystem depends on maintaining an equilibrium — the right amount of rain in the right season, the right amount of soil washed down the mountain, and so on — the health of the human body depends on maintaining balance within its different systems.

Western medicine also recognizes the importance of balance within a human body. The term used is *homeostasis*: the ability of the body to maintain its biochemistry within specific ranges by adjusting to the demands placed upon it by internal and external circumstances. But Chinese medicine's definition of balance is far greater than any biochemical response. *Maintaining and restoring balance is at the heart of diagnosis and treatment in Chinese medicine.*

Say you found yourself subject to frequent headaches, for example. You could take a pain reliever like Tylenol or Advil, but that's treating the symptom, not the cause. Western doctors might try to discover what is causing your headaches, perhaps ordering an MRI to assess if the pain might be symptomatic of a bigger problem, like a brain tumor. You might receive further treatment based on the doctor's diagnosis — or you might just get a prescription for a stronger painkiller.

In contrast, a TCM practitioner would treat your headache by endeavoring to discover the imbalance that is creating the symptom. You'd be asked a range of questions about the location and quality of the pain, your diet, stress levels, exercise patterns, sleep habits, and so on. The TCM practitioner would read your pulse and look at your tongue to check the state of your organs and meridians. Based on these findings, you'd receive a diagnosis of deficiency or excess in one or more energetic systems. You'd be given prescriptions of herbs, acupuncture, and dietary changes designed to bring your organs and energy meridians back into balance. Once balance was restored to your body, your headaches would go away. And you'd probably find that your overall health and well-being improved as well. This illustrates the fundamental difference between Western and Eastern medicine. Traditional Chinese medicine doesn't treat a kidney or a lung or an ovary; instead, it addresses the energetic health underlying those organs, then it gently coaxes the body to function in the most efficient manner.

How does this apply to human reproduction and, specifically, fertility? Rather than looking at infertility simply as a problem with an ovary or a specific hormone, TCM teaches us that fertility is a woman's natural state from the time of menarche until she reaches menopause. Subfertility results from imbalances within the network of organs, hormones, and energy systems within a woman's body. These imbalances stop her body from doing what it was meant to do: potentially conceive a child every time her ovaries release an egg. A TCM practitioner will investigate every aspect of a woman's health history and habits to determine which organs and meridians are out of balance, and then prescribe a regimen of acupuncture, herbs, exercise and/or dietary changes to restore equilibrium to her body. When a woman's body is restored to balance, the hormones needed for conception and pregnancy are produced the way nature intended.

One of the beauties of Eastern medicine is that there is no separation of mind, body, emotions, and spirit, and TCM therapy is based upon ministering to them all. I believe this approach is more in alignment with the body's own design. I also believe that because TCM focuses on restoring balance to the entire body, it can serve as a valuable adjunct to Western medical technology.

Nowadays some Western scientists are becoming interested in researching and measuring the effects of TCM. There have been a growing number of studies (in China and Europe especially) investigating the efficacy of treatments such as acupuncture and herbal prescriptions for many reproductive problems. Indeed, in 1996 the World Health Organization (WHO) of the United Nations endorsed acupuncture treatment for a wide range of conditions, including reproductive problems like impotence, infertility, PMS, pelvic inflammatory disease (PID), vaginitis, irregular period or cramps, and morning sickness. Today researchers are becoming increasingly interested in this age-old healing technique. A December 2002 study at Weill Medical College of Cornell University on the role of acupuncture in the treatment of female infertility stated, "There is sufficient evidence of acupuncture's value to expand its use into conventional medicine and treatment of female infertility."

In this chapter we'll explore the fundamentals of TCM so you will understand the diagnoses and recommendations found in the rest of this book. We'll talk about the different components of our reproductive system — hormones like estrogen and progesterone; structures like the uterus, follicles, and ovaries; and processes like ovulation, menstruation, and menopause — viewed through the lens of traditional Chinese medical diagnosis.

I ask you to read this chapter with an open mind. Women understand the idea of the human body as an ecosystem because we ourselves are an "environment" within which (hopefully) a child can be conceived and grow to term. If you listen from the deepest part of your awareness, I believe you will experience the truth of this ancient and wise tradition of healing.

ENERGY, OPPOSITES, AND BALANCE: THE BASIS OF TCM

Being and non-being create each other.
Difficult and easy support each other.
Long and short define each other.
High and low depend on each other.
Before and after follow each other.

— *TAO TE CHING* BY LAO TSU (TRANSLATED BY STEPHEN MITCHELL)

The key to Chinese medicine is found in the ancient philosophy of the Tao. The Tao sees everything in the universe as an interplay of opposites: light and dark, male and female, growth and decay, birth and death. This is defined by the concept of Yin and Yang, two opposites that create the universe and are present in everything. Each energy has a kernel of the other buried within it, as you can see in the following illustration.

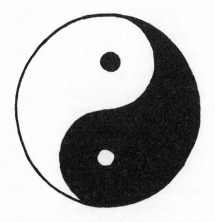

Figure 3.1: Yin and Yang (Tai Chi)

To draw an example from nature, the shortest day of the year is also the point when the days begin to lengthen; the longest day of the year marks the point when the amount of daylight begins to decrease. Each day contains the seed of its opposite.

The characteristics of Yin and Yang are likened to water and fire. Yin, like water, is yielding, receiving, cold, slow, dim, passive, and heavy; Yang, like fire, is hot, quick, burning, bright, light, and aggressive. Yin and Yang are often defined as "feminine" and "masculine" energy, respectively, but this does not mean that all women are completely Yin and all men are completely Yang. While certain energies may be connected to certain physical functions, it is the *balance* between the energies that is truly important. All women have Yang energy, and all men have Yin energy. Each energy must contain a portion of its opposite.

Yin and Yang hold each other in check with what the Chinese call "mutual restraint." The ancient "Treatise on the Essential Law of Disease Occurrence" says: "When Yin is even and Yang is firm, a relative equilibrium is maintained, and health is guaranteed." However, the interplay between Yin and Yang is constantly shifting. Within the human body, we affect the balance of Yin and Yang by what we eat, how we feel, our activities, our emotions, even our thoughts. Much of the time, we maintain this stability without thinking. We act during the day (Yang) and sleep at night (Yin). We exercise, which increases our Yang energy, and then we rest, falling into Yin. We eat hot, spicy foods (Yang) and drink something cold (Yin). We balance periods of intense mental effort (Yang) with relaxation (Yin). Even our emotions right themselves — fear (Yin) is followed by relief and often laughter (Yang), anger (Yang) is followed by calm (Yin).

The guidelines for maintaining harmony in a human body are based upon the laws of the natural universe. Discord arises when there is (1) too much of something — an excess or repletion — or (2) too little of something — a deficiency or vacuity. Symptoms produced by Yin/Yang discrepancies are often categorized into pairs: heat and cold, damp and dry, acute and chronic. An excess of Yang energy, for example, often manifests as heat, while an excess of Yin will manifest as cold. An excess of one energy causes a relative deficiency in the other. If you are experiencing fever, for instance, this usually indicates too much Yang. But you could have too much Yang because your Yin energy is weak, allowing Yang to over-produce.

Let's see how this balance plays out in a woman's reproductive system. Estrogen, the dominant hormone during the follicular phase of the menstrual cycle, is Yin. Various tissues throughout the body, including the ovaries and our fat cells, produce this hormone. Under the Yin influence of estrogen, reproductive tissue flourishes. Estrogen generates a plush uterine lining, causes cervical changes, and produces fertile cervical mucus during ovulation. It prepares the "cave" of the uterus to accept the fertilized egg and nurture the evolving embryo.

As women approach menopause, estrogen levels drop, and we experience night sweats, hot flashes, and vaginal dryness. Because our Yin (in the form of estrogen) is deficient, the Yang (hot energy) of our body rises to the fore, producing these symptoms. To eliminate the symptoms of Yin deficiency, synthetic estrogen supplementation is common among menopausal women. However, one of the side effects of this treatment is a predisposition to cancers of the breast and uterus. Traditional Chinese medicine says that these cancers are pathological accumulations of excess damp (Yin) because there isn't enough Yang Qi to move the extra Yin. The synthetic supplementation, which was trying to supply the missing Yin energy, has shifted the imbalance from deficiency to excess, and disease is the result.

Yang energy is connected to the production of testosterone and progesterone. Progesterone, a hormone secreted by the corpus luteum of the ovary after ovulation, is Yang in nature, as it heats, transforms, and invigorates. Luteal phase defect, a common cause of subfertility, occurs when the corpus luteum does not release adequate levels of progesterone to transform the endometrial tissue so it can hold a fertilized ovum. Most hormonal stimulation used in Western reproductive medicine stimulates Yang energetic functions.

Thyroid hormone is also Yang in nature. Those diagnosed with excess thyroid hormone become overly anxious, very hot, and have difficulty sleeping (excess Yang). Hypothyroidism (too little thyroid hormone) produces the sensation of cold and sluggish Yang energies.

Just as we need a balance of Yin and Yang to live, we need the proper equilibrium of Yin and Yang for our reproductive system to function normally. But instead of flooding the body with supplemental hormones, TCM uses the body's own energy to stimulate production of endorphins and hormones. Traditional Chinese medicine treatments simply remind the body of what it was meant to do.

QI: THE ENERGY OF LIFE

The root of the way of life, of birth and change is Qi . . .

— *JHANGSHI LEIJING*

The basis of all traditional Chinese medicine is energy. This energy is the force that enlivens every cell. Every living organism in creation is simply energy that has taken form ($E = mc^2$). Our bodies are made up of energy that flows in patterns of electricity. All of our cells and tissues conduct and transfer energy through protein molecules, giving us life. This energetic source flows throughout every aspect of our body, invigorating our organs and powering the processes that link them as well. This electromagnetic force directs every chemical and hormonal release.

The Chinese call this universal energy "Qi." As described in the classic Chinese medical text *Leijing,* "the source wherefrom the sun, moon and stars derive their light, the thunder, rain, wind and cloud their being, the four seasons and the myriad things their birth, growth, gathering and storing: all this is brought about by Qi. Man's possession of life is completely dependent upon this Qi."

In the human body, Qi manifests in several different ways. First, Qi is a kind of bioelectrical force that flows throughout the body, carried by an extensive network of channels called "meridians." These channels are invisible to the naked eye, yet they have been mapped over the course of thousands of years of observation and experimentation by Oriental physicians. The application of force (acupressure) or insertion of a needle (acupuncture) at different points along these meridians produces measurable, demonstrable effects on different parts, organs, and systems within the body.

Second, this fundamental form of source Qi is converted in the body to several different substances and fluids that make the body run. The four vital substances of the body are Qi (which is both energy and a fluid), Yin, Yang, and Blood. The fluids include Essence and Moisture. Each fluid and substance works within the different Organ systems of the body, helping to carry energy throughout the system. These fluids and substances are intimately involved in converting what we take in from our external environment — air, water, and food — into the different forms of nourishment our bodies need. Then these fluids and substances transport the nourishment to our organs, cells, and systems, and take away any waste products, eventually transporting them out of the body.

Third, Qi takes form as all the different organs and systems. Traditional Chinese medicine looks at organs in a very different way from Western medicine. Although the names of the organs (lungs, kidneys, spleen, uterus, and so on) may be familiar, the functions attributed to the energetic systems of the organs are expanded. For example, in TCM the Liver is intimately related with the

Blood. Thus, whenever there is a problem with menstruation, a TCM practitioner would suspect some kind of Liver system involvement. Other Organs directly affecting fertility include the Spleen and Kidneys.* We'll review the functions of each Organ system later in this chapter.

Qi not only makes up the organs and the fluids in the body but also flows to and through them, carried by the meridians. This means that specific acupuncture points can be used to treat specific organs. For instance, Lung Qi moves through a channel that runs into the chest, down the inside of the arms, and to the fingertips. Using acupuncture or acupressure on these points will affect the flow of Qi through the meridian and in turn affect the functioning of the Lung system. That's why it's possible to treat a wide variety of conditions using different combinations of points.

The Qi that flows through our bodies is the same Qi that creates every other part of the universe. Plants, animals, air and water resonate with the same frequency as our individual energies. Therefore, if someone takes an herb, has an acupuncture treatment, or changes her lifestyle or living environment, then the Qi present in all those things will cause a change in the internal Qi.

---

*To distinguish between what Western medicine means by certain words, like *blood, kidney,* and *liver,* and the TCM versions of the same organs, systems, and substances, references to the Chinese organs, systems, or fluids will be capitalized.

❦ THE MERIDIANS

> *The Tao gives birth to One.*
> *One gives birth to two.*
> *Two gives birth to three.*
> *Three gives birth to ten thousand things.*

> — *TAO TE CHING*

To benefit from TCM treatments, you don't need to understand how acupuncture works. But for those who require more information, science has provided several theories describing how the lines of energy running throughout the body (meridians) affect systems and organs that on the surface appear to have no relation. One theory — which I find interesting for obvious reasons — has to do with the development of the embryo. When a woman's egg is fertilized it becomes a zygote. Then the single cell divides horizontally into two cells and is called a blastomere. The two cells divide again vertically into four, then eight, in a process called cleavage (fig. 3.2).

As cleavage continues, the dividing cells align themselves tightly against one another to form a compact ball known as a morula. At the next stage of development, the blastocyst stage, the multiplying cells separate further. A thin outer layer forms, called the trophoblast, which later becomes the fetal part of the placenta. The other cells form an inner cell mass, which becomes the embryo (fig. 3.3).

As the embryo continues to develop, certain cells start to coalesce along what look like fold lines. These fold lines mark the separation of one group of cells from another; they also mark the connection between groups of related cells. As cells

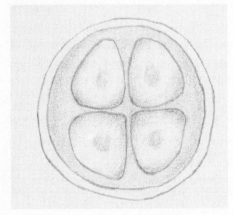

Figure 3.2: Cleavage

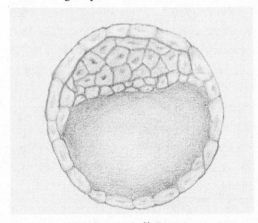

Figure 3.3: Cell Division

continue to differentiate along fold lines, they become the organs and organ systems.

Why is this important? Because remnants of the embryonic folds remain in our bodies even after the organ systems are formed, and modern researchers in Chinese medicine believe that the embryonic folds become energy meridians. These embryonic folds serve as "channels of connection" between apparently separate parts of the body. Think of the embryonic folds like an electrified fence. The folds keep what's on one side of the fence separated from what's on the other side. At the same time, if you were to put a jolt of electricity into one end of the fence, the energy would travel very quickly and efficiently from point A (where the energy went in) to point B (the other end of the fence). Even if point A and point B were a long way from each other, the fence (embryonic fold) would serve as a very efficient conduit for energy. This explains why points in the feet or along the arms can affect the function of the kidneys or lungs or ovaries.

An acupuncture point is an area on the skin where the electromagnetic current that runs throughout the body comes close to the surface, so it makes sense that those spots would be sensitive to electrical energy from outside the body. Anything you do to decrease or enhance the flow of electromagnetic energy throughout the body will have the greatest effect at the acupuncture points.

As electrical energy flows from one place to the other, it encounters resistance that builds up from the channels it's flowing through. To make energy flow more smoothly, you must do everything you can to decrease resistance. Let's go back to our electric fence analogy. To transmit energy through the fence, you'd want to find a way of enhancing the flow of energy from one end of the fence to the other by decreasing resistance. And what's the best conductor of electrical energy? Metal.

Here's what this means in terms of acupuncture and the meridians. Say you have a meridian where the electrical energy isn't flowing as well as you'd like. If you put a metal needle (an excellent conductor of electricity) into an acupuncture point (where the meridian runs close to the surface of the body), you are decreasing resistance while promoting the flow of energy along that meridian. Since the meridian connects a whole series of tissues and organs, stimulating an acupuncture point on the leg, for instance, can regulate the energy in the Spleen. The improved flow doesn't just put more energy into a specific organ; instead, it normalizes the flow of energy throughout the system. If there's too much energy, it allows the excess to drain; if there's too little energy, it allows more to flow into that particular area or organ.

The effects of acupuncture on the body's electromagnetic field have been studied extensively over the past twenty years in both the East and the West. Certain studies on acupuncture's ability to relieve pain also demonstrate how acupuncture can help improve fertility. These studies indicate that pressure exerted by an acupuncture needle triggers the release of prostaglandins, which stimulate production of chemicals in the nerve endings, which in turn transmit a message to the hypothalamus. Located at the base of the brain, the hypothalamus is the regulatory control center for all hormonal activity. It is of special interest to us because it also controls the discharge of gonadotropin-releasing hormones (GnRH), which govern ovulation, menstruation, and pregnancy. Acupuncture affects the functioning of the hypothalamus and the release of hormonal substances throughout the body — both necessary aspects of the treatment of many causes of infertility.

The Eastern explanation of the effects of acupuncture on the body is far simpler: *acupuncture balances the whole body system.* Think of a large field that gets its water from a network of canals. If one of the canals is blocked at any point, the blockage would not only keep the water from flowing to certain parts of the field but also cause other parts to get too much water as things back up. Acupuncture is like removing the blockage from an energetic "canal." When the right points are stimulated, energy that has been blocked will flow freely again. The parts of the body that have been starved for energy will receive it, and the parts of the body where energy has been building up will return to proper levels.

There are twelve major meridians in six pairs that run throughout the body and link directly to certain organ-related energy systems:

1. Kidney/Urinary Bladder system
2. Liver/Gallbladder system
3. Spleen/Stomach system
4. Heart/Small Intestine system
5. Lung/Large Intestine system
6. Pericardium/Triple Warmer (the internal energetic source of life heat)

Later in this chapter we'll discuss how and why these organs are linked together. But deeper than these Organ system meridians are what is called the *Extraordinary meridians:*

1. Penetrating meridian (Chong Mai)
2. Conception meridian (Ren Mai)
3. Governing meridian (Du Mai)
4. Girdle meridian (Dai Mai)

The Penetrating, Conception, and Governing meridians control the energies that determine growth, maturity, and aging. They also affect the hormonal aspects of reproduction. Together these three meridians represent the hypothalamic–pituitary–ovarian (HPO) axis — the energies that are released when a girl reaches menarche and diminish when a woman enters menopause. The Extraordinary meridians also govern embryological development, genetic constitution, age, and decline.

THE PENETRATING MERIDIAN

The Penetrating meridian is called the "sea of the twelve channels" since it communicates with the other meridians. It is also said to represent the "sea of Blood." In women it originates in the Uterus and presides over the function of menstruation. It controls our hormonal cycles. It also is related to the psychoneuroendocrinological system, or the interdependence of the mind, emotions, and hormones. From the Penetrating meridian arise the Conception and Governing meridians, which direct the Yin and Yang energies of the body.

THE CONCEPTION MERIDIAN (YIN)

The Conception meridian is said to be the "sea of all Yin meridians." This means it regulates the Yin energies of the body, those associated with female nature: cool, dark, moist, and nurturing. From the Conception meridian come the Yin energies that supply the Lungs, Liver, Spleen, Kidneys, Heart, and Pericardium (the covering around the Heart). The production of estrogen (a Yin hormone) is also connected to the Conception meridian.

THE GOVERNING MERIDIAN (YANG)

The Governing meridian is the "sea of all Yang meridians." Yang energies are more male in nature: strong, hard, warm, bright, and energetic. The Yang energies govern the Urinary Bladder, the Gallbladder, the Stomach, the Triple Warmer, and the Small and Large Intestines. The Governing meridian oversees the production of testosterone and progesterone, two Yang hormones.

THE GIRDLE MERIDIAN

The Girdle meridian encircles the body horizontally at the waist. In TCM it's described as a belt that cannot be too tight or too loose. It connects the Penetrating and Conception meridians with the Kidney, Liver, and Spleen channels. We drain excesses like profuse vaginal discharge through the Girdle meridian. The Girdle meridian also restrains vaginal leakage, including miscarriage.

THE ORGANS

Heaven has five musical sounds, humans have five Yin Organs . . .

— *NEI JING*

The six paired meridians are directly related to specific Organ systems. While often considered to perform the same functions as

they do in Western medical thought, in TCM these Organs have additional responsibilities. Take a woman's menstrual cycle, for instance. If there were problems with a woman's cycle, Western medicine would look to her hormones or uterus for the cause. In TCM, however, menstrual difficulties could be caused by problems with either the meridians or the Organs other than the Uterus. According to the *Su Wen (Questions and Answers About Living Matter)*, written by Liu Wan Su, a woman cannot have a period unless she has a "communicating" Conception meridian and a "full" Penetrating meridian.* She also has to have enough Essence in her Kidneys, and enough Blood supplied by the Liver and Spleen. Treating menstrual problems with TCM, therefore, may involve the Penetrating and Conception meridians, and/or the Kidneys, Liver, or Spleen. Treatment would endeavor to balance the Blood, the Essence, or the proportion of Yin/Yang energy.

While it's important for our general health that all Organ systems are balanced, the Lung/Large Intestine and Pericardium/ Triple Warmer systems are only tangentially involved with reproduction and fertility, and therefore I will not cover them here. However, in addition to the six paired organ systems, TCM has designated other organs as Extraordinary or "curious" (like the Extraordinary meridians described above). One of these is the Uterus; another is the Brain. Both the Brain and the Uterus are governed by the Kidneys, which oversee the reproductive aspects of the Extraordinary meridians. (We will be putting this information into a more concrete context as we look at diagnosing and treating specific causes of infertility in later chapters.)

THE KIDNEY SYSTEM AND REPRODUCTION

In Western medicine the kidneys are two bean-shaped organs located on each side of the lower back. They are responsible for fluid and acid balance, metabolism, and elimination of waste products. But in TCM the Kidney system is accountable for our genetic makeup. It dictates growth and development. It determines when women menstruate and when they go into menopause. The Kidneys are responsible for bone and teeth formation and overall brain function. And yes, the Kidneys also control water balance and elimination.

When the organ systems are being formed in the embryo, the ovaries, testicles, uterus, fallopian tubes, and, to some extent, the adrenal glands are all developmentally related. In TCM, the Kidney system connects and encompasses the reproductive system, the skeletal system, the neurological system, and the endocrine system. In traditional Chinese medicine the emotion of fright is damaging to the Kidneys as well as to the adrenals. Fright is said to "scatter the Qi," and when Qi is scattered, it cannot hold an embryo in the uterus. This describes one

---

*The *Su Wen* is one of two books that make up the *Nei Jing*, the seminal Chinese medical text. One focuses more on natural medicines, while the other focuses more on acupuncture energetics.

way in which stress (fear) can impair proper functioning of the reproductive system.

The symptoms associated with menopause — profuse sweating, loss of bone density, emotional turmoil — are all related to changes in a woman's hormonal levels. But in TCM, these symptoms are usually treated with remedies that tonify the Kidneys, such as stimulating points on the Kidney meridian. With this treatment many women find relief from night sweats, feel better mentally, and restart menses. Occasionally a woman who has been told she is going into menopause and has no chance of becoming a mother actually becomes pregnant once her Kidney system has been put back into balance.

Stimulating the Kidney system can also restore normal levels of FSH. According to Western reproductive medicine, the main determinant of reproductive "youth" is FSH, which is produced by the pituitary gland. In the course of a normal monthly cycle, the release of FSH stimulates a woman's ovaries to produce estrogen and begin follicular development. Early in a woman's cycle this particular hormone should be low (below 10 international units [IU] per liter). If this particular hormone is elevated above 10 IU on day 3 of a woman's cycle, this tells the gynecologist that the woman's ovaries are not responding appropriately, a condition that prompts the ovaries to send a message to the brain that the pituitary gland needs to produce more FSH. A woman with elevated FSH levels will be diagnosed as having "ovarian failure." However, as I have seen

time and again in my clinic, if a woman has sizeable, pink (i.e., healthy) ovaries, by treating her Kidney system with herbs and acupuncture, TCM can stimulate her ovaries to respond normally to FSH, produce higher levels of estrogen, and develop healthy follicles and eggs.

Chinese medicine considers the Kidneys the root and support of all the other organs. As one of the ancient texts states, "the Kidneys are the residence of Yin and Yang . . . the channel of death and life." Unlike the other Organ systems, the Kidneys rarely exhibit an excess of anything; disorders are almost always a result of some kind of deficiency. Therefore, most of the treatments offered are designed to tonify or build up the Kidneys' energies through diet, herbs, and acupuncture.

The Kidneys are also where we store our Essence, the genetic material we receive from our parents and pass on to our offspring. The process of aging depletes our Essence. That's one of the reasons that menopausal symptoms can be alleviated when the Kidney system is tonified or stimulated, thus augmenting the Essence. A second type of Essence stored in the Kidneys is produced by the Spleen from the food, air, and water we take in. Because an unhealthy diet and unwholesome lifestyle exhaust the Essence, making changes in your diet and lifestyle can have a direct effect on the Kidney system. And because the Kidneys are located in the lower back, menstrual difficulties accompanied by lower back pain suggest Kidney involvement.

THE SPLEEN, DIGESTION, AND IMMUNOLOGICAL SYSTEMS

The Western concept of the spleen encompasses its role in the production and destruction of blood and immune cells. In TCM, however, the Spleen system (which includes aspects of the pancreas) governs most energetic processes in the body. The Spleen transforms the food we eat into Qi, Blood, and other types of usable energy, so it must be functioning optimally for a healthy menstrual cycle. The Spleen is also responsible for producing certain hormones, such as thyroid hormone and progesterone, as well as for aspects of the circulatory and immunological systems. A malfunctioning Spleen system often causes thyroid abnormalities, autoimmune problems, allergies, digestive disturbances, and bleeding disorders. Menstrual difficulties can also be caused by a Spleen imbalance.

Spleen energy manifests in the gastrointestinal system and also is markedly affected by what we eat. Immoderate sugar and refined carbohydrate consumption damages the Spleen, and damp, greasy foods clog up its works. When our Spleen system is strong, we have a lot of physical energy; when it's weak, we feel tired and depleted.

The emotion associated with the Spleen system is worry. The Chinese believe "overthinking" can inhibit the energetic processes of the Spleen. This explains why excessive worry causes digestive disturbances like stomach ulcers and irritable bowel syndrome. We have so much information that it clogs up our minds, yet all too often we think far more than we act, producing a backup of energy that causes disharmony between the Spleen (thinking), the Heart (spirit), and the Kidneys (will). Exercise is beneficial to the proper functioning of the Spleen.

Because the Spleen is linked with digestion and elimination, the Spleen system is implicated when menstruation is accompanied by loose stools. The Spleen also is involved in many cases of luteal phase defect in which spotting precedes menstruation (see chapter 9).

THE HEART, THE SPIRIT, AND THE UTERUS

The Chinese concept of the Heart encompasses the mind and spirit as well as the Blood and circulatory system. The Heart endows us with personality and allows us peace. The Heart is ministered to whenever there are shattered emotional and spiritual issues. The Heart also provides Blood for the Uterus. If there are emotional upsets, this may influence the Uterus's ability to nourish a developing fetus. The Uterine Vessel, called the Bao Mai, provides the link between the Heart and the Uterus. The *Su Wen* says, "When the period does not come it means the Uterine Vessel is obstructed." For functional purposes, however, the Penetrating meridian is treated first when disorders of the Uterus and Heart arise.

THE LIVER/GALLBLADDER SYSTEM AND STRESS

The liver is a large, dark-red gland in the upper part of the right side of the abdomen, just beneath the diaphragm. In both Western and Eastern medicine, the liver's main functions include storage and filtration of blood, and metabolic activities including the metabolism of hormones. But Chinese medicine says that the Liver is also involved in the smooth flow and distribution of Blood, emotions, and Qi. Liver Qi is responsible for all transformations in the body, including ovulation.

The Liver is important in reproduction largely because of its role in menstruation. During the premenstrual period, the Liver shifts the Blood flow from other body parts to the Uterus. Right before menstruation, when the Liver is busy directing the body to menstruate, it has a tendency to neglect its other functions — such as keeping the Qi and emotions flowing smoothly. As a result, the emotional energy becomes blocked, and depression, anger, sadness, or weepiness may be experienced. There may be headaches, breast pain, cramps, and a variety of other physical and emotional symptoms. At this time any Liver obstruction will cause Qi and Blood to "back up" or stagnate. If the channels remain closed, the flow of energy to the Uterus will be impeded, and then menses is associated with pain and cramping.

Liver imbalances that cause energetic obstructions confine the energy of this important system to a very small space. This confinement of energy creates a large amount of heat, which ascends up the Gallbladder meridian and can cause premenstrual migraine headaches. (In fact, migraines were once referred to as "the megrims," or bouts of biliousness, a disease associated with the gallbladder.)

When diagnosing patterns preventing conception, it is absolutely essential to address blockages in the Liver and Gallbladder. If the Liver system is not functioning smoothly, neither is the hormonal system. The Uterus itself can become a toxic environment, hostile to implantation. Liver Qi stagnation causes hormones like estrogen to build up in the body. Estrogen dominance is implicated in conditions like endometriosis, fibroids, polycystic ovarian syndrome, and cancer. Most women with these diseases are diagnosed with an element of Liver Qi stagnation.

In addition to governing all transformations and discoursing Qi and emotion, the Liver is responsible for Blood conservation (storage). When the Blood (which is Yin) is depleted (through loss of blood, an overactive lifestyle, too much stress, exercise, and lack of rest and self-care), the Liver loses its ability to smooth the emotional energy. Even small annoyances may become exaggerated to the level of frustration and anger, blocking already pent-up emotional energy. Such emotional blockages can impede the Liver's transformation functions, like ovulation and menstruation. Here again, stress affects our ability to reproduce. As the emotional basis of Liver Qi stagnation is said to be unfulfilled desires, this condition is apparent in most women who have trouble conceiving.

Alcohol consumption damages the energetic function of the Liver. Therefore, women who are diagnosed with an overabundance of stagnant Liver Qi should not consume alcohol when they are trying to get pregnant.

THE UTERUS

The Chinese word for uterus literally means "palace of the child." Although the Uterus is an independent organ, it is intimately connected with the rest of the body. Both the Conception meridian and Penetrating meridian are said to originate in the Uterus.

The Uterine Vessel is the conduit between the Heart and Uterus and provides Blood to the Uterus. There are further networks of blood supply responsible for connecting and communicating between the Uterus and the other organs. One such network connects the Kidneys to the Uterus. This is the energetic pathway by which the Kidney Essence nourishes the Uterus and thickens the uterine lining. (This relationship represents the pituitary's message to the ovary to produce estrogen, and the Uterus's responsive growth of its lining.) If the Uterus does not receive Essence from the Kidneys by way of this network, and Blood from the Heart by way of the Uterine Vessel, conception cannot occur.

❧ HOW TCM TREATMENTS WORK

Illnesses may be identical but the persons suffering from them are different. Physicians therefore must carefully take into account the differences among people . . .

— HSU TA-CH'UN (1757)

Reproductive health, like all health, is about balance and relativity. The most important distinction a TCM practitioner can make is correctly identifying the *pattern,* which underlies any process of disease. As Joseph Needham (1900–1995), a great Western historian of Chinese science, wrote, "The key word in Chinese thought is *Order* and above all *Pattern.*"

Traditional Chinese medicine describes the female reproductive system as a network of energy systems with complementary organs and hormonal responses. This network responds to stress, chemicals, lack of exercise, poor eating, and excess emotions, all of which can put the body off balance. Even a slight aberration can throw the entire system off so that it no longer functions smoothly. Yet, just as the body responds to negative influences, it also responds to gentle direction to return to balance.

In Eastern medicine, there is *always* a reason one part of the system does not function as it should. There will be expressions of the underlying imbalance, and when the root problem is treated, these manifestations will disappear. If you go to a practitioner of TCM for treatment, he or she will review your symptoms and, based on observations, diagnose where your body is out of balance: whether there is too much heat or cold, dryness or moisture, deficiency or excess, vacuity or repletion. Prescriptions include acupuncture, herbs, diet, lifestyle changes, or a combination of all four to bring your system back to its proper functioning.

Below and on the following page you'll find a chart summarizing the basic meridians and Organ systems of TCM and their functions. But even if you have some difficulty with the finer points of TCM, remember the basic tenets of Chinese medicine:

◆ the body's internal environment operates in many of the same ways as other ecosystems in nature
◆ an imbalance at any point in the system can cause symptoms and disease
◆ restoring the body to balance is the goal of treatment.

I believe this foundation will provide you with a new source of health and hope in your quest to heal your body and restore your fertility.

Meridians and Organ Systems and Their Functions

Meridians	Functions
Penetrating meridian	• Communicates with other meridians • Presides over menstruation and hormonal cycles • Source of Conception and Governing meridians
Conception meridian	• Regulates Yin energy • Supplies Kidney, Liver, Spleen, Heart, Pericardium, and Lung Organ systems • Connected with production of estrogen
Governing meridian	• Regulates Yang energy • Supplies Urinary Bladder, Gallbladder, Stomach, Small and Large Intestines, and Triple Warmer • Oversees testosterone and progesterone production
Girdle meridian	• Encircles the body horizontally at the waist • Binds the Penetrating, Conception, Kidney, Liver, and Spleen channels • Used to drain excess vaginal discharge • Restrains vaginal leakage, including miscarriage

Organ Systems	Functions
Kidney	• Contains our genetic makeup • Controls the reproductive system and a woman's hormones • Connects reproductive, skeletal, neurological, and endocrine systems • Stores Essence, one of the key energies of the body
Spleen	• Governs energy production, metabolism, digestion, and elimination • Converts nutrients and Qi into Blood • Essential for healthy menstrual cycle • Affects thyroid hormone production • Sustains the luteal phase
Heart	• Governs mind and spirit • Controls Blood and circulatory system • Provides Blood for the Uterus
Liver	• Controls smooth flow and distribution of Blood • Responsible for all transformations in body, including ovulation • Provides Blood for menstruation • Affects expression of emotions, calms emotional energy • Stores Blood
Uterus	• "Palace of the child" • Connected with rest of body, especially the Heart and Kidneys • Source of Conception and Penetrating meridians

4

"Why Can't I Get Pregnant?"

A Questionnaire of Discovery

Natures differ,
and needs with them.
Hence the wise men of old
did not lay down
one measure for all.

— Chuang Tse (fourth century b.c.e.)

Most women who have been diagnosed as infertile have been through test after test to determine what's "wrong" with them. They come into my office with diagnoses like "polycystic ovarian syndrome (PCOS)," "fallopian tube blockage," and so on. They are usually frustrated with the invasiveness and impersonal quality of Western medicine when dealing with this most personal aspect of their life.

I'm happy to take a look at charts and listen to step-by-step accounts of a patient's Western medical treatment. However, Western-based diagnosis is merely an indication to me of potential areas of investigation. Many of the questions I ask patients assess symptoms seemingly unrelated to the reproductive organs — whether the feet are cold, for example, or if the mouth gets dry. My questions are designed to uncover excesses and deficiencies in the flow of Qi throughout the body, to determine which Organs are involved, and to find out how the different systems are interacting to throw the patient's body out of balance. As we emphasized in chapters 2 and 3, according to TCM, *all illness is a result of deficiencies and excesses in the body's energy.* Traditional Chinese medicine focuses more on restoring balance to the body than treating individual conditions. Any diagnosis, therefore, will involve every aspect of a woman's life.

THE CORNERSTONES OF TCM DIAGNOSIS: LOOKING, LISTENING, AND TOUCHING

One of the primary responsibilities of the physician is accurate diagnosis. In Western medicine, diagnosis is based on information from three different sources: interview (patient reports), observation, and clinical tests. However, any diagnosis must be confirmed by scientific testing to be considered valid. These tests are often invasive and expensive, and may or may not indicate a clear cause for the problem.

Traditional Chinese medicine relies upon the symptoms the patient reports combined with the doctor's observation of the patient during the initial and subsequent visits. When a woman comes to see me, I begin by reviewing the extensive questionnaire she fills out either in my waiting room or before her visit (see fig. 3.4).

In many cases, I can guess a patient's diagnosis by simply reading her answers. But any theory I have must be confirmed by looking, listening, and feeling — the "tests" used in TCM for thousands of years.

LOOKING

Observing a patient always provides a wealth of clues. Western doctors look at the patient's color, breathing patterns, movements, and so on. Practitioners of TCM will do the same, only TCM doctors will draw different conclusions from their observations than their Western counterparts.* Is the patient's complexion red or flushed, indicating an excess of heat within the body? (Remember, heat doesn't necessarily equal fever.) Does she look pale or seem sluggish? This may mean a deficiency of Yang energy. Experienced TCM practitioners can read the complexion and tone of the skin with ease, but we also look at the body's overall tone and shape (firm and muscular, obese, thin), as well as observe the condition of the eye (clear, yellow, rheumy, swollen).

*To a Western doctor, a yellow complexion means jaundice. To a TCM practitioner, a yellowish tinge to the skin may point to Liver pathology or excess dampness, depending on other symptoms.

Eastern Harmony
ACUPUNCTURE & HERBAL CLINIC

Women's Fertility History

CONFIDENTIAL

Eastern Harmony Acupuncture & Herbal Clinic ■ 4611 Montrose Blvd, Suite A201 ■ Houston, TX 77006   Phone: 713-529-1610   Fax: 713-529-6870
www.easternharmonyclinic.com

NAME (LAST, FIRST, MIDDLE)	DATE

Age at which menses began _____

Are your periods painful? ☐ Yes ☐ No

  How many days does the pain last?_____

How many days do you normally bleed?_____

How heavy is the bleeding? ☐ Light   ☐ Normal   ☐ Heavy

What color is the blood? ☐ Light red ☐ Red   ☐ Dark red ☐ Purple
☐ Brown   ☐ Black

Is there clotting? ☐ Yes ☐ No

Do you have premenstrual tension? ☐ Yes ☐ No

Does your face break out before or during your period? ☐ Yes ☐ No

Do your breasts become tender premenstrually? ☐ Yes ☐ No

Do you bleed or spot between periods? ☐ Yes ☐ No

Are your menstrual cycles spaced irregularly? ☐ Yes ☐ No

How many days are there from from one period to the next?_____

Date of last menstrual period_____

	Number	Years
How many pregnancies have you had?	____	_____
How many children do you have?	____	_____
How many abortions have you had?	____	_____
How many miscarriages have you had?	____	_____
How many times has a D&C been performed?	____	_____

Have you ever had an abnormal pap smear? ☐ Yes ☐ No

Have you ever had a cervical biopsy,
operation, cauterization or conization? ☐ Yes ☐ No

Have you ever had a venereal disease? ☐ Yes ☐ No

Do you get yeast infections regularly? ☐ Yes ☐ No

Have you ever been diagnosed with a chlamydial infection? ☐ Yes ☐ No

Do you have chronic vaginal discharge? ☐ Yes ☐ No

Do you have any sores on your genitalia? ☐ Yes ☐ No

Have you ever had pelvic inflammatory disease? ☐ Yes ☐ No
Were you treated for it? ☐ Yes ☐ No

How_____

_____

Date of last Pap smear_____

Have you ever been diagnosed with uterine fibroids or polyps? ☐ Yes ☐ No

Have you ever been diagnosed with endometriosis? ☐ Yes ☐ No

Have you been diagnosed with pelvic adhesions? ☐ Yes ☐ No

Have you been diagnosed with any pelvic abnormalities? ☐ Yes ☐ No

Have you taken any medications for
gynecological conditions other than contraceptives?

Medication	Reason	How long
_____	_____	_____
_____	_____	_____
_____	_____	_____
_____	_____	_____
_____	_____	_____
_____	_____	_____
_____	_____	_____
_____	_____	_____
_____	_____	_____
_____	_____	_____

Have your cycles changed since they began? ☐ Yes ☐ No

How? _____

Do you ovulate on your own? ☐ Yes ☐ No

On what day of your cycle?_____

Do your breasts get tender at/during ovulation? ☐ Yes ☐ No

Do you get premenstral low back pain? Yes   No

Do your bowel movements become loose at the beginning of your period?

  ☐ Yes ☐ No

Eastern Harmony
ACUPUNCTURE & HERBAL CLINIC
Women's Fertility History *Continued*

Have you had fertility treatments? ☐ Yes ☐ No

　If yes, when and where?_____

　By whom?_____

　What types?_____

Have you taken medication to help you ovulate? ☐ Yes ☐ No

　When _____ How long?_____

Have your fallopian tubes been evaluated medically? ☐ Yes ☐ No

　What were the results?_____

Have you had any tubal operations? ☐ Yes ☐ No

Have you had any hormone laboratory tests performed? ☐ Yes ☐ No

　What were the results?_____
_____

Do you have a single partner
with whom you have been trying to conceive? ☐ Yes ☐ No

　How long have you been married or living together?_____

　Has he had a fertility workup? ☐ Yes ☐ No

　What were the results?_____

　Is your partner supportive of your wish to conceive? ☐ Yes ☐ No

Have you taken oral contraceptives? ☐ Yes ☐ No

　When _____ How long?_____

Have you ever had an IUD? ☐ Yes ☐ No

　When _____ How long?_____

Have you ever taken DepoProvera? ☐ Yes ☐ No

　When _____ How long?_____

How long have you been trying to conceive? _____

Have you had a diagnosis relating to infertility? ☐ Yes ☐ No

　What was it?_____

How is your sexual energy? ☐ Low ☐ Normal ☐ High

Do you douche regularly? ☐ Yes ☐ No

　With what?_____

Do you use vaginal lubricants? ☐ Yes ☐ No

Are you more than 20% over your ideal body weight? ☐ Yes ☐ No

Are you more than 20% below your ideal body weight? ☐ Yes ☐ No

Do you have a stressful occupation? ☐ Yes ☐ No

Do you exercise regularly? ☐ Yes ☐ No

Do you have excessive facial hair? ☐ Yes ☐ No

Do you have excessively oily skin? ☐ Yes ☐ No

Have you experienced excessive loss of head hair? ☐ Yes ☐ No

Have you noticed discharge from your nipples? ☐ Yes ☐ No

Was your mother exposed to
diethylstilbestrol (DES) when she was pregnant with you? ☐ Yes ☐ No

Have you been exposed to any
known environmental toxins or hormones? ☐ Yes ☐ No

Are you presently taking steroids? ☐ Yes ☐ No

COMMENTS/NOTES

Figure 3.4: Women's Fertility History Questionnaire

One of the most important diagnostic means used by TCM practitioners is observation of the patient's tongue, which is considered the "map of the body" since its overall shape and condition correspond to the wellness of systems and internal organs. I note the tongue body to see if it is small or large, swollen or shrunken. I look at the color (a pale tongue means deficiency, a red one points to an excess of heat, and so on) and for any cracks or blemishes that appear on the surface, signifying problems with specific Organs. Another aspect of my examination is to assess the tongue's coating. (I request that my patients refrain from brushing their tongue before they come to see me.) A healthy person's tongue will have a thin, moist, white coating. A thick white coating indicates too much cold, while a yellow-tinged coating suggests too much heat.

Based on the meridians of energy running through the body, the questions I ask determine whether the problem is too much or too little energy, Blood, or fluid reaching the Organs linked to reproduction (which include the Kidneys, Liver, Spleen, and Heart) or to the hormonal balance of the body. Remember, the Organs in Chinese medicine are more like energy systems than specific units in the body. Thus, a patient can have a condition of excess — too much dampness caused by Qi that is not moving — that prevents energy from flowing through a system like the Spleen, which will then become relatively deficient and also depress the overall flow of Qi energy throughout the body. It's like the common cold: some colds affect the nose and sinuses, others settle in your chest, still others make your joints ache, and the really bad ones include all of these symptoms. In the same way, excess or deficiency has an impact on your entire body, but depending on your symptoms, it's clear that certain Organs are more affected than others.

I categorize my observations of the patient according to the patterns of imbalance I have diagnosed and treated in thousands of women over the years. But my perception must be confirmed by two other means of diagnosis: listening and touching.

LISTENING

In the course of my first interview with a patient, I spend most of my time listening and observing. For many of my patients, the freedom to express themselves openly and to be heard with compassion are two of the most important parts of the healing process. And I *want* to hear them. To diagnose their condition properly, I need to know not only about their physical symptoms but also about their emotions, their lifestyle, their relationships, and so on. The more I know about the total patient, the more informed and accurate my diagnosis.

While my patients are talking, I listen and look for evidence of underlying imbalances. I also ask a lot of questions about their menstrual cycle, where most hormonal problems will manifest. I ask about the flow, the quantity, when the breasts are tender, how they feel during ovulation and menstruation, sleep patterns, vision changes, quality of life, etc. I ask about timing of menstruation (periods that arrive earlier than usual may refer to heat, which causes the Blood to move too fast; irregular cycles can mean the Liver Qi is imbalanced), and the color and consistency of menstrual blood (thin, pale blood means deficiency; clotted, purplish blood can indicate obstruction). I ask about amount, color, and timing of vaginal discharge, as changes in fluid can signify problems with moisture distribution in the Organs.

If a woman has been treated for infertility by Western medical doctors, I ask about her responses to the drugs or hormones she received. I'll ask questions such as "The last time you went through an in vitro cycle, how did you respond? How many follicles did you produce? How much time passed before the eggs were retrieved? How was your lining?" If the woman responds, "I only had two follicles," or "My lining wasn't thick enough," she won't know what that means in terms of TCM — but I will.

Once I start to get a sense of the underlying pattern, I focus my questions in that direction. Patterns of imbalance manifest as conditions of either deficiency or excess, or more often as a combination of the two. So I begin to ask questions based on the patterns that are showing up. It's very common for my patients to say, "How did you know?" when I query them about symptoms they didn't tell me about, symptoms that seem to have no relation to infertility. They think I am psychic, when in truth all I am doing is

confirming my diagnosis of the underlying pattern.

For example, I might ask, "Is your energy lower after you eat a meal? Are your hands, feet, or nose cold very often? Do you find yourself sweating a lot even if you're not exerting yourself? Are your menstrual cramps accompanied by a bearing-down sensation in your uterus?" None of these indications seem to have much relation to fertility or to the Spleen, yet they are classic symptoms of a Spleen Qi deficiency. Questions like "Do you think you're prone to anger? Do you have difficulty falling asleep at night? Do you ever wake up with a bitter taste in your mouth? Are you irritable and bloated premenstrually? Is the menstrual blood thick and dark or purplish in color?" all point to Liver Qi stagnation.

Like every other physician's, my job is to identify patterns so I can provide the most accurate diagnosis possible. I listen to the patient's answers openly and objectively, and make a diagnosis based upon my experience. One final test remains: touching.

TOUCHING

When we think of taking the pulse, we usually think of how quickly, slowly, or evenly the heart is beating. Traditional Chinese medicine, however, teaches practitioners to read the pulse at three varying depths at three different wrist locations, using three fingers. Various pulse points on each wrist are related to different Organ systems. Varying degrees of pressure are applied — light, to read the pulses on the surface of the wrist; medium, to reach the pulses below the surface; and heavy, to read the deep pulses.

Traditional Chinese medicine practitioners assess both the rate and the quality of the pulses. A bounding, solid pulse indicates an excess in the system. A taut pulse is associated with Liver or Gallbladder imbalance. A rough pulse can indicate either Blood stagnation or deficiency. A deep, slippery pulse is a clear sign of pregnancy. My patients are often amazed when I take their pulse and tell them they're pregnant even before they've dared to hope themselves — and long before they've taken a pregnancy test. I can tell when a person is ovulating because the Kidney Yin pulse tends to rise

from its usual deep level to the surface, bubbling up like a fountain during ovulation. After ovulation the pulse settles down again. By reading pulses I also can tell how my patients are responding to the hormones they are given during IVF cycles. (If their systems are being overloaded, I can offer specific treatments to help the body metabolize the excess hormones.)

A TCM practitioner uses the three diagnostic tools, looking, listening, and touching, to home in on a patient's diagnostic pattern. But no one knows your own body like you do. Simply by answering the questions in this chapter, you can begin to get a sense of the underlying patterns of deficiency and excess that are affecting your health and fertility.

YOUR VOYAGE OF DISCOVERY: WHAT ARE YOUR PATTERNS?

In terms of a woman's fertility, there are four Organ systems — Kidney, Spleen, Heart, and Liver — and four vital substances — Yin, Yang, Qi, and Blood — that are most likely to be suffering from imbalance caused by excess, deficiency, or stagnation of energy. *All TCM treatments for infertility are based upon restoring balance and health to these systems and vital substances.* The following questions will allow you to assess your Chinese diagnostic category. I have grouped the questions according to the

Organ affected and the symptoms associated with each condition.

The patterns diagnosed rarely occur alone; there is usually some degree of overlap. Having just one of the symptoms listed in a particular category may not be significant. However, if you seem to fit 25 percent or more of the identified signs, it is likely that you suffer from this pattern. Subsequent chapters will associate these patterns with specific reproductive impairments and give suggestions for treating these conditions and restoring balance to the body.

Understand also that these diagnoses address long-term conditions, not just daily variations. In the same way your pulse will be higher after you've been jogging or when you're nervous, sometimes you may exhibit all of the signs and symptoms of all the patterns. But what's important is identifying the symptoms that occur on a regular basis, because these will indicate any underlying imbalances.

Answer yes or no to each of the following questions. Don't worry about what the symptoms mean; just note whether you experience them. If you have more than one-fourth to one-third yes responses in any diagnostic category, then you may have an element of this imbalance in your system. You may have more than one kind of imbalance operating at the same time, so don't be surprised if you have 50 percent yes answers for more than one diagnostic category. Note the abbreviation(s) for your category or categories, then find pertinent treatment principles marked throughout the rest of the book.

DIAGNOSIS

	Yes	No
KIDNEY YIN DEFICIENCY (**Ki Yi−**)		
Do you have lower back weakness, soreness, or pain, or knee problems?	☒	☐
Do you have ringing in your ears or dizziness?	☒	☐
Is your hair prematurely gray?	☐	☐
Do you have vaginal dryness?	☐	☐
Is your midcycle fertile cervical mucus scanty or missing?	☐	☐
Do you have dark circles around or under your eyes?	☐	☐
Do you have night sweats?	☐	☐
Are you prone to hot flashes?	☐	☐
Would you describe yourself as afraid a lot?	☐	☐
Does your tongue lack coating? Does it appear shiny or peeled?	☐	☐

DIAGNOSIS

	Yes	No
KIDNEY YANG DEFICIENCY (**Ki Yan−**)		
Do you have lower back pain premenstrually?	☒	☐
Is your low back sore or weak?	☒	☐
Are your feet cold, especially at night?	☒	☐
Are you typically colder than those around you?	☒	☐
Is your libido low?	☒	☐
Are you often fearful?	☒	☐
Do you wake up at night or early in the morning because you have to urinate?	☐	☐

	Yes	No
Do you urinate frequently, and is the urine diluted and/or profuse?	☐	☐
Do you have early morning loose, urgent stools?	☐	☐
Do you have profuse vaginal discharge?	☐	☐
Does your menstrual blood tend to be dull in color?	☐	☐
Do you feel cold cramps during your period that respond to a heating pad?	☑	☐
Is your tongue pale, moist, and swollen?	☐	☐

DIAGNOSIS

	Yes	No

SPLEEN QI DEFICIENCY (**Sp–**)

	Yes	No
Are you often fatigued?	☐	☐
Do you have poor appetite?	☐	☐
Is your energy lower after a meal?	☐	☐
Do you feel bloated after eating?	☐	☐
Do you crave sweets?	☑	☐
Do you have loose stools, abdominal pain, or digestive problems?	☑	☐
Are your hands and feet cold?	☑	☐
Is your nose cold?	☑	☐
Are you prone to feeling heavy or sluggish?	☑	☐
Are you prone to feeling heaviness or grogginess in the head?	☐	☐
Do you bruise easily?	☑	☐
Do you think you have poor circulation?	☐	☐
Do you have varicose veins?	☑	☐
Are you lacking strength in your arms and legs?	☐	☐
Are you lacking in exercise?	☐	☐
Are you prone to worry?	☑	☐
Have you been diagnosed with low blood pressure?	☑	☐
Do you sweat a lot without exerting yourself?	☐	☐
Do you feel dizzy or light-headed, or have visual changes when you stand up fast?	☑	☐
Is your menstruation thin, watery, profuse, or pinkish in color?	☐	☐
Are you more tired around ovulation or menstruation?	☐	☐
Do you ever spot a few days or more before your period comes?	☐	☐
Have you ever been diagnosed with uterine prolapse?	☐	☐
Are your menstrual cramps accompanied by a bearing-down sensation in your uterus?	☐	☐
Are you often sick, or do you have allergies?	☐	☐

	Yes	No
Have you been diagnosed with hypothyroid or anemia?	❏	❏
Do you have hemorrhoids or polyps?	❏	❏
Does your tongue look swollen, with teeth marks on the sides?	❏	❏
Do you have a pale, yellowish complexion?	❏	❏

DIAGNOSIS

	Yes	No
BLOOD DEFICIENCY (Bl−) *(not necessarily equated with anemia)*		
Are your menses scanty and / or late?	❏	❏
Do you have dry, flaky skin?	☒	❏
Are you prone to getting chapped lips?	☒	❏
Are your fingernails or toenails brittle?	❏	❏
Are you losing hair on your head (not in patches, but all over)?	❏	❏
Is your hair brittle or dry?	❏	❏
Do you have diminished nighttime vision?	❏	❏
Do you get dizzy or light-headed around your period?	❏	❏
Are your lips, the inner side of your lower eyelids, or tongue pale in color?	❏	❏

DIAGNOSIS

	Yes	No
BLOOD STASIS (Bl X) *(often associated with blood deficiency symptoms; see Bl−)*		
Is your menstrual flow ever brown or black in color?	❏	❏
Do you feel midcycle pain around your ovaries?	❏	❏
Do you have painful, unmovable breast lumps?	❏	❏
Do you experience periodic numbness of your hands and feet (especially at night)?	❏	❏
Do you have varicose or spider veins?	☒	❏
Do you have red hemangiomas (cherry-red spots) on your skin?	❏	❏
Does your complexion appear dark and "sooty"?	❏	❏
Do you have chronic hemorrhoids?	❏	❏
Does your menstrual blood contain clots?	☒	❏
Have you been diagnosed with endometriosis or uterine fibroids?	❏	❏
Is your lower abdomen tender to palpation (resisting touch)?	☒	❏
Can you feel any abnormal lumps in your lower abdomen?	❏	❏
Do you have piercing or stabbing menstrual cramps?	❏	❏
Does your tongue look dark?	❏	❏
Do you have dark spots on your tongue?	❏	❏
Are the veins beneath your tongue twisty and tortuous?	❏	❏

	Yes	No
Do you have dark spots in your eyes?	❑	❑
Have you been diagnosed with any vascular abnormality or blood clotting disorder?	❑	❑

DIAGNOSIS

	Yes	No
LIVER QI STAGNATION (Lv Qi X)		
Are you prone to emotional depression?	☑	❑
Are you prone to anger and/or rage?	❑	❑
Do you become irritable premenstrually?	☑	❑
Do you feel bloated or irritable around ovulation?	☑	❑
Does it feel as if your ovulation lasts longer than it should?	❑	❑
Are your breasts sensitive/sore at ovulation?	❑	❑
Do you experience nipple pain or discharge from your nipples?	❑	❑
Do you have a lot of premenstrual breast distention or pain?	❑	❑
Have you been diagnosed with elevated prolactin levels?	❑	❑
Do you become bloated premenstrually?	❑	❑
Are your pupils usually dilated and large?	❑	❑
Do you have difficulty falling asleep at night?	☑	❑
Do you experience heartburn or wake up with a bitter taste in your mouth?	❑	❑
Are your menses painful?	❑	❑
Do you feel your menstrual cramps in the external genital area?	❑	❑
Is the menstrual blood thick and dark, or purplish in color?	❑	❑
Is your tongue dark or purplish in color?	❑	❑

DIAGNOSIS

	Yes	No
HEART DEFICIENCY (Ht–) *(often associated with heat)*		
Do you wake up early in the morning and have trouble getting back to sleep?	❑	❑
Do you have heart palpitations, especially when anxious?	❑	❑
Do you have nightmares?	❑	❑
Do you seem low in spirit or lacking in vitality?	❑	❑
Are you prone to agitation or extreme restlessness?	❑	❑
Do you fidget?	❑	❑
Is the tip of your tongue red?	❑	❑
Is there a crack in the center of your tongue that extends to the tip?	❑	❑
Do you sweat excessively, expecially on your chest?	❑	❑

DIAGNOSIS	Yes	No
EXCESS HEAT (^H)		
Is your pulse rate rapid?	☐	☐
Are your mouth and throat usually dry?	☐	☐
Are you thirsty for cold drinks most of the time?	☐	☐
Do you often feel warmer than those around you?	☐	☐
Do you wake up sweating or have hot flashes?	☐	☐
Do you break out with red acne (especially premenstrually)?	☐	☐
Do you have a short menstrual cycle?	☐	☐
Do you have vaginal irritation or rashes?	☐	☐

DIAGNOSIS	Yes	No
DAMPNESS (D)		
Do you feel tired and sluggish after a meal?	☐	☐
Do you have fibrocystic breasts?	☐	☐
Do you have cystic or pustular acne?	☐	☐
Do you have urgent, bright, or foul-smelling stools?	☐	☐
Does your menstrual blood contain stringy tissue or mucus?	☐	☐
Are you prone to yeast infections and vaginal itching?	☐	☐
Do your joints ache, especially with movement?	☐	☐
Are you overweight?	☐	☐
Do you have a wet, slimy tongue?	☐	☐

DIAGNOSIS	Yes	No
DAMP HEAT (DH)		
Do you have signs of heat and/or dampness as indicated above?	☐	☐
Do you have foul-smelling, yellow, or greenish vaginal discharge?	☐	☐
Are you prone to vaginal and/or rectal itching during your luteal or premenstrual phase?	☐	☐

DIAGNOSIS	Yes	No
COLD UTERUS (CW)		
Do you fit the Kidney Yang deficiency (Ki Yan−) category?	☐	☐
Do you fall into the Blood stasis pattern?	☐	☐
Does your lower abdomen feel cooler to the touch than the rest of your trunk?	☐	☐

These diagnoses will make more sense to you as we explore the different categories of reproductive problems. Individuals differ, and so must their treatments. The TCM therapy you choose must be based upon the underlying patterns, not just the symptoms you exhibit. As you read the chapters on diet and lifestyle, acupuncture, and herbal medicine, remember your diagnostic category abbreviation and try the associated suggestions for treatment. You may find your symptoms resolving quickly, or you may see changes happen gradually over a number of months.

Remember, only rarely will an individual fall completely into one category. For example, it is not unusual for someone to experience Spleen Qi deficiency (**Sp–**) with Liver Qi stagnation (**Lv Qi X**). Such a woman might be tired during most of the month and have cold hands and feet (Spleen Qi deficiency), while around her period she might become angry, irritable, bloated, have difficulties sleeping, and get bad cramps (Liver Qi stagnation). Someone with Kidney Yin deficiency (**Ki Yi–**) associated with Blood deficiency (**Bl–**) might have vaginal dryness and low back pain combined with dry, flaky skin, scanty or late menses, and brittle nails. The same woman might show symptoms of Blood stasis (**Bl X**), including varicose veins, hemorrhoids, and a tender lower abdomen, and even signs of excess heat (**^H**), such as rapid pulse, hot flashes, and dry mouth. Kidney Yang deficiency (**Ki Yan–**) may be experienced along with Spleen Qi deficiency (**Sp–**) and excess dampness (**D**). A woman experiencing all three could feel cold, have low libido and low overall energy, be prone to worry, have fibrocystic breasts, get lots of yeast infections, and be overweight.

An imbalance in one Organ or a systemic imbalance of excess or deficient heat, dampness, or cold will affect every element of the body in one way or another. *Any one element of imbalance will have multiple effects.* For example, Blood and Kidney Yin (Essence) share a common source. Yin is transformed into Essence, which is necessary for creating, transforming, and engendering the Blood. The Liver (which stores Blood) and the Kidneys (which store Essence) arise from the same root. Therefore, if one becomes weak or insufficient, the other will tend to become weak or insufficient as well. It is very common to see symptoms of Blood and Kidney Yin deficiency in the same patient. Each pattern must be addressed in order for health to be restored.

The good news is that treating any or all of these conditions involves very specific, simple remedies available to women everywhere. In preceding chapters, I have tried to help you gain a theoretical understanding of Chinese medicine. But just as it is unnecessary for you to understand exactly how an aspirin works for it to relieve your headache, you don't have to understand all the details of Chinese diagnosis for its medicines and treatments to work. Simply (1) remember which imbalance your symptoms indicate, (2) look for the suggestions made in the rest of this book to treat that imbalance, and (3) apply those suggestions using your own common sense.

No matter what your individual condition or combination of conditions, TCM can help you bring your system back into balance, restore you to greater health and well-being, and prepare your body to conceive healthy children and carry them to term. Along the way, you'll probably find you feel much better as well — you'll have increased energy, your emotions will be more even, and you'll approach life with a much better perspective.

PART II

THE ANCIENT CHINESE PROGRAM FOR REPRODUCTIVE WELLNESS

The Valley Spirit never dies.
It is named the Mysterious Female.
And the Doorway of the Mysterious Female
is the base from which Heaven and Earth sprang.

It is there within us all the while;
draw upon it as you will, it never runs dry.

— *TAO TE CHING*

This section from the *Tao Te Ching* encapsulates what I believe is true about the heart and spirit of women. Mysterious and ancient, our spirit is the mother of all creation, bringing forth both the heavens and the earth. Even if we sometimes feel this spirit is hidden, it is always within us. When facing the challenges of infertility, we can draw upon its life-giving potential. This spirit wants to give life, to be healthy, to harbor children; our job is simply to help our bodies do what they were meant to do.

Bringing the body into alignment with this ancient drive has been the focus of my practice for years, and I have used every technique available. I drew upon elements from all my medical training, as well as from everything I had ever learned in my studies of TCM and other "alternatives," yet I wasn't satisfied until I evaluated every technique through one filter: *Did it help my patients get pregnant?* As time passed, I discovered that TCM techniques are *the* most effective in restoring my patients to health and fertility.

Traditional Chinese medicine addressed infertility long before the Christian era began. The earliest records of gynecological writings are found in inscriptions on bones and tortoiseshells dating from the Shang dynasty (1500–1000 B.C.E.). One of the first significant written Chinese medical texts, *Book of Mountains and Seas* (from the Warring States period, 475–221 B.C.E.), describes the use of medicinal plants to treat infertility. The famous *Yellow Emperor's Classic of Internal Medicine* (*Nei Jing*) provides for the treatment of amenorrhea (absence of menstruation) and menorrhagia (abnormally heavy or long menstrual periods). The same author's *Plain Questions* describes the hormonal changes that occur throughout a woman's life cycle and attributes these fluctuations to certain energy meridians, which have since been linked to the HPO axis. Today, elements of TCM, such as acupunc-

ture, Chinese herbs, certain forms of exercise, and dietary prescriptions, are being tested and proven effective in clinical trials throughout the world.

Every woman's reason for not conceiving is unique and personal to her. It may even vary from one menstrual cycle to the next. Traditional Chinese medicine seeks not only to restore balance and health to every aspect of a woman's body, but also to redirect the body's attention and energy back to the reproductive system so the woman may bring forth life.

The program outlined in the following chapters, however, is not necessarily the same as that recommended by a typical doctor of Oriental medicine. In my drive for results, my approach to healing always has been flavored by my Western medical training. I tell my patients I practice a hybridization of Chinese medicine. There are certain elements of TCM upon which I rely heavily (like tonifying the Kidney system) and those I draw upon only rarely (like clearing Lung heat) based upon how well they treat infertility. This program is not based on ideas about how to treat infertility; it's based on experience.

You may be wondering about my success rate. At my clinic I define success simply: if my patients get pregnant after coming to me and following my program, that's a success. Many of my patients find they get pregnant naturally after they follow my regimen. Other women, after a few months on my prescriptions, get frustrated and return to their reproductive endocrinologists, and lo and behold, the same IUIs or IVFs that didn't work before now result in pregnancy. Still other women come to me with undiagnosed fertility challenges that I diagnose using TCM principles. I put them on a program designed to restore their health, and then eventually may suggest they consult a doctor who specializes in their condition. These women, too, often have a higher chance of becoming pregnant simply because they have been diagnosed accurately and treated appropriately with a combination of Western medicine and TCM. I would consider all of those successes because the TCM prescriptions helped these women get pregnant. Based on these criteria, my success rate is somewhere around 75 percent.

Many of the 25 percent who are not successful have not followed through with their treatment plans. Traditional Chinese medicine is not a quick fix; restoring the body to health takes time. If you are reading this book and wish to apply TCM to your own condition, *you must give yourself at least three months for the treatments to have full effect.*

The good news is you don't have to wait that long to get tangible physical results! Over the first few months of treatment, you should look for specific changes, some of which may occur quickly. Are your symptoms improving? Are your breasts less tender at ovulation? Are your cycles becoming more regular? Is your flow better? Are you experiencing fewer mood swings before menstruation? Whatever your symptoms, you should experience improvement in

them as your body restores itself to hormonal health. Maybe that's all the proof you need that TCM is working for you. But if you need more proof, or if you have been diagnosed with specific conditions by your Western medical doctor, please feel free to have yourself tested or retested by your Western physician. All I ask is that you remember that some conditions have been a long time in the making, and it may take a while for the body to unmake them. Give the body time; use how you feel to gauge your progress in the program. Are you feeling healthier? More normal hormonally? Is your reproductive system starting to respond as it's supposed to during the course of a monthly cycle? Use your subjective response as your most accurate gauge.

In my experience, pregnancy comes when certain symptoms either appear or disappear. The sudden appearance of fertile cervical mucus is one such symptom. So at each visit I am diligent in asking patients how they are responding to therapy. If there hasn't been improvement, I know I have to adjust my treatment. Give your body a chance to heal itself, and look for progress. Have there been positive changes in your cycle? Is your sense of health and well-being getting stronger? In some cases it's also possible that one condition resolves and another one appears. You may clear the excess heat in your system, for example, but then need to build up your deficient Yin energy. If your symptoms are not changing, you may wish to revisit chapter 4 for a fresh diagnosis and try some of the other suggestions for similar patterns.

Infertility can be cured only when we combine treatment with patience, action with hope, results with a willingness to recognize true healing. And remember always, the Mysterious Female resides within you. With gentle nurturing, you can reclaim the blessing of your fertility.

5

Step One: Preparing the Reproductive System — Balancing Opposing Energies

If there is heat, cool it;
If there is cold, warm it;
If there is dryness, moisten it;
If there is dampness, dry it;
If there is vacuity, supplement it; and
If there is repletion, drain it.

This description is taken from the *Nei Jing*, and it illustrates the foundation of all healing in TCM. First, you must discover patterns of imbalance in the body. Then you must correct the imbalances in two ways: (1) where there is too much of anything, reduce it, and (2) where there is too little of something, replenish it. For our bodies to function properly, all our organs need balance. Acupuncture, herbal medicine, and dietary and lifestyle changes can help restore the balance of Yin and Yang, dampness and dryness, heat and cold, deficiency and excess.

Our monthly cycle is a complex interplay of almost every system in the body. If any part is off kilter by even a tiny amount, it can affect our fertility. For example, most women know hormones play a significant role in our cycle. If there's not enough estrogen early on in the cycle, the eggs won't mature adequately. If there's too much estrogen later in the cycle, the uterine lining won't develop properly. Many hormonal problems are the result of slight imbalances in the delicate endocrine system. Modern diagnostic techniques may not detect any clinical abnormality or functional problem, yet this undetectable irregularity may be the root cause of our inability to conceive.

The recognized causes of female infertility (in order of decreasing incidence) are:

1. hormonal factors and ovulatory dysfunction,
2. fallopian tube abnormalities,
3. uterine and cervical factors, and
4. unexplained infertility.

Most of these problems can be healed naturally, or at least improved upon, using three elements of TCM: diet and lifestyle, acupuncture, and herbs.

DIET AND LIFESTYLE

Our nutritional habits and routines often need revising for full recovery to take place. Unfortunately, the common lifestyle in Western society brings inherent fertility problems. Stress, coffee or other stimulants, alcohol, nicotine, sweets, chemicals, hormones, and other byproducts of our affluent lifestyle can all leave deep imprints in our reproductive capacity. Making changes in what, when, and how we eat and drink, as well as adding certain forms of exercise, massage, meditation, and other self-care techniques, can contribute significantly to enhancing our fertility. Chapter 6 will cover many ways to use lifestyle changes to increase your odds of bearing a healthy child.

ACUPUNCTURE

Research has shown that by influencing hormonal pathways, acupuncture assists our own internal energies to restore endocrine harmony. The main meridians influence the internal organs, and the Extraordinary meridians control the reproductive organs and the HPO axis, which is responsible for ovulation and sperm production. In chapter 7 you will discover the complex yet precise relationship between acupressure and acupuncture points and your Organs and energetic systems. You'll learn how you can balance your system, improve circulation, and restore function to impaired reproductive organs by massaging these acupoints on a regular basis.

❦ HERBS

There is conclusive evidence that herbal therapy has been practiced throughout history. The Chinese, Greeks, and Egyptians have used herbs for centuries to enhance fertility, with diverse effects. Herbs may act on the ovulatory phase or may regulate the secretion of mucus; they may stimulate the uterus or assist in the production of adequate progesterone. However, unlike Western drugs, which try to provide chemically based substitutes for the body's natural hormones, Chinese herbs are designed to help the body produce the proper levels of hormones on its own. Chinese herbs act on the endocrine system by stimulating hormone production, altering the rate of hormone metabolism, or changing the response of hormone receptors. Many of the ingredients in Chinese herbal formulas may have little

or no hormonal effects, but the effect of the *whole* formula will substantially increase hormone levels. In chapter 8, I'll review a wide variety of Chinese herbs used to balance hormonal levels and enhance fertility.

In this chapter we will examine the different parts of a woman's reproductive cycle using both the Western and Eastern views. You'll begin to learn which deficiencies and excesses are associated with problems during specific phases of your menstrual cycle, and you'll receive some basic guidance for rebalancing your energy throughout the month. Then, in later chapters, you'll discover more detailed recommendations for restoring harmony to your hormonal pathways and enhancing your fertility based on both your Western and Eastern medical diagnoses.

❦ A NEW (OLD) VIEW OF OUR FERTILITY

According to the *Nei Jing*, women should be capable of pregnancy from the onset of menstruation until menopause. When we reach menarche, the energy in our Conception and Penetrating meridians overflows, and we have our first period. Every month until we become pregnant or reach menopause, the same cycle of rising and falling energy occurs within certain Organs and meridians. In most cases this process takes approximately twenty-eight days, or the amount of time

from one full moon to the next. The menstrual cycle can be broken down into phases, just like the phases of the moon. Phase I may be thought of as the new moon, Phase II (ovulation) as the full moon, and Phase V as the dark of the moon.

A woman's menstrual cycle is a dynamic process of hormonal fluctuation. Producing an egg, allowing fertilization, developing a suitable environment for implantation, and maintaining a pregnancy require a series of complex and interrelated events. To distinguish which patterns can interrupt the balance of the reproductive system, however, we must first understand how a properly harmonized hormonal monthly cycle should occur.

While you read the following sections, compare your own experience to the description of a normal cycle. Take notes on how your cycle differs from this account. Remember the patterns you identified in chapter 4 and pay particular attention to the ways in which your symptoms appear each month. This information can help pinpoint imbalances in your overall energy or specific Organs. Then you can refer to chapters 6, 7, and 8 for guidelines on how to restore your system to health.

The key to natural conception is a healthy, normal monthly cycle. Here's a general guideline for tracking and assessing your own.

EVALUATING YOUR MONTHLY CYCLE

1. Using the principles of Chinese medicine, assess your condition based on the suggestions in this chapter and the questions in chapter 4. Note where you believe you are experiencing deficiency or excess, and in which Organ systems.

2. Copy the basal body temperature (BBT) chart at the end of this chapter. Record your temperature with a digital thermometer every morning upon awakening. (Before rising, rolling around, getting a drink of water,

talking — anything — pop the thermometer in your mouth, read your temperature, and record it.) Note your temperature on each day of your cycle and then create a graph. A typical graph will show a slight drop in temperature just prior to ovulation, followed by a rise of about half of one degree Fahrenheit, a result of rising progesterone after ovulation (see fig. 5.1, on page 59). Temperature (and progesterone) should remain elevated for twelve to fourteen days and then drop, signaling the onset of menses. If conception occurs, your temperature should remain elevated and even jump to a third level on the graph.

3. Notice any changes in vaginal mucus during the month: it should be wet and slippery, like egg white, around ovulation. Note these changes on your BBT chart.

4. Note alterations in the cervix. Heightened estrogen levels around ovulation cause it to soften and move up and away from the vagina while the cervical opening enlarges. To check your cervix, reach into the vaginal canal with your finger. The tip of your finger will hit the tip of the cervix. You should be able to notice subtle variations in the cervical texture and placement over time. Note these changes on your BBT chart as well.

Because a woman's BBT typically rises by four-tenths of a degree to a degree when she ovulates, taking your basal temperature throughout the month is one of the best ways to keep track of your progress through the phases of your own cycle. If your body is not showing a "normal" curve on the BBT graph, the right diet, exercise, acupressure

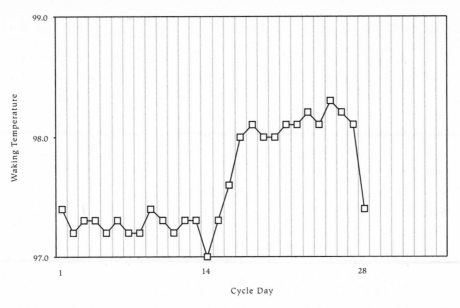

Figure 5.1: Basal Body Temperature (BBT) Graph — Normal 28-Day Cycle

or acupuncture, and herbal formulas can correct this. See pages 70–76 for a list of conditions seen in each stage of the menstrual cycle, as well as recommendations for ways to normalize each stage.

Keeping a BBT chart will help you determine if, when, and how smoothly ovulation is occurring, and it can also track temperature irregularities so that you can diagnose imbalance. Temperatures that are too high during the follicular phase indicate excess

heat, just as temperatures that are too low during the luteal phase indicate deficiency. Erratic temperature fluctuations are consistent with Liver Qi stagnation (**Lv Qi X**).

Another helpful habit is to keep a daily journal of symptoms that occur at various phases throughout the cycle. The more information you have to correctly assess your diagnostic pattern, the closer you will be to resolving your barriers to conception.

THE PHASES OF A WOMAN'S CYCLE

In Chinese medicine, different energies dominate each phase of the menstrual cycle:

Phase I: *Kidney Yin* and *Blood* energies govern the follicular phase.

Phase II: *Liver Qi* and *Blood movement* control ovulation.

Phase III: *Kidney Yang* and *Spleen Qi* energies manage the luteal phase.

Phase IV: *Liver Qi* helps the premenstrual transformation.

Phase V: *Blood* is allowed to flow. Menstruation is a time of rest for all energies.

To regulate the reproductive cycle, we work with the phases' dominant energies to bring the cycle back into balance. For example, if you fit the Kidney Yin deficiency category (**Ki Yi–**), with symptoms like vaginal dryness and scant or missing cervical mucus, you should apply treatments for the deficiency especially during the follicular phase, when Yin energies are most needed. Keep in mind, though, your primary pattern diagnosis should always be addressed no matter what phase you're in. (See the Checklist of Symptoms and TCM Indications on pages 70–76, as well as the information in chapters 6, 7, and 8 for specific treatments to help enhance each phase of your menstrual cycle and address your overall patterns of imbalance.)

The following sections describe the biological processes that occur during each phase of the menstrual cycle and explain the TCM diagnoses of problems in each phase. In some cases, I have included sample BBT graphs showing the temperature patterns that accompany each phase.

PHASE I: THE YIN PHASE

Phase I is known as the follicular, or proliferative, phase, or the hypothermal (low temperature) phase. After menstruation, the hormones, uterine lining, and ovaries prepare to surge in their cyclic development. This is a time of renewal, when the whole reproductive system begins a new cycle.

Phase I is governed by Yin energy. Indeed, the Yin hormone estrogen sends signals to the Uterus to make the "cool, moist, dark cave" ready to encourage growth within it. In preparation for expelling its egg, the ovary selects a dominant follicle and nurtures its growth. The uterine lining develops (Yin, Essence, and Blood), becoming at least 8 to 10 millimeters in thickness. Finally, hospitable cervical fluid is produced. The cervix opens up (a Yin function) and discharges this wet, clear, stretchy mucus (Yin fluid), which allows sperm to survive and pass through. (During other times of the cycle, cervical fluid is hostile to sperm.) Follicular development and egg production are fortified by Yin and produce more Yin and Blood. We encourage and maximize the energies of Phase I by supplementing the Kidney Yin and nourishing the Blood.

Phase I typically lasts between twelve and fifteen days, and for optimum fertility, it shouldn't be shorter than ten or longer than seventeen days. If this phase is too short, the egg doesn't have time to mature, and the uterine lining doesn't have time to thicken enough to support implantation. A short Phase I means there is abnormal heat of some sort, either insufficient heat (caused by too little Yin) or excessive heat (caused by too much Yang).

If Phase I is too long, it may mean a woman's estrogen production is low, compromising egg quality and delaying ovulation. Phase I may be prolonged if Kidney Yin production is insufficient to trigger the transformation of Yin energy into Yang, or if there is not enough Kidney Yang or Spleen Qi available to perform the transformation.

A high BBT during Phase I indicates heat, often caused by Kidney Yin deficiency (**Ki Yi–**). In these cases we would attempt to prolong the follicular phase by tonifying Kidney Yin and clearing excess heat. This will result in lower FSH and higher estrogen levels. Conversely, a low BBT indicates an insufficiency of Kidney Yang (**Ki Yan–**). Treatment should be given during Phase I to nourish Yin and Blood and to support the transformation of Yang energy, which will induce ovulation.

PHASE II: OVULATION — A PROCESS OF TRANSFORMATION

Contrary to what most women think, ovulation is a process, not an event. Traditional Chinese medicine says the Liver sets ovulation in motion. Toward the end of the follicular phase, as estrogen peaks and Yin energy reaches its apogee (when maximum Yin produces a dip in temperature before ovulation), Liver Qi is triggered to begin the transformation of Yin energy (estrogen) into Yang energy (progesterone). This process encourages gonadotropin-releasing hormone (GnRH) from the brain to trigger the pituitary gland to emit both luteinizing hormone (LH) and FSH. A whole series of other hormones are also produced at this time.

As these hormones are released, a cascade of events occurs over the next couple of days. In the ovary, the follicle, now swollen to a diameter of 20 millimeters (about the size of a grape), bursts and discharges its egg into the abdominal cavity. Then the fingerlike ends of the fallopian tube (the fimbriae) sweep the egg inside, providing a clear path to the uterus.

There should be minimal pain at ovulation. If you experience pain, however, it is advisable not to use anti-inflammatory medications like Advil or Midol, which can inhibit prostaglandin release and prevent follicular rupture. Pain at ovulation indicates Blood stasis (**Bl X**). Bloating indicates Liver Qi Stagnation (**Lv Qi X**).

Once the egg is released by the ovary, the cervix starts to firm up and close. The egg then travels down the fallopian tube toward the uterus, looking for the sperm to penetrate its outer layer and spur on the process of new life.

During ovulation, Yin (from growth during the follicular phase) must be abundant enough to convert into Yang. Qi and Blood must flow freely to allow this change to occur. To assure free-flowing Qi in Phase II, you must also address any problems present during Phase I (see Checklist of Symptoms and TCM Indications on pages 70–76 for treatment guidelines).

PHASE III: THE YANG PHASE

In Western medicine Phase III is called the luteal phase, and it should last about fourteen days. As the egg travels through the fallopian tube, the follicle that released the egg becomes a corpus luteum, or "yellow body," which looks like a shriveled yellow prune. The corpus luteum releases progesterone, a hormone governing this third phase (also known as the hyperthermal, or high temperature, phase).

Like fuel for the body's incubator, progesterone is warming and therefore Yang in nature. It has one primary purpose: to prepare the endometrium of the uterus for safe implantation of a fertilized egg. Progesterone triggers small blood vessels in the uterus to supply the uterine lining with more blood

flow. During the window of implantation (about five to seven days after ovulation), certain proteins appear on the surface of the now receptive endometrium and allow the developing blastocyst to adhere and embed within the uterine lining. Further hormonal, vascular, and glandular development must proceed for the imbedded embryo to develop.

During the Yang-dominated luteal phase your BBT should remain elevated an average of at least four-tenths of one degree over the follicular phase baseline temperature for fourteen days. This phase is governed by Kidney Yang and Spleen Qi. Many causes of "luteal phase defect" (a short or ineffective luteal phase) are the result of deficient Kidney Yang (**Ki Yan–**) and/or Spleen Qi (**Sp–**). When a luteal phase defect is present, progesterone production is low. Supplementing Spleen Qi (**Sp–**) or Kidney Yang (**Ki Yan–**) will raise the body's production of and response to progesterone. There should be no premenstrual spotting (which indicates Qi deficiency, Blood stasis, or pathological heat) or extreme breast tenderness (which suggests Qi stagnation) in the absence of pregnancy.

If there is a pregnancy, the embryo will release human chorionic gonadotropin (hCG), which signals the corpus luteum to increase its production of progesterone, thus maintaining a thick, hospitable uterine lining for the embryo. Often, a woman's basal temperature will then rise again. However, if there is no embryo secreting hCG, the corpus luteum does not produce more progesterone, and it undergoes a programmed demise. Progesterone levels (and temperatures) drop, and the uterine lining is shed.

On the BBT graph, a biphasic, slow, step-like pattern is indicative of Qi stagnation caused by Blood stasis (**Bl X**) or Kidney Yang deficiency (**Ki Yan–**) (fig. 5.2).

This means the Qi isn't doing its job of transforming Yin into Yang because there either isn't enough fresh Blood being produced by the Spleen, or there isn't enough Yang energy in the Kidneys. Often this stepwise pattern also indicates Qi stagnation in the Liver (**Lv Qi X**). You can bring the body back into balance by helping the Blood to flow freely (see Checklist of Symptoms and TCM Indications on pages 70–76). A sawtooth, erratic pattern in the temperature graph (fig. 5.3) is also a clear indication of Liver Qi stagnation (**Lv Qi X**).

Since Liver Qi is responsible for all transformations of Yin into Yang, and for all transitions from Phase I to Phase III of your cycle, a Liver with stagnant Qi (**Lv Qi X**) will obviously have a detrimental effect on your fertility. If the sawtooth temperature pattern occurs throughout the month, it means the stagnant Qi needs to be rectified the entire time. If the pattern appears only between ovulation and menstruation, the Qi needs to be harmonized only during the luteal phase. Pathologically elevated levels of certain hormones like prolactin and estrogen will often manifest as signs of Liver Qi stagnation (**Lv Qi X**) as well as a sawtoothed BBT. Resolv-

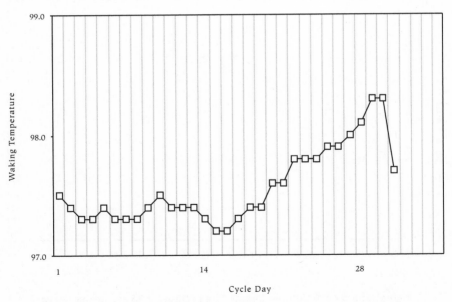

Figure 5.2: BBT Graph — Qi Stagnation Caused by Kidney Yang Deficiency
(**Ki Yan–**) or Blood Stasis (**Bl X**)

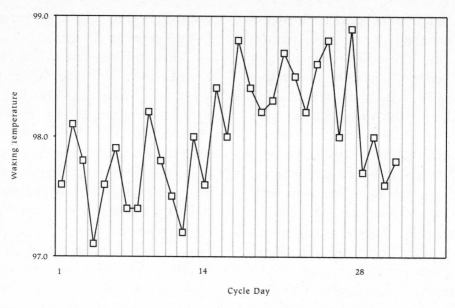

Figure 5.3: BBT Graph — Liver Qi Stagnation (**Lv Qi X**)

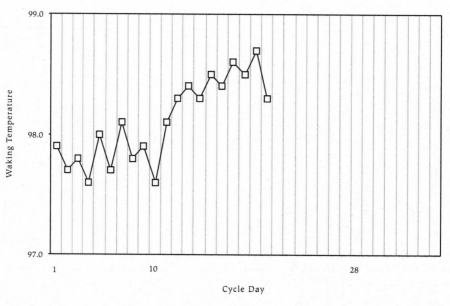

Figure 5.4: BBT Graph — Luteal Phase Shorter Than Twelve Days

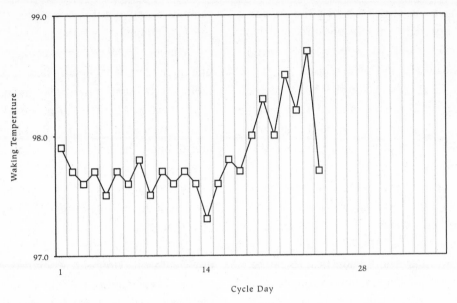

Figure 5.5: BBT Graph — Shortened Luteal Phase with Liver Qi Stagnation
(**Lv Qi X**) and Excess Heat (**^H**)

ing Liver Qi stagnation will help the body metabolize excess hormones.

A luteal phase shorter than twelve days (fig. 5.4) indicates a dysfunction. The most common reasons for a shortened luteal phase are Qi or Yang deficiency. However, it's also possible a Yin deficiency has allowed the Yang energies to become too dominant. Without adequate Yin (cooling) energies to moderate the frenetic action of the Yang, the luteal phase may be disturbed by heat.

Remember, for a cycle to be healthy, the body's energies must be in balance — Yin and Yang, heating and cooling, and so on.

A biphasic, steplike, slow-rising basal temperature during a shortened luteal phase, as shown in fig. 5.5, may indicate

Liver Qi stagnation (**Lv Qi X**), which produces excessive heat.

Liver Qi stagnation (**Lv Qi X**) causing excess heat (**^H**) may also raise overall temperatures in Phase I (the hypothermal, or low temperature, phase) and Phase III (the hyperthermal, or high temperature, phase). To lower excess heat, use foods, herbs, and acupressure to cool the body as described in chapters 6, 7, and 8.

PHASE IV: THE PREMENSTRUAL PHASE

Without fertilization and implantation, your body moves into the premenstrual phase. Here the Yang transforms back into Yin, and once again the Liver Qi directs the conversion. Depending on your constitution, this phase may last anywhere from two to seven days and overlap the luteal phase.

As the Liver Qi converts Yang energy into Yin, the corpus luteum ceases its progesterone production. Your basal temperature falls, and your period begins. For this transformation to occur smoothly, however, both Qi and Blood must be flowing freely throughout the body. If these vital energies are blocked, there will be premenstrual symptoms such as irritability, pain, constipation or diarrhea, headaches, bloating, night sweats, insomnia, depression, edema, nausea, appetite changes, nosebleeds, mouth sores, vaginal irritation, dizziness, clumsiness, muscle aches, and so on. During the premenstrual phase, the Liver Qi should be harmonized (see Checklist of Symptoms and TCM Indications at the end of the chapter). This will help eliminate many premenstrual symptoms while restoring health and balance to the body.

PHASE V: THE BLOOD PHASE

This phase is considered the resting, shedding stage, and it begins on the first day of bleeding. (Spotting doesn't count; day 1 begins when the blood actually starts to flow.) Enzymes liquefy the uterine lining (endometrium), allowing it to shed. Basal body temperature usually drops on the first day of menstruation, but some women with endometriosis find that their temperature

remains elevated during the period (and we must clear heat if this is the case).

The menstrual period, especially for the first three days of a woman's flow, is the hormonal zero point, when no principal hormone prevails. After three days, the hormonal cycle begins again, but until then it's important to allow the body to rejuvenate. In the same way the season of winter or the period between midnight and dawn is a time of rest, menstruation is the reproductive system's period of rest.

This is also a time to take a break from any treatment. Unless a woman is experiencing severe cramps, I ask her not to schedule any appointments at my clinic during the first three days of her period. I also suggest she make menstruation a time of reprieve from all fertility pursuits. According to TCM, women should not exercise or undertake many activities (including intercourse) during the first three days of their period. While modern life rarely allows us the privilege of complete rest, you will feel much better if you take it easy as much as possible when you're menstruating. Relax, stay warm, and allow your body, your mind, your emotions, and your spirit a much-needed time-out.

Like your temperature, menstruation is an extremely important indicator for any TCM practitioner who wishes to correctly diagnose and treat disorders of fertility. We can gain a wealth of information about the state of the entire endocrine milieu by assessing the menstrual blood. It is a monthly report card of a woman's reproductive status because it mirrors the state of her ovaries' hormonal activity. If a woman is healthy and her cycle normal, the menstrual flow should be smooth and neither scanty nor excessive. The color should be red, not brown or black, and the consistency should not be watery. Clots should be minimal to none. The bleeding should last approximately four to six days, then stop rather abruptly without spotting. There should be no pain, either uterine or abdominal cramping or lower back discomfort (Kidney involvement). If there is pain, it is important to note the quality of the pain. Is it sharp or stabbing in nature (Blood stasis), or is it a dull, heavy aching (Qi deficiency)? Is there bloating or distention (Qi stagnation)? Does the application of heat or pressure ease the pain (indicating deficiency)? All of these factors will help you diagnose where and how your system is imbalanced.

If the blood flow is scanty in amount or lasts for only a day or two, this usually indicates there is not enough Blood to nourish the uterine lining. This often corresponds to a lack of estrogen during the follicular phase (Phase I), and Blood (and Yin) should be nourished during this time. If the blood is pink and watery, this is a possible sign of Spleen Qi deficiency (**Sp–**). In this case, both Qi and Blood need to be boosted. If the blood is scant and brownish in color, the Blood needs to be tonified and invigorated.

If the menstrual blood flow is abnormally profuse, lasts beyond seven days, or occurs at times other than menses, we must determine the source of the abnormal bleeding. According to TCM there are only three causes of any type of abnormal gynecological bleeding. First is Qi deficiency (an overall relative lack of Qi). When menstruation is excessive in amount (menorrhagia), extends beyond its normal time (metrorrhagia), or both (menometrorrhagia), there may be insufficient Qi to control the menstrual cycle. In this case there will be other signs of Qi deficiency, such as fatigue, cold hands and feet, digestive complaints, and poor circulation. It is relatively simple to supplement the Qi using herbs such as ginseng, Atractylodes, and Astragalus. (See chapter 8 for a comprehensive guide on using herbs to tonify the Qi.)

Second, abnormal flow can be caused by Blood stasis (not enough movement of the Blood) (**Bl X**). When you cut yourself, the blood flows red, and menstrual blood should be red as well. However, obstructed blood will tend to stagnate and oxidize; hence it will no longer be red in color nor appear fresh. The Chinese phrase for "static Blood," *xue yu*, is akin to the concept of sediment. If the menstruate is dark, clotty, and accompanied by pain, it is likely due to Blood stasis (**Bl X**). This condition must be resolved if the Uterus is to become nontoxic and allow conception. The old Blood has to be eradicated before new, fresh Blood can take its place. We know treatment is progressing when the Blood flows fresh and unimpeded.

The third and last cause of abnormally heavy flow is excess heat (caused either by too much Yang or too little Yin). If the menstrual cycle is shorter than the average twenty-eight days, the blood is bright red and profuse, and other signs of heat are present, the Blood will need to be cooled. If your pattern indicates the presence of Liver Qi stagnation (**Lv Qi X**) as well, the Liver Qi will need to be cleared for the excess heat to be resolved. If symptoms of Yin deficiency (like night sweats, hot flashes, and vaginal dryness) accompany the heat, Yin must be supplemented as well, or the heat will return.

When menstruation does not occur at all (amenorrhea), it is because of either deficiency (not enough Blood) or excess (something blocking menstruation from occurring), or a combination of both. The origin will be apparent from the pattern diagnostic checklists in chapter 4. If Blood is not sufficient, you will need to tonify it. If menstruation is blocked as a result of Blood stasis (**Bl X**), we must get it moving. See the Checklist of Symptoms and TCM Indications on pages 70–76.

PELVIC BLOOD FLOW

In addition to addressing the proper functioning of the menstrual cycle, we must also discuss the state of the ovaries and Uterus when we evaluate fertility. To function correctly, these organs need adequate blood supply. The endometrium must be thick enough to be receptive for the developing embryo. Indeed, poor blood flow through the uterine artery correlates with lower pregnancy rates. Ovarian health and function are also affected by both hormonal state and blood supply. Therefore, anything we can do to improve blood flow to the uterus and ovaries can help increase our fertility.

In 1996, a groundbreaking study conducted in Sweden and published in *Fertility and Sterility* reported that acupuncture reduced constriction in uterine arteries, thereby increasing the blood flow to the reproductive organs. This effect was found to improve dramatically the outcome of ART. *Acupuncture is the only known technique to directly increase vascular response.* The acupuncture treatments used in the Swedish study suppressed the sympathetic nervous system response at the spinal-cord level, reducing the local "fight or flight" response in the pelvis. When the sympathetic response was reduced, blood flow improved to the uterus and ovaries. In all of the women on whom acupuncture was performed, the constriction of the uterine arteries was lessened by 21 percent after eight treatments, dramatically increasing their blood flow. If you have been diagnosed with poor ovarian response or a meager uterine lining, you may be able to improve this with exercises and acupuncture treatments that help increase blood flow to your uterus and ovaries (see chapters 6 and 7).

Many progressive reproductive clinics in the United States use the findings of this study to diagnose and treat infertility patients. They perform Doppler studies to evaluate the flow of blood through the uterine arteries to the pelvic organs. If the results show diminished blood flow, patients are sent to receive acupuncture until the pelvic blood supply improves.

HOW TO TAKE CONTROL OF YOUR FERTILITY

By now, you should be starting to understand how Chinese medicine views problems with your menstrual cycle and how to correct any imbalances that may be preventing you from getting pregnant. For instance, instead of simply adding more estrogen to the system during Phase I, as Western medicine might suggest, TCM builds up the Yin energy throughout the entire body by supplementing the Kidneys and tonifying the Blood. It also decreases any excess Yang that might be inhibiting the Yin needed in Phase I. It directs these balanced energies to the reproductive system, which in turn will affect the other phases of the menstrual cycle in positive ways, restoring the natural cyclical fluctuations of our hormonal processes.

The Persian mystic poet Rumi once wrote:

When the time comes for the embryo to
*   receive the spirit of life,*
At that time the sun begins to help.
This embryo is brought into movement, for
*   the sun quickens it with spirit.*
From the other stars this embryo received
*   only an impression, until the sun shone*
*   upon it.*

How did it become connected with the
*   shining sun in the womb?*
By ways hidden from our senses:
the way whereby gold is nourished,
the way a common stone becomes a garnet
*   and the ruby red,*
the way fruit is ripened,
and the way courage comes to one distraught
*   with fear.*

— TRANSLATED BY KABIR AND
CAMILLE HELMINSKI

This expresses the mystery of how life begins inside each one of us and makes clear the connection between what happens in our bodies and in nature — fruit ripening on the tree, crystalline rock turned into precious stones, the sun warming and quickening the earth. Western medicine's scientific analyses are certainly valuable, but they lose the sense of the whole, of the need for us to be in tune with our true nature to bring forth life. When we use the treatments of TCM, we are declaring our desire to be in alignment with nature. We are putting our trust in our body's innate wholeness and seeking ways to help the body remember what it was meant to do — experience the ebb and flow of procreative energy, feel the womb prepare itself to hold a child, sense the start of a new life when conception takes place, and hold this new life safely until it is ready to be born. This is what a woman's body does. All we need to do is help our bodies find their natural balance once again.

Checklist of Symptoms and TCM Indications

Make note of any symptoms during the course of your menstrual cycle, then check this list for your TCM category/diagnosis and suggestions for rebalancing your system. Don't worry about understanding the treatments at this time; simply record them, and when you review the next three chapters, pay particular attention to the prescriptions for your specific imbalance.

Phase/Symptom	Condition	Treatment
Phase I: The Yin Phase	Kidneys need to be supplemented; Blood needs to be nourished. **Related pattern:** Kidney Yin deficiency (**Ki Yi–**)	• Supplement Kidney Yin with fruit, chlorella, spirulina, seaweed, eggs, royal jelly, and wheat germ. • Nourish blood with Angelica (Dang Gui). Perform exercises to improve Blood flow to pelvic organs. • Get plenty of rest; avoid too much external stimulation (parties, drugs, loud or agitating noises). • Do not smoke or drink coffee. • Stay away from all stimulants, including herbal weight-loss or "energy" formulas.
Prolonged Phase I	Not enough Yin produced to transform into Yang **Related pattern:** Kidney Yin deficiency (**Ki Yi–**)	• Supplement Kidney Yin with acupuncture and herbs. • Stimulate acupoints Ki 3, Sp 6, Zigong, ear intertragic notch, Ren 3, and Ren 4. • Supplement with herbs like Angelica (Dang Gui) if you exhibit signs of Blood deficiency, or consider the patent herbal formula Six Ingredient Rehmannia Decoction (Liu Wei Di Huang Tang), which nourishes Kidney Yin.
Prolonged Phase I	Not enough Kidney Yang **Related pattern:** Kidney Yang deficiency (**Ki Yan–**)	• Tonify Kidney Yang with warming herbs like Epimedium (Yin Yang Huo) and Morinda (Ba Ji Tian). • Stimulate acupoint Ki 7. • Warm the lower abdomen with a hot water bottle or heating pad.

Phase/Symptom	Condition	Treatment
Prolonged Phase I	Not enough Spleen Qi **Related pattern:** Spleen Qi deficiency (**Sp–**)	• Supplement Qi with herbs such as ginseng (Ren Shen) and Astragalus (Huang Qi). • Stimulate acupoints St 36, Ren 6, Sp 6. • Avoid refined carbohydrates, sugar, and dairy products.
Polycystic ovarian syndrome diagnosis	**Related pattern:** Dampness (**D**)	• Follow Spleen advice above. Keep carbohydrate level low; don't eat yams. • Stimulate acupoints St 40 and Sp 9. • Take Two Cured Decoction (Er Chen Tang) or Six Gentlemen Decoction (Liu Jun Zi Tang), and Gleditsia (Zao Jiao Ci).
Shortened Phase I	Abnormal heat caused either by deficiency or excess **Related pattern:** Excess heat (**^H**)	• To lower heat, take cooling herbs like Phellodendron (Huang Bai), red peony (Chi Shao), or the Chinese patent formula Anemarrhena, Phellodendron, and Rehmannia Pill (Zhi Bai Di Huang Wan), which supplements the Kidney and clears heat. • Avoid hot-natured foods or medicines, like pepper and Clomid. • Stimulate acupoints Sp 10, LI 11, UB 17.
High BBT	**Related pattern:** Kidney Yin deficiency (**Ki Yi–**)	• Supplement Kidney Yin by stimulating acupoints Ki 3, Sp 6, Ren 3, and Ren 4. • Supplement with Six Flavor Pill with Rehmannia (Liu Wei Di Huang Wan).
High BBT	**Related pattern:** Excess Heat (**^H**)	• Clear the Liver with Lv 2 and Lv 3. • Rectify Liver Qi with herbs such as Bupleurum (Chai Hu). • Clear heat if present (see recommendations for clearing heat listed under "Treatment" in "Shortened Phase I" above).
Low BBT	Insufficient Kidney Yang **Related pattern:** Kidney Yang deficiency (**Ki Yan–**)	• Tonify Kidney Yang with warming herbs like Vitex, or chaste tree berry, (Man Jing Zi) and Eucommia (Du Zhong). • Stimulate acupoint Ki 7. • Warm the lower abdomen with a hot water bottle or heating pad.

Phase/Symptom	Condition	Treatment
Phase II: Ovulation	Phase is triggered by Liver Qi transforming Yin (estrogen) into Yang (progesterone). **Related pattern:** Liver Qi stagnation **(Lv Qi X)**	• Ensure enough Liver Qi to power transformation. • Unobstruct Liver Qi with black cohosh (Sheng Ma). • Stimulate acupoints Lv 3, Lv 14.
	Blood needs to be free-flowing and clear. **Related pattern:** Blood stasis **(Bl X)**	• Ensure adequate Blood during the follicular phase by stimulating acupoint Sp 6. • Invigorate the blood with Sp 8, Sp 10, and UB 17. • Supplement with herbs like Leonurus (Yi Mu Cao) and Leonurus seed (Chong Wei Zi).
Painful ovulation	**Related pattern:** Blood stasis **(Bl X)**	• Invigorate static Blood by stimulating acupressure points like Sp 10 and UB 17. • Acupressure point ear intertragic notch should be massaged to encourage proper circulation. • Blood-invigorating herbs like peach kernel (Tao Ren) also can relieve ovulatory pain.
Sore breasts and irritability at ovulation	**Related pattern:** Liver Qi stagnation (**Lv Qi X**)	• Massage acupuncture points Lv 2, Lv 3, LI 4, and ear triangular fossa. • Supplement with herbs like black cohosh (Sheng Ma) or Bupleurum (Chai Hu). • Meditate, do yoga or Qi Gong breathing exercise.
Phase III: Yang Phase (luteal phase)		
Diagnosis of luteal phase defect	Yang or Qi deficiency **Related patterns:** Kidney Yang deficiency (**Ki Yan–**) Spleen Qi deficiency (**Sp–**)	• Tonify Yang and Qi with points Ki 7, St 36, Ren 6, Du 4, UB 23, UB 52. • Eat fresh pineapple for the enzyme bromelain, which helps implantation. • See treatments recommended in chapter 9 for luteal phase defect.
Uterine lining out of phase with day of cycle	**Related patterns:** Cold Uterus (**CW**) Kidney Yang deficiency (**Ki Yan–**) Blood stasis (**Bl X**)	• Invigorate and warm the Uterus with lower abdominal massage, femoral massage, hot water bottle, heating pad. • Use herbs like Curculigo (Xian Mao) and the herbal formula Warm the Menses Decoction (Wen Jing Tang).

Phase/Symptom	Condition	Treatment
Shortened Phase III	**Related patterns:** Excess heat (**^H**) Kidney Yin deficiency (**Ki Yi–**) Liver Qi stagnation (**Lv Qi X**)	• Eat cooling foods like fruits. • Use the herbal formula Anemarrhena, Phellodendron, and Rehmannia Pill (Zhi Bai Di Huang Wan). • Stimulate acupoint Ki 3 to nourish Yin. • Take Stellaria (Yin Chai Hu). • Stimulate acupressure points Lv 2, LI 11, Sp 10, and UB 40 to cool the body. • Meditate. • Breathe. • Avoid hot, spicy, and greasy foods. • Do not take hot baths, saunas, or Jacuzzis.
Slow, biphasic, stepwise formation on BBT graph	Qi stagnation caused by Blood stasis or Kidney Yang deficiency **Related patterns:** Liver Qi stagnation (**Lv Qi X**) Blood stasis (**Bl X**) Kidney Yang deficiency (**Ki Yan–**)	• Invigorate Blood with exercises like femoral massage. • Stimulate acupoints like Sp 10 and St 36, based on pattern diagnosis. • If Blood is deficient and stagnant, the Chinese patent formula Four Substances Decoction with Safflower and Peach Pit (Tao Hong Si Wu Tang) would be appropriate. • Supplement Yang in Kidneys with herbs like Epimedium (Yin Yang Huo), Eucommia (Du Zhong), or Dipsacus (Xu Duan). • Rectify Qi by not overeating. • Massage acupoints Lv 3 and Lv 14.
Erratic, low and high temperatures, fatigue, inadequate luteal phase	Qi or Yang deficiency together with Liver depression **Related patterns:** Spleen Qi deficiency (**Sp–**) Kidney Yang deficiency (**Ki Yan–**) Liver Qi stagnation (**Lv Qi X**)	• Supplement Spleen Qi by stimulating acupoints Sp 6, St 36, Ren 6. • Stimulate Kidney Yang points Ki 7 and Ren 4. • Rectify Liver Qi by stimulating Lv 2, Lv 3, and Lv 14. • Take herbs like black cohosh (Sheng Ma) and herbal formula Rambling Powder (Xiao Yao San).
Low temperatures during Phase III	Yang deficiency **Related patern:** Kidney Yang deficiency (**Ki Yan–**)	• Stimulate Kidney Yang points Ki 7 and Ren 4. • Eat walnuts and non–hormonally treated organ meats. • Supplement with L-arginine. • Take the herbal formula Eight Ingredient Pill with Rehmannia (Ba Wei Di Huang Wan).

Phase/Symptom	Condition	Treatment
Erratically high temperatures with emotional symptoms	Spirit disharmony, Liver and Heart fire. **Related patterns:** Excess heat (**^H**) Liver Qi stagnation (**Lv Qi X**) Heart deficiency (**Ht−**)	• Harmonize the Liver and clear excess heat by stimulating Lv 2. • Clear Heart fire with herbs like Scutellaria (Huang Qin). • Stimulate spirit-calming points like ear triangular fossa, Yintang, UB 42, and Ht 7.
Sawtooth erratic pattern on BBT graph	**Related pattern:** Liver Qi stagnation (**Lv Qi X**)	• If sawtooth pattern occurs throughout the month, Qi needs to be unobstructed continuously. If erratic temperature occurs only in Phase II, rectify only then. • Use herbs like black cohosh (Sheng Ma). • Stimulate acupoint Lv 3. • The Chinese herbal formula Rambling Powder (Xiao Yao San) helps resolve Liver Qi stagnation. • Lv 3, Lv 8, and Lv 14 may be massaged, but avoid the lower abdominal and uterine points (including Li 4 and Sp 6), which are contraindicated during pregnancy and therefore during the luteal phase.
Biphasic, step form, slow-rising BBT during shortened Phase III	**Related patterns:** Liver Qi stagnation (**Lv Qi X**) Excess heat (**^H**)	• Rectify Liver Qi (see recommendations above). • Clear heat with herb Stellaria (Yin Chai Hu). • Stimulate acupoint Lv 2.
Elevated overall temperature in any phase	**Related patterns:** Liver Qi stagnation (**Lv Qi X**) Excess heat (**^H**)	• Unobstruct the Liver by stimulating acupoint Lv 3. • Clear Heat by stimulating acupoint Lv 2. • Take Stellaria (Yin Chai Hu). • Slow down. • Meditate. • Get adequate exercise and rest.
Phase IV: **The Premenstrual** **Phase**	Liver Qi directs the transformation of Yang back into Yin. **Related pattern:** Liver Qi stagnation (**Lv Qi X**)	• Rectify Liver Qi. • Get adequate physical exercise. • Avoid situations you find frustrating, as any stagnated emotional tension can inhibit the Qi mechanism. • Laugh. • Breathe deeply and relax. • Do not overeat. • Try to avoid heavy, hard-to-digest foods like nuts, peanut butter, butter, animal fats, too

Phase/Symptom	Condition	Treatment
		much meat, and too much bread. • Avoid foods with preservatives or chemicals. • Augment with Qi-rectifying herbs like Cyperus (Xiang Fu), citrus peel (Chen Pi), and black cohosh (Sheng Ma), or the formula Rambling Powder (Xiao Yao San).
	Qi and Blood must be flowing smoothly throughout the body.	• Eat a healthy diet with organic produce and small amounts of organic animal products. • Exercise moderately. • Meditate daily. • Always remember to breathe.
	Liver Qi needs to be harmonized	• Stimulate acupuncture points Lv 3, Lv 8, Lv 14.
Premenstrual symptoms: irritability, pain, constipation, diarrhea, headaches, bloating, night sweats, insomnia, depression, edema, nausea, appetite changes, nosebleeds, mouth sores, vaginal irritation, dizziness, clumsiness, muscle aches, etc.	Blocked Qi and Blood **Related patterns:** Liver Qi stagnation (**Lv Qi X**) Blood stasis (**Bl X**)	• Herbs like Bupleurum (Chai Hu), black cohosh (Sheng Ma), Citrus peel (Chen Pi), and herbal formula Rambling Powder (Xiao Yao San) all rectify Liver Qi. • Herbs like Leonurus (Yi Mu Cao) move static Blood. • Acupoints Lv 2, Lv 3, Lv 8, and Lv 14 move stagnant Liver Qi. • Stimulate acupoints Sp 10 and UB 17 to move the Blood.
Phase V: **The Blood Phase**	Yin and Yang in balance	• Rest for first three days. • No TCM treatments unless there is severe pain.
Blood flow scanty or only lasts for a day or two	Not enough Blood to nourish uterine lining; lack of estrogen in Phase I **Related pattern:** Blood deficiency (**Bl−**)	• Nourish Blood and Yin during Phase I with Angelica (Dang Gui), white peony (Bai Shao), and nettles.
	Related patterns: Blood deficiency (**Bl−**) and Qi deficiency (**Sp−**)	• Qi and Blood need boosting throughout the cycle. • Stimulate acupoints Sp 6, St 36, Ren 4, and Ren 6. • Take herbs like Avena sativa and the herbal formula Eight Treasures Decoction (Ba Zhen Tang).

Phase/Symptom	Condition	Treatment
Blood is pink and watery	**Related pattern:** Spleen Qi deficiency (**Sp–**)	• Supplement the Qi throughout the cycle. • Avoid sugar, refined carbohydrates, starches, dairy products, cold drinks, and raw foods. • Supplement with herbs like gingseng (Ren Shen), Astragalus (Huang Qi), and Atractylodes (Bai Zhu).
Blood is scant and brownish in color	Blood needs tonifying and quickening **Related patterns:** Blood deficiency (**Bl–**) Blood statis (**Bl X**)	• Angelica (Dang Gui) and Four Substances Decoction with Safflower and Peach Pit (Tao Hong Si Wu Tang) tonify and invigorate Blood. • Perform exercises like the femoral massage to enhance blood flow to the Uterus during Phase I. • Apply castor-oil packs to lower abdomen (after menstruation and before ovulation only).
Menstrual flow abnormally profuse or lasts beyond seven days	Qi deficiency/insufficient Qi to control menstrual cycle (often accompanied by fatigue, cold hands/feet, digestive complaints, poor circulation, etc.) **Related pattern:** Spleen Qi deficiency (**Sp–**)	• Supplement using herbs such as ginseng (Ren Shen), Atractylodes (Bai Zhu), and Astragalus (Huang Qi) throughout cycle. • Use the Spleen Qi diet, avoiding refined carbohydrates, sweets, and dairy products.
Heavy flow appears dark and clotty, and is accompanied by pain	**Related pattern:** Blood stasis (**Bl X**)	• Use herbs like peach kernel (Tao Ren), safflower (Hong Hua), frankincense (Ru Xiang), and Achyranthes (Huai Niu Xi). • Use sanitary napkins rather than tampons. • See suggestions in chapter 13.
Blood bright red and profuse, cycle shorter than 28 days	Excess heat (caused by too much Yang or too little Yin) **Related pattern:** Excess heat (**^H**)	• Cool the blood with herbs like red peony (Chi Shao) and moutan (Mu Dan Pi) throughout cycle.
No menstruation at all (amenorrhea)	Deficiency of Blood **Related pattern:** Blood deficiency (**Bl–**)	• Use tonifying herbs like Angelica (Dang Gui), Polygonatum (He Shou Wu), nettles, white peony (Bai Shao), and cooked Rehmannia (Shu Di Huang) • You may also need to tonify Spleen Qi, and Kidney Yin and/or Yang throughout cycle. See earlier recommendations.

Month(s) _____ Year _____ Last 12 Cycles: Shortest _____ Longest _____ This Cycle's Length _____

Cycle Day	1	2	3	4	5	6	7	8	9	10	11	12	13	14	15	16	17	18	19	20	21	22	23	24	25	26	27	28	29	30	31	32	33	34	35	36	37	38	39	40	41	42	43	44	45
Date																																													
Day of Week																																													
Intercourse																																													
Time Temp Taken																																													

Waking Temperature grid (99 down to 97⁹, repeated across all 45 cycle days)

Cycle Day	1	2	3	4	5	6	7	8	9	10	11	12	13	14	15	16	17	18	19	20	21	22	23	24	25	26	27	28	29	30	31	32	33	34	35	36	37	38	39	40	41	42	43	44	45
Cervical Fluid																																													
Vaginal Sensation																																													
Cervix																																													
Cervical Fluid Description																																													
Hormone Levels																																													
Follicle Sizes																																													
OPK/LH Surge																																													
Ovulatory Pain																																													
Fertility Medication																																													
Miscellaneous																																													
Cramps																																													
Bloated																																													
Headaches																																													
Sore Breasts																																													
Emotional																																													

Figure 5.6: Basal Body Temperature Chart

6

Step Two: Diet and Lifestyle — Taking Care of Your Body Gently and Naturally

The doctor of the future will give no medicines, but will interest his patients in the care of the human frame, in diet, and in the causes of disease.

— THOMAS EDISON

Until relatively recently, many women smoked, drank alcohol, and ate whatever they chose while trying to conceive, and even during pregnancy. They never worried or wondered about the effects of stress or medications on their ability to get pregnant. Things are different today. As soon as we start trying to have a baby we're told to quit alcohol and caffeine, take extra folic acid and calcium, reduce our stress, keep our weight within narrow parameters, exercise moderately, and so on. While all these directives can be frustrating and sometimes hard to follow, they address a critical area of fertility: the effects of diet and lifestyle on our ability to conceive.

When faced with my own fertility challenges, like many other desperate women I was obsessed with making sure I did everything possible to help my body conceive and carry a child. I altered my diet, cut out all forms of animal products, and choked down a shot of wheatgrass every day. Nothing artificial, inorganic, refined, or processed crossed my lips or was used on my body. I meditated to keep my stress low. I exercised when I could, but nothing too strenuous just in case I was already preg-nant. I held my breath when a car drove by. Lifestyle was one of the few things I could control, I thought; therefore, I would make whatever changes might move me one hair-breadth closer to pregnancy.

I also started incorporating elements of the Chinese medicine I was studying. Chinese medicine is based on the idea of balancing every aspect of the body, including diet and lifestyle. The *Nei Jing* describes how different foods can be used to treat deficiencies and excesses of Yin and Yang. And while acupuncture and acupressure are two forms of treating energy flow within the body, other treatments like massage and exercise can form important parts of a Chinese medical prescription. And since Chinese medicine is designed to recognize the interrelation of body, mind, and spirit, recommendations for practices such as meditation, visualization, focused breathing, and other relaxation techniques are also common.

This chapter is designed to show you how to take better care of your body, mind, and spirit using TCM dietary principles. The care suggestions are once again put in both Western and Eastern terms, with specific guidelines for TCM-diagnosed conditions that affect fertility, like Kidney, Liver, or Spleen deficiencies, Yin or Yang excess or deficiency, and so on. There are also some general guidelines to increase your health and well-being so you can get pregnant naturally or support any Western ART.

A Chinese proverb states "When the soil is well prepared, the harvest will be bountiful." Any gardener will tell you that the quality of the soil is what influences the productivity and health of the plant. Preparing the soil isn't the most glamorous job: it takes time to turn the soil and balance the pH, and if done naturally, it can involve smelly things like manure and compost. In the same way, changing our diet and lifestyle can at times be unglamorous. We have to say no to such addictions as coffee or cigarettes or even excess worry. We may not be able to stay out late because we need our sleep. We may have to skip the convenience of a Starbucks breakfast or a McDonald's lunch and prepare healthful food instead. We may have to forsake a couple of hours of TV to spend time meditating or exercising. But I believe you will find such lifestyle changes offer two compensations. First, you will discover a much greater feeling of health and vitality within yourself when you start really taking care of the needs of your body, mind, and spirit. Second, you can be certain that you are doing everything possible to prepare the first and most important "home" for your future son or daughter — your own body.

❧ HOW NUTRITION MAKES A DIFFERENCE

Those who take medicine and neglect their diet waste the skill of the physician.

— CHINESE PROVERB

Women facing fertility challenges are often told that certain vitamins and dietary adjustments can restore hormonal functioning, reduce FSH levels, and ultimately help them get pregnant. Yet many women try to cut out processed meats, refined sugars, and dairy products for a few weeks or supplement their diets with large doses of vitamins and don't notice a bit of difference. It is well documented that body fat content has an effect on our fertility (too high or too low a body fat content accounts for 12 percent of infertility cases in the United States); lesser known is how much of a role nutrition plays in our reproductive health.

The Chinese tradition recognizes food as the main source of energy. The Spleen converts food into usable energy (including Qi, Blood, and Essence). Each food has different energetic qualities. For example, hot, spicy foods are more Yang in nature, while sweet foods are more Yin. Some foods build up the Blood; others help draw heat and dampness from the body. The different tastes — sweet, spicy, sour, bitter, salty, and aromatic — have certain effects when taken in moderation. However, if any of these tastes predominate, they can create imbalance in the body. The effects of overindulging in some of these

tastes are recognized in Western medicine, too. In Chinese culture, salty flavors are considered necessary for the Kidneys, but too much salt is said to obstruct the flow of the Blood. In Western medicine, too much salt causes water retention, affecting the kidneys, and also can create problems with the circulation of the blood.

In the Chinese tradition, a meal isn't just an accumulation of calories but an opportunity to supply our Organs with the balanced tastes and energies needed for health. When the body is out of balance, food is one way to make up for deficiency and drain excess from the system.

According to TCM philosophy, the *shen* (translated as Kidney and spirit) governs the reproductive system. If you are having problems conceiving, there is often a deficiency in the shen energy. Symptoms of Kidney deficiency include lower back pain, weak legs, dry mucous membranes, night sweats, cold feet, irregular menses, low libido, increased urinary frequency, and nighttime urination, to name a few. (During menopause, a woman's Kidney Essence, or shen, decreases, and many of the same symptoms occur.) A doctor of Oriental medicine would suggest taking herbal supplements to increase the shen and also would recommend a diet containing foods that nourish the Kidneys, such as walnuts, black sesame seeds, barley, tofu, black soybean, wheat germ, seaweeds, various beans, organ meats, and wheatgrass.

Kidney Essence, or shen, encompasses Kidney Yin and Yang, and both Kidney Yin (**Ki Yi–**) and Kidney Yang (**Ki Yan–**) deficiencies can be helped with dietary changes that supplement the Essence. A patient with Kidney Yin deficiency should avoid too much exercise, external heat, and hot, spicy foods. Someone with Kidney Yang deficiency should not consume ice-cold drinks, especially during menses, as these would lower the heat in a body that is already heat deficient. She also should eat lightly steamed vegetables instead of raw ones, which require more Qi (which is Yang in nature) to digest.

The goal of every dietary prescription is to bring the body back into balance. Here are some general dietary recommendations I make to my patients who are trying to get pregnant.

1. Eat alkaline rather than acidic foods.

Many contemporary sources advocate eating alkaline foods like noncitrus fruits, vegetables, sprouts, cereal grasses (wheatgrass, barley grass), and herbs like black cohosh and valerian root to help provide the entire reproductive system with the right pH for conception and implantation. Acidic foods (like meat, dairy products, and most grains) produce acidic environments. Acidic cervical mucus may become hostile to sperm, which requires an alkaline environment to survive. Since saliva can have an alkalizing effect, it is also recommended that you chew your food thoroughly and refrain from drinking liquids with your meal. Let your own salivary enzymes digest the food, rather than washing it down with fluids.

I don't advocate strict vegan diets, but you should make sure the bulk of your diet comes from organic plant sources. Bioflavonoids, found in many fruits and vegetables, also help in the formation of healthy blood vessels, helping the uterus prepare for implantation and prevent miscarriage.

2. Get plenty of essential fatty acids, preferably from unprocessed plant sources and deep-sea fish.

The essential fatty acids linoleic acid and alpha-linolenic acid are essential to every living cell in the body. They are also key in ovulation, specifically in the process of follicular rupture (releasing the egg) and collapse (allowing the development of the corpus luteum). Good sources of essential fatty acids are fish, fish oil, nonhydrogenated cold-pressed oils such as flaxseed and pumpkin-seed oils, eggs, soy products, raw nuts and seeds, and dark-green and winter vegetables like broccoli, cauliflower, beets, carrots, kale, collards, cabbage, turnips, rutabaga, and Brussels sprouts.

Be aware, however, that with long-term exposure to heat and light, essential fatty acids found in vegetable oils may become trans fatty acids, which are toxic. Trans fatty acids can impair the proper functioning of the immune and reproductive systems. Other sources of trans fatty acids are shortening, margarine, lard and animal fat, and hydrogenated vegetable oils, which are found in many processed foods. Do your best to stay away from trans fatty acids in your diet. Store oil in a cool, dry place, and once it's open, use the oil within a couple of months.

Another key fatty acid, omega-3, is found in deep-sea fish oil. Omega-3 fatty acids have been found to clean the blood of fat deposits, reduce clotting, and encourage blood flow to the tissues, including the uterus. Omega-3 fatty acids also boost the immune system and have been found to reduce certain immune cells (NK, or natural killer, cells) which prevent the embryo's implantation in the uterus. The omega-3 fatty acids eicosapentaenoic acid (EPA) and docohexaenoic acid (DHA) are also essential in fetal brain development.

🐉 NOTE: Be aware that elevated levels of mercury can be found in many deep-sea fish. Some companies do ensure purity standards for their fish, guaranteeing low or no toxic metals.

---

3. **Eat organic foods and hormone-free meats whenever possible.** In natural-food circles, organic foods are touted as necessary for optimum hormonal functioning because many of the pesticides, chemicals, and hormones used to treat produce and animal products contain synthetic estrogen-like substances, which occupy estrogen receptor sites and have negative effects on our organ and endocrine systems. However,

Chinese medicine provides an additional reason for choosing organic food: food loses its Essence and Qi as it moves away from its source. We all have experienced the truth of this: we know fruit off a tree tastes much fresher than fruit from a grocery bag, and vine-ripened tomatoes taste much better than those ripened on the counter.

The processing most food undergoes eliminates much of the natural nutrition present in the original fruits, grains, and vegetables. When we eat refined pasta and white bread, we are consuming mostly processed leftovers; little of the original substance of the wheat is left. Processed fruit juices consist of mostly sugar, and sugar damages the Spleen, which controls digestion. Frozen meals are packed with sodium, which depletes the Kidneys. Most of the canned, prepared foods that form the basis of the typical American diet contain preservatives and minuscule original food value.

Overall improvements to dietary health can be made by consuming more of a macrobiotic diet, including mostly fresh, organic produce supplemented with small amounts of hormone-free meat and animal products. The typical Asian diet is macrobiotic — meals consist mostly of fresh, lightly sautéed vegetables, rice, and small amounts of meat for flavoring.

You also might want to consider how you prepare your foods. Traditional Chinese cuisine advocates chopping vegetables and meat to allow for the release of more energy when they are eaten, and lightly cooking vegetables rather than eating them raw to make them more easily digestible. It's also a good idea to stay away from the microwave. Microwaving food affects its structure and, according to some, decreases the Qi energy available in the food. Cooking on top of the stove or in the oven is preferable.

4. Add more cruciferous vegetables like cabbage, broccoli, Brussels sprouts, and cauliflower to your diet. Cruciferous vegetables contain di-indolylmethane (DIM), a compound that stimulates more efficient use of estrogen by increasing the metabolism of estradiol (one form of estrogen produced by the body). Excess estradiol is associated with breast pain, weight gain, breast and uterine cancer, moodiness, and low libido. Adding DIM sources to your diet allows the estradiol to break down into the beneficial 2-hydroxy estrogens, which don't have estradiol's negative effects.

5. Supplement your diet with a natural, high-potency multivitamin and mineral complex with iron, folic acid, and B vitamins. The vitamins and minerals important for reproductive health (vitamins A, C, E, B complex, zinc, and selenium) enhance fertility yet are lacking in the usual Western, highly processed diet. If these nutrients were adequately supplied through the diet, many fertility problems could be avoided. Other supplements you might wish to try include the following:

◆ *Bee pollen and/or royal jelly* is regenerative and tonifying. Bogdan Tekavcic, M.D., a Yugoslavian gynecologist, conducted a study in which the majority of women who were given bee pollen with royal jelly showed improvement or disappearance of their menstrual problems, while there was no change in the placebo group. Another study showed bee pollen significantly improved sperm production in men. Bee pollen, which is worker bee food, is rich in vitamins, minerals, nucleic acids, and steroid hormones, and improves health, endurance, and immunity. Royal jelly is modified pollen fed only to the reproducing queen bee, whose job it is to produce more infant bees. This nutritive tonic might be considered the bee equivalent of fertility drugs. Rich in amino acids, vitamins, and enzymes, royal jelly helps the queen lay millions of eggs and live longer than the worker bee.

◆ *Blue-green algae* is the origin of life-giving nourishment on this planet. Micro-algae contains chlorophyll, amino acids, minerals, vitamins, and steroid building blocks. Chlorella is freshwater green algae; spirulina is saltwater blue-green algae. Chlorella and spirulina nourish the endocrine, nervous, and immune systems; tonify Qi, Blood, and Essence; regulate metabolism; and repair tissue.

◆ *Wheatgrass* is tonifying and curative. It nourishes Qi, Blood, and Essence, enhances immunity, and restores hormonal functioning. Other cereal grasses like barley grass function the same way.

- *Vitamin B6* helps the body metabolize excess estrogen, produce adequate progesterone, and lower elevated prolactin levels. A Harvard study treated women with galactorrhea (lactation not associated with childbirth or nursing)/amenorrhea syndrome with 200 to 600 milligrams of vitamin B6 daily. Within three months all the women in the study had normal menstrual cycles and had stopped lactating.
- *Coenzyme Q-10* assists mitochondrial function, the powerhouse of each cell.
- *Folic acid* is extremely important in cellular division. I am a proponent of supplementing your diet with folic acid for months before you conceive and throughout pregnancy. You should be aware that the adult daily minimum requirement for folic acid advocated by the Food and Drug Administration (FDA) is well below the amount we actually should take. If you have a history of abnormal cell division, such as cervical dysplasia, you should eat foods with high folic acid content, like dark-green leafy vegetables and natural orange foods — oranges, cantaloupe, yams, and sweet potatoes — in addition to your folic acid supplement.

6. Eliminate caffeine, nicotine, and alcohol. Caffeine, nicotine, and other stimulants should be avoided, especially if you have Yin, Blood, or Heart deficiency with heat symptoms. The *American Journal of Epidemiology* reports nicotine is ten times more concentrated in the uterine fluid than it is in plasma. Nicotine ages the ovaries and makes the eggs resistant to fertilization. Alcohol is particularly damaging if you fall into the damp, heat, or Liver Qi categories of disharmony. One study reported that *any* alcohol consumed during an IVF cycle reduced its chance of success by 50 percent.

Tea, especially green tea, is not as problematic as coffee. It contains about 20 percent less caffeine, and fewer volatile oils. Coffee constricts vessels while tea opens them. Green tea (and, to a lesser extent, black tea) has an antioxidant benefit coffee does not share. If you require assistance "revving up" in the morning, use green tea.

7. If at all possible, avoid unnecessary medications and drugs, including over-the-counter preparations. Even non-steroidal anti-inflammatories (NSAIDs) like ibuprofen can block the synthesis of prostaglandins and therefore inhibit ovulation.

If you have scanty cervical mucus, you should avoid decongestants, antihistamines, and excess supplemental vitamin C. You may, however, use guaifenesin, an expectorant that thins all mucus secretions, including cervical fluid that is too thick. (While guaifenesin can be found in over-the-counter cough medicines like Robitussin, I prefer using natural sources such as beech wood, which you can buy at the health-food store and which contain no additives.) Avoid vaginal lubricants other than egg whites.

8. Avoid junk food, excessive stress, too little sleep, too much exercise, or anything taxing to the immune system. In general, you should give your body every chance to be at its strongest and healthiest so that it can nourish your child. Late hours, bad food, or excessive stress of any kind means your body has to dedicate its precious resources to keeping you healthy instead of making a baby. Live healthfully until you conceive and carry your child to term.

A SPECIAL NOTE FOR MEN: Men who are having fertility problems should make similar dietary adjustments. Avoid environmental estrogens and dietary sources of free radicals including saturated fats, hydrogenated oils, and trans fatty acids. Stop or reduce all unnecessary medications, especially antihypertensives, antineoplastics, and anti-inflammatory drugs, which can impair sperm production.

Increase consumption of legumes and soy (which is high in phytoestrogens and phytosterols), and include vitamins C, E, and B12, beta-carotene, folic acid, and zinc, and herbs such as ginseng, which increases production of testosterone and helps with sperm production. Supplement with the amino acids L-arginine and L-carnitine, which are especially associated with enhancing sperm production. (Chinese medicine classifies arginine as a Kidney Yang tonic, while carnitine nourishes the Yin and Blood.)* This regimen will improve not only sperm but overall health.

LIFESTYLE CHANGES: TAKE GOOD CARE OF YOUR BODY, MIND, AND SPIRIT

Food is only one aspect of our lives affecting our fertility. Any chemicals we take in — through our skin, from the air we breathe, the water we drink, even the cleaning products we use — can produce minute yet important changes in our biochemistry. The same is true of the lives we live. If we don't get enough rest, we can deplete our systems of valuable nutrients, because our bodies have to work harder to keep in balance. If we don't exercise, everything can get flabby, including the systems carrying Blood and Qi throughout the body. If we are experiencing a lot of stress in our lives, the biochemical

---

*It is possible that arginine and carnitine also can be helpful for increasing a woman's fertility. An article in the July 1999 *Human Reproduction Journal* described an Italian study in which numerous women classified as "poor responders" to ovarian stimulation were given oral L-arginine, an amino acid and dietary supplement that tonifies the Kidneys. In the L-arginine–treated group, a lower cancellation rate and an increased number of eggs collected and embryos transferred were observed. The study concluded that "oral L-arginine supplementation in poor responder patients may improve ovarian response, endometrial receptivity and pregnancy rates."

storm released by our emotions definitely can affect our fertility.

Women today have been told time and time again that it's important to prepare themselves physically before they conceive. It is as crucial for us to take a clear-eyed, dispassionate look at the effects of our lifestyle on our reproductive health and to make any necessary changes to help us get pregnant. That includes examining the effects of one of the most difficult aspects of our life to face: the amount of stress we experience. Unfortunately, a diagnosis of infertility and subsequent medical treatments for the condition can create immense levels of physiological and psychological stress — which can present a significant barrier to conception.

STRESS: THE FERTILITY KILLER

Stress is defined as an inability to respond appropriately to the environment. The resulting physical response can manifest as myriad nervous system complaints including insomnia, restlessness, nervousness, or a general state of agitation. In some cases the immune system becomes compromised, resulting in everything from an increased susceptibility to colds and flu to hormonal imbalances and chronic disease states.

Stress puts the body into a "fight or flight" mode, which increases the cortisol hormones and other neurochemicals and selectively redirects the blood flow to the brain, the eyes, and the musculoskeletal sys-

tem. This adaptive mechanism allows us to escape from danger. However, most of the stressors we experience in twenty-first-century life do not require the "fight or flight" response, yet our bodies haven't adapted as our environment has changed. Our stress response may be triggered by an endless number of situations — overwork, environmental pollution, emotional factors, worry, and so on. Far too many of us live with high stress levels most of the time. Unfortunately, the stress response preferentially redistributes blood flow *away* from the gastrointestinal, endocrine, and reproductive systems, all of which are nonessential to the "fight or flight" response. Day in and day out, our bodies still need to eat, relax, and reproduce, but under stress these systems won't get the blood flow they need to function efficiently. Blood quits flowing to the stomach, hence we get ulcers and have a wide range of digestive complaints. Blood overnourishes certain parts of the endocrine system and starves others, so we don't produce the right balance of hormones needed for a healthy menstrual cycle. And the poor uterus and ovaries are ignored altogether! In addition, the hormone adrenaline, which is released by the adrenal glands during conditions of stress, inhibits the utilization of progesterone, one of the key hormones of reproduction.

In October 2001 an important study of the effects of stress on conception was published. Doctors at the University of California, San Diego, examined the success rates of a group of women undergoing gamete intrafallopian transfer (GIFT) or IVF (two forms of ART). The study concluded that women with the highest rated life stress levels were 93 percent less likely to become pregnant and achieve a live birth than women who scored lower on the stress scale.

Interestingly enough, in China there is no counterpart to the English word *stress*. The closest physical phenomenon is a state called Liver Qi stagnation (**Lv Qi X**). This describes a condition noted for contracted blood vessels, tight muscles, and a hyperactive sympathetic nervous system. The people who receive this diagnosis are usually those we would describe as being under stress. Yet the Chinese say the most common reason for Liver Qi stagnation is "unfulfilled desires." (I don't know of any greater unfulfilled desire than trying and failing to have a child.) Techniques like Qi Gong breathing, meditation practices, and acupuncture/acupressure focus on resolving the effects of stagnated emotions. In some cases psychological support from therapy or infertility support groups can be helpful in releasing the stuck emotions. Meditation and guided-imagery CDs or tapes help reduce stress. Sites such as www.AnjiOnline.com provide visualizations and meditations specifically for supporting reproductive health.

Oriental medicine has been extremely effective in helping the body deal with stress, depression, and insomnia; it can balance the hormonal system and regulate the menstrual cycle. Remember, in the Chinese medical tradition there is no separation between mind, body, and spirit. Whatever treats the body helps the mind, and whatever heals the spirit will also help restore balance to the physical being. Fortunately, all three elements of the wellness program described in this book will help you mitigate the effects of stress on your body, mind, and spirit. As you add these elements to your health regimen, you will find your stress levels dropping and, as my patients have discovered again and again, you will create an environment in which conception can occur naturally.

First, step away from any guilt you may feel about how you have been living up to this point. Begin by relaxing. Believe your journey has been perfect (even with all of its shortcomings) up to this point. Resolve to make whatever changes you can to support greater health for your mind, body, and spirit. The greatest gift you can give your potential child is to love, honor, and accept yourself.

STRENGTHENING YOUR REPRODUCTIVE SYSTEM WITH EXERCISE AND MASSAGE

Taking good care of yourself should involve some kind of massage, meditation, or other physical indulgence. Chapter 7 will define specific acupoints that when stimulated help resolve patterns of imbalance and relieve overall stress levels. While general massages will make you feel more relaxed and pampered, there are specific techniques to help redirect your body's attention and energy to your reproductive organs. Here are a few exercises you can do to improve the blood flow to the uterus and ovaries.

FEMORAL MASSAGE

This exercise increases blood flow to pelvic organs, providing more nourishment to the uterus and ovaries. (This massage may be more effectively performed by a partner.)

1. Compress (by applying pressure with your fingertips) the large artery just beneath the crease in your groin between your thigh and lower abdomen (see fig. 6.1). This is the femoral artery, which comes from the iliac artery. The iliac artery has branches that supply blood to the uterus, fallopian tubes, and ovaries. (The ovaries have an additional Blood supply, which branches off the arterial section that supplies the Kidneys.)

2. You should be able to feel with your fingertips when the pulsation in the artery stops. Hold the pressure for 30 to 45 sec-onds. The blood is now backing up and increasing the pressure in the iliac arteries, forcing more blood into the pelvic arteries and flooding the pelvic organs with more blood.

3. Release the pressure and let the blood flow normally. When the hold is released, you should feel a sensation of warmth rushing down your leg as the blood supply returns to the lower extremity.

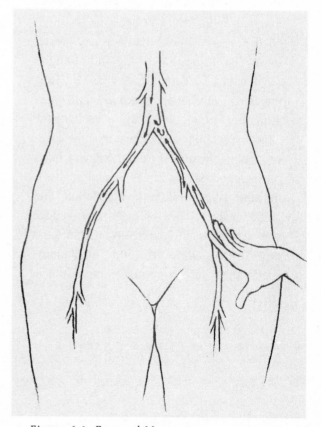

Figure 6.1: Femoral Massage

4. Repeat on the opposite side. Perform this femoral massage sequence three times in a row, twice a day, up to ovulation (or the day before embryo transfer, not beyond).

🔖 NOTE: Do not perform this exercise if you are or might be pregnant. If you have high blood pressure, heart disease, circulatory problems, or a history of strokes or detached retinas, do not practice this technique.

QI GONG BREATHING

This ancient Taoist exercise utilizes the basic life force — the breath — for relaxation and enhances the body's focus on the reproductive organs. We literally breathe life into and through the uterus.

1. Put the tip of your tongue on the roof of your mouth, just behind the top front teeth.

2. Breathe in through your nose, deeply, and concentrate on bringing your breath from your nose and down the midline of your body, between the breasts, down the abdomen, and eventually down to the region two inches below your navel (fig. 6.2). This is called the *Dan Tien*. Let the breath energy pool here. Push out your belly as you inhale.

3. At the end of inhalation, bring the focus from the area below your navel down through the uterus and to the muscles around the vagina. Perform a Kegel exercise, squeezing the pelvic floor muscles encircling the vagina as if you were attempting to stop a flow of urine.

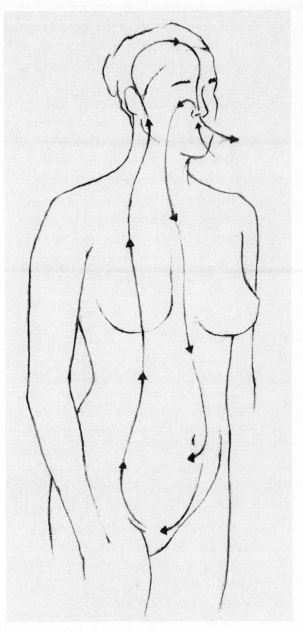

Figure 6.2:Qi Gong Breathing

4. Release the Kegel and begin the exhalation. During exhalation, let the focus of your attention travel from the tip of the coccyx up the spine to the top of the head, then down the midline of the head and out the nose.

5. Repeat steps 2, 3, and 4 until they become one smooth, continuous movement.

Do this exercise anytime and anywhere, as often as possible, *other than* during menstruation or pregnancy. You can perform Qi Gong breathing while you are in traffic, during times of stress, or while watching TV or cooking. The more you do it, the more natural this form of breathing will become.

FOOT SOAK

Most women with Kidney deficiency symptoms have cold feet, especially at night. Soaking the feet in warm water for ten to twenty minutes per day improves the circulation to the lower half of the body and warms the feet. This treatment dilates the blood vessels in the lower half of the body and increases the blood flow to the pelvic organs as well. All the meridians of the body passing through the uterus go down to the feet, and soaking the feet helps improve the circulation of Qi and Blood, not to mention the relaxing effect of a warm foot soak!

LYMPHATIC MASSAGE

While the lymph glands are not technically a part of the reproductive system, they are responsible for cleaning the blood and removing toxins from the body. Therefore, they are an important component in keeping our reproductive organs healthy and clean. Lymph nodes lie along the sides of the femoral and iliac arteries in the lower abdomen, so we will focus the massage there. Lymphatic massage may be performed at any time. It is recommended to use it once a day.

1. Lie on your back and apply a pumping motion to the lower abdomen with your whole hand, massaging upward toward the heart. Try to make the lower belly undulate.

2. Press and release quickly, over and over again, making a wavelike pattern to change the pressure gradient within the lower abdomen and pump the lymphatics.

3. Lying on your back with your feet straight out, have your partner repeatedly pump the balls of your feet and toes up toward the head and back down until your abdomen experiences the wavelike motion.

PHYSICAL EXERCISE

Exercise helps relieve stress and oxygenate the tissues. Too much exercise, however, depletes Yin. This depletion of Yin shows up as a lack of estrogen from too little body fat. But even when body fat content is adequate, if the body focuses too much of its energy on the musculoskeletal system, it will be at the expense of the reproductive system. I have seen many women who work out daily, aerobically and with weights, until you can literally see the lack of Yin in their appearance — masculine, sculpted (Yang) muscles replace (Yin) curves. Even this relative Yin/Yang imbalance may be enough to deprive the reproductive system of its needed essence. If you experience *any* of the symptoms of Kidney Yin deficiency, please sacrifice the hard body for a while.

PILATES

Pilates strengthens the core and firms up the center. This makes for hard abdominal muscles but does not allow the pelvic organs enough room to breathe. I have had to ask quite a few women who consistently do Pilates to back off the abdominal exercises to allow the blood flow to resume to the lower abdominal organs. The same holds true for excessive sit-ups. When you're trying to get pregnant, it's not the time to be working on a six-pack set of abs.

YOGA

Yoga is a wonderful form of exercise. It is relaxing, energizing, and wonderful for unblocking energetic obstructions. But I advise my patients to take their yoga classes before acupuncture treatments, not right afterward. (Yoga distributes energy throughout the body, and the goal of an acupuncture treatment is to direct the energy to specific locations and Organs.) Do not do inversion techniques during menstruation, especially if you have endometriosis. The energetic focus should be downward during menstruation rather than upward. Women who have signs of Yin deficiency should not do Bikram yoga. It is too hot and further depletes the body of its precious (little) Yin fluid.

DIANA'S "HEALTHY" LIFESTYLE

Diana came to see me after numerous failed cycles of stimulated intrauterine inseminations and one IVF. After the last disappointment, her doctor told her she had poor-quality eggs and would never conceive using her own. At age thirty-eight, Diana was already experiencing hot flashes, night sweats, vaginal dryness, and overall irritability. She was afraid she was going into menopause. Diana described herself as healthy and had a sculpted, athletic body. She mostly ate meat, worked out either aerobically or with weights every day, and couldn't understand why her system was aging prematurely. I could — her Yin energies had become depleted.

I asked Diana to cut down on her exercise. Her body had been using up all its energy to feed the musculoskeletal system at the expense of her reproductive system. I also asked her to incorporate more Yin foods like fruits and vegetables into her diet and to

supplement with a few herbs. Every week, I treated her with acupuncture to strengthen her Kidney Yin. I stimulated Ki 3, Sp 6, Ren 3, Ren 4, upper and lower ear points, and, when heat was present, Sp 10.

Although Diana did not conceive naturally because her husband had severe sperm issues, when they decided to try another IVF, she stimulated very well and conceived.

❧ WHAT CAN YOU DO TO HELP YOURSELF? RECOMMENDATIONS ACCORDING TO YOUR DIAGNOSTIC CATEGORY

Your ability to conceive is profoundly influenced by the complex interaction between you and your environment. By adding lifestyle elements recommended by TCM to your day, you will be working consciously to enhance your ability to conceive.

Just as TCM assesses each patient individually and adjusts treatments accordingly, it also makes individual dietary recommendations to balance energies and restore health. Each of the conditions described in chapter 5 has foods and lifestyle choices that will help it come into balance. To refine your diet and make it more specific to your individual pattern or condition, follow these suggestions.

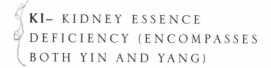

KI– KIDNEY ESSENCE DEFICIENCY (ENCOMPASSES BOTH YIN AND YANG)

1. Do not drink caffeine or take any stimulant, herbal or otherwise, including herbal weight-loss or "energy" formulas.
2. Avoid alcohol.
3. Take supplements such as dehydroepiandrosterone (DHEA) (a hormone building block that declines with age) and glandular supplements (including placenta) for short periods only.
4. Take time each day for rest and relaxation.
5. Avoid too much external stimulation (parties, drugs, loud music, too much sex).
6. Do not smoke.

7. Eat as much as possible of the following foods:
   - black beans and legumes
   - kelp
   - parsley
   - spirulina, chlorella, or blue-green algae
   - wheat germ
   - wheatgrass
   - string beans
   - mulberry
   - millet
   - non–hormonally treated organ meats
   - oysters, clams, lobster, crayfish
   - tofu
   - raspberries
   - walnuts
   - wild rice
   - pork, venison
   - chestnuts
   - black sesame seeds
   - Lycium fruit
   - adzuki beans
   - yams
   - gelatin
   - corn

KI YI– KIDNEY YIN DEFICIENCY

1. A diet for Kidney Yin deficiency should be rich in the following foods:
   - wheat and wheat germ, bulgur, tofu, millet, barley, rice, amaranth
   - asparagus, black beans, kidney beans, red beans, string beans, mung beans, peas and chickpeas, bean sprouts, eggplant, and beets
   - seaweed, chlorella, and spirulina
   - fruit such as apples, bananas, raspberries, blackberries, grapes, lemons, mangoes, mulberries, melons, and pineapple (The enzyme bromelain, found in fresh pineapple, augments the endometrial-adherent molecules necessary for implantation.)
   - shellfish like clams, oysters, and mussels
   - eggs
   - duck, organ meats such as kidneys, brains, and hearts (all from organic, non-hormonally treated sources)

2. Avoid the use of dry, pungent, acrid spices (pepper, curry, horseradish, etc.).

3. Increase dietary sources of phytoestrogens like those found in soy and flaxseed oil.

4. Do not overexercise. Too much physical exertion depletes Yin. Even though the thought of becoming flabby or putting on weight seems daunting, you may have to choose for a while between a hard body and a baby.

5. Do not take saunas or do Bikram yoga, as excess heat may further deplete the Yin.

KI YAN– KIDNEY YANG DEFICIENCY

1. Adhere to the dietary suggestions for Kidney Essence deficiency.
2. Eat warm, nourishing foods.
3. Consume one to three servings of hormone-free meat or animal products each day. Vegan diets are not healthy for the Kidney Yang deficient. Include lobster, lamb, shrimp, and animal kidneys.
4. Include gingerroot, black beans, adzuki beans, lentils.
5. Include grains like oats, spelt, sweet brown rice, and quinoa.
6. Eat walnuts.
7. Fruits should include citrus peel, dates, and cherries.
8. Eat vegetables that are Yang in nature, including parsnips, parsley, mustard greens, winter squash, cabbage, kale, onions, leeks, chives, garlic, and scallions.
9. Cook with peppers and warming spices and herbs such as anise, ginger, cinnamon, cloves, fennel, basil, rosemary, dill, caraway, and cumin.
10. Stay warm. Take warm baths, warm your feet, and warm your lower abdomen with a heating pad or hot water bottle, especially before ovulation.
11. Exercise moderately.
12. Supplement with L-arginine.

SP QI– SPLEEN QI DEFICIENCY*

1. Consume mostly organic vegetables, sautéed or lightly cooked.
2. Do not eat raw, cold foods. Don't consume ice-cold beverages, or put ice in your drinks. Avoid ice cream and Popsicles. Don't eat food straight out of the refrigerator.
3. Avoid energetically "cold" fruits like mangoes, watermelon, pears, and persimmons. "Cold" vegetables include cucumbers, lettuce, celery, and spinach.
4. Do not eat refined carbohydrates like white bread or pasta. Avoid any food made with white flour. Simple starches are converted to glucose immediately after ingestion and become sugar as far as the body is concerned, which damages the Spleen.
5. Eat grains like rice, Job's tears (coix), oats, and sorghum.
6. Eat yams, pumpkin, and pumpkin seeds *unless you have PCOS.* (While some fertility diets advocate it, massive yam consumption can actually delay or prevent ovulation if you have PCOS because the high starch and sugar content in yams exacer-

*Because the Spleen is directly involved in the digestion of all food, the typical Chinese diet incorporates the principles of eating to support the Spleen. Very little cold, raw food is eaten, very little bread or pastry, and almost no dairy products.

bates the impaired glucose metabolism that occurs with this condition.)

7. Eat beef, chicken, goose, ham, herring, rabbit, mackerel, and sturgeon.

8. Eat cherries, coconut, dates, figs, grapes, molasses, potatoes, and shiitake mushrooms.

9. Avoid sugar and sugar substitutes and any concentrated sweets including honey and maple syrup.

10. Do not drink fruit juice; the sugar content is too high. Eat fruits only in their whole form.

11. Avoid damp-creating foods like milk and milk products such as cheese or ice cream.

12. Get adequate rest and sufficient exercise.

13. Do not exercise excessively during menstruation.

14. Perform meditative techniques to help relieve the mind of undue worry. Some people find biofeedback exercises helpful. "Biodots" — feedback stickers somewhat akin to mood rings — turn colors when your blood vessels constrict, allowing you to moderate your own stress level.

BL– BLOOD DEFICIENCY

1. Include the following foods in your diet:
   - apricots, blackberries, raspberries, grapes

- mulberry
- eggs
- organic meats
- spirulina
- turnip, watercress, spinach, dark leafy greens
- Blood-nourishing foods like hormone-free liver and bone marrow

2. Don't smoke cigarettes.

3. Rest during your period.

BL X BLOOD STASIS

1. Consume moderate amounts of soy and soy products (like tofu); however, if you also suffer from concomitant damp or cold symptoms, don't eat soy at all. Soy is cool and sweet, and therefore dampening in nature.

2. Buy only organic fruits and vegetables.

3. Avoid refined, hydrogenated oils.

4. Use only unprocessed plant sources of essential fatty acids, such as raw nuts and seeds, and dark-green vegetables.

5. Use oils rich in both linoleic and alpha-linolenic fatty acids, like flaxseed, pumpkin-seed, and chiaseed oils, but *only* if they are recently cold-pressed and refined. Supplement with oils from fish, evening primrose, linseed, black currant, or borage seeds.

6. Include dietary spirulina.

7. Avoid sources of arachidonic acid,

which comes from animal meats, dairy products, eggs, peanuts, and seaweed.

8. Avoid animal products, except fish.

9. If you cannot eliminate animal products, make sure they are organic and have not been hormonally treated. Synthetic estrogen feeds both endometriosis and fibroids, which are caused by Blood stasis.

10. Eat walnuts, chestnuts, chives, crabs, hawthorn berries, peaches, mustard leaf, onions, scallions, dark greens, saffron, and cold-climate crops like cabbage, broccoli, Brussels sprouts, beets, turnips, cauliflower, and carrots.

11. Foods especially good for resolving Blood stasis include lemons, limes, onions, kelp, Irish moss, and bladder wrack (the last three are forms of seaweed).

12. Include antioxidants (vitamins C, E, beta-carotene, selenium, zinc) and superantioxidants like those in pycnogenol or oligomeric proanthocyanidins (OPC) found in grape seed extract, pine bark extract, red wine extract, bilberry extract, and citrus bioflavonoids. See www. alwaysbuying.com.

❧ NOTE: Don't overwhelm your body with massive doses of vitamin C, however, as too much acid can lower the cervical pH.

---

13. Avoid cold foods right out of the refrigerator or freezer.

14. Do not put ice in your drinks.

15. Do not swim in cold water or have intercourse during menstruation.

16. Use feminine hygiene pads rather than tampons. Tampons do not allow adequate expulsion of blood and may aggravate endometriosis backflow.

17. To purify the blood, add grapes, raspberries, lemons, limes, tomatoes, cucumbers, celery, beets, watercress, vinegar, and salt to your diet.

18. During menstruation, add extra seaweed and spirulina.

19. If you experience abnormal uterine bleeding, eat abalone, black fungus, chicken, squid, and vinegar.

CW COLD UTERUS

*(The diagnosis of cold uterus includes signs of Kidney Yang deficiency [**Ki Yan–**] and Blood stasis [**Bl X**]. The lower abdomen feels cool to the touch.)*

1. Adhere to the Kidney Yang deficiency and Blood stasis suggestions described earlier.

2. Between menstruation and ovulation, apply warmth (a hot water bottle or heating pad) to the lower abdomen.

LV QI X
LIVER QI STAGNATION

1. Do not overeat. Try to avoid heavy, hard-to-digest foods like nuts, peanut butter, butter, animal fat, too much meat, and too much bread.
2. Avoid foods with preservatives and chemicals.
3. Sit down when you eat.
4. Eat frequent small meals. This keeps the blood sugar levels more stable and inhibits adrenaline release.
5. Use spices that move the Qi, like peppermint, rosemary, spearmint, turmeric, and thyme.
6. Supplement your diet with zinc (especially premenstrually).
7. Chew foods adequately.
8. Do not drink alcohol or caffeine. Do not smoke cigarettes.
9. Incorporate the Spleen Qi deficiency dietary principles listed earlier.
10. Get adequate physical exercise.
11. Avoid harboring anger and resentment. Feelings of frustration and internal emotional tension need to be resolved as soon as possible, as any stagnated emotion can inhibit the Qi mechanism.
12. Laugh. Watch funny shows or movies to release any stuck internal feelings.
13. Breathe deeply and relax.
14. Too much estrogen creates Liver Qi stagnation. To help the liver metabolize the excess estrogen, stop eating hormonally treated animal products.

HT– HEART DEFICIENCY

1. Avoid coffee, caffeine, natural or artificial stimulants, and, of course, tobacco.
2. Include foods that nourish the Blood and the Yin. Eat mung beans, beets, and corn.
3. Take time each day for rest and deep relaxation.
4. Meditate. Breathe.
5. Perform Qi Gong techniques to quiet the spirit.
6. Listen to meditative tapes before bed.

^H EXCESS HEAT

1. Do not consume alcohol.
2. Avoid spicy foods.
3. Avoid greasy foods.
4. Do not take hot baths, saunas, or Jacuzzis.
5. Include cooling, Yin-tonifying foods. Burdock root, plums, pears, tomatoes, and pomegranates all clear heat from the body.

D DAMPNESS

1. Avoid greasy, fried foods.
2. Avoid sugar, sweets, fruit juices, and refined carbohydrates.

3. Do not consume milk or dairy products, including ice cream.

4. Do not overindulge in soy products, which are dampening in nature.

5. Avoid wheat, which is more damp in nature than barley or rice. (Rice is also diuretic and may help clear excess fluids, which is helpful in eliminating dampness from the body.)

6. Don't eat bananas, chocolate, or nuts.

7. Do not consume alcohol.

8. Include drying foods such as Job's tears, which has a diuretic effect. Other diuretic foods include alfalfa, parsley, radishes, summer melons, celery, carrots, cabbage, cranberries, cucumbers, lettuce, and kelp.

9. If you have damp heat signs, eat a lot of green vegetables containing indole-3-carbinol, which helps the Liver rid the body of the negative (damp heat) effects of excess estrogens.

One final reminder: Anything can be harmful if used in the wrong way or in too great an amount. This includes food, water, and any of the other recommendations in this book. Please use these suggestions in moderation and stick to the prescription fitting your particular pattern. You're going to get much better results if you approach your body with care and appreciation. Remember, we are speaking of a lifestyle, not a quick fix; by definition, a lifestyle can be lived comfortably over the long term.

The *Tao Te Ching* says,

What is rooted is easy to nourish.
What is recent is easy to correct.
What is brittle is easy to break.
What is small is easy to scatter.

Prevent trouble before it arises.
Put things in order before they exist.
The giant pine tree
grows from a tiny sprout.
The journey of a thousand miles
starts from beneath your feet.

The diet and lifestyle changes you make may be very small to start with, like the sprout that becomes the giant pine tree. But by eating and living to encourage fertility, you are putting down deep roots for your health and well-being. Remember, what is rooted is easy to nourish. And when your body, mind, and spirit feel nourished, they will be ready to welcome and nourish your precious child.

JAN'S DIET WAS ATTACKING HER SPLEEN

Jan, a twenty-eight-year-old veterinarian, had been married to Lyle for four years, and for four years they had been trying to conceive. Her medical questionnaire listed her major health concerns as "infertility, poor ovarian reserve, and elevated FSH." Jan also had been diagnosed with ulcerative colitis, a disease in which the immune system attacks the colon, for which she was taking steroids. Jan and Lyle had undergone numerous medicated insemination cycles and one unsuccessful IVF. After failing a subsequent Clomid challenge test, they then journeyed to a clinic that specialized in treating women diagnosed with elevated FSH, where they underwent another disappointing IVF cycle.

Jan arrived at my clinic with very little hope. She knew her chances of having a child with Lyle were almost nil, so they were petitioning to adopt. She was becoming concerned about her overall health and whether she would be a healthy mother for her adopted child.

Jan's menstrual cycle was thirty-three days long, with a very short, light-pink period and quite a bit of pain. She experienced scant midcycle cervical fluid and usually had vaginal dryness and burning pain with intercourse. She was often extremely tired "because of my ulcerative colitis," she said (but my mind jumped over her excuse and went right to blaming the Spleen). Jan reported that she always had cold hands and feet, bruised easily, had premenstrual lower back pain, and craved sweets. Her

tongue was thin and red with no coating, and her pulse was very weak. My diagnosis was Spleen Qi deficiency with some Kidney Yin deficiency, causing heat.

Because she was on steroids and still experiencing excruciating pain and diarrhea, she did not think her digestive system could absorb any herbs. But I knew that Jan's severe autoimmune problem could benefit from diet alone.

We discussed the TCM view of the Spleen governing the immune and digestive systems. I told her the main dietary causes of a damaged Spleen were wheat flour, sweets, and dairy products. Jan ate a typical American diet, although she didn't drink much milk because it aggravated her bowel. She agreed to cut out all refined carbohydrates, especially those made from wheat flour.

Jan called me three and a half months after our consultation and told me her bowel and menstrual symptoms had improved dramatically after she changed her eating habits. She also was five weeks pregnant, naturally.

7

Step Three: Clearing Your Energy with Acupuncture and Acupressure

It is astounding . . . how much energy the body is capable of pouring out and then replenishing. That is a magical act, because you never really understand where all that energy comes from.

— Robert Bly

In the spring of 2002, a headline appeared on the science pages of many newspapers and on Internet health sites: "Acupuncture could help women undergoing fertility treatment conceive." *Fertility and Sterility*, a journal published by the American Society for Reproductive Medicine, reported on a study by German researchers investigating the effects of acupuncture on women undergoing IVF. The researchers stimulated acupuncture points that were meant to "relax the uterus according to the principles of traditional Chinese medicine." Meridians were selected in an effort to create "better blood perfusion and more energy in the uterus." Ear points were used to stabilize the endocrine system, and points designed to promote patients' general relaxation and well-being also were chosen. The women in the treated group received one acupuncture session before embryo transfer and one afterward.

Ultrasound testing six weeks after embryo transfer revealed that almost twice as many women from the acupuncture group than from the untreated group became pregnant. The two groups and their embryos were quite similar in all respects. The researchers weren't quite sure why acupuncture helped increase the chances of successful implantation, but they declared that more study was definitely warranted.

Another study by Cornell University, published in the December 2002 issue of *Fertility and Sterility*, reported, "The peripheral impact of acupuncture in improving uterine artery blood flow and hence endometrial thickness . . . provides encouraging data regarding its potential positive effect on implantation." The study concluded, "Because acupuncture is nontoxic and relatively affordable, its indications as an adjunct in assisted reproduction or as an alternative for women who are intolerant, ineligible, or contraindicated for conventional hormone induction of ovulation deserves serious research and exploration."

To me, these results were not surprising. I have been collecting articles on studies of acupuncture and fertility issues for years. More important than studies, however, are the results my patients and I have seen. For years I have used acupuncture in my clinic to treat many different fertility problems. Almost every stage of a woman's cycle and pregnancy can benefit from the balancing effects of working with the meridians to promote the flow of Qi through the body and to bring the Organs up to the highest level of health.

THE PRINCIPLES OF ACUPUNCTURE

Acupuncture is applied in order to supply what is lacking and drain off excessive fullness.

— *NEI JING*

As you learned in chapter 3, acupuncture allows practitioners of TCM to tap in to the energy system that enlivens the body. Based on archaeological evidence, it's believed that the earliest precedents of acupuncture date as far back as 1000 B.C.E. Thousands of years ago, sharpened stones and rudimentary needles made of flint were used to penetrate precise points on the skin, yielding consistently predictable results. These points were then charted into meridians, or energy pathways, which have complex and fascinating physiological effects on Organ systems. The accumulated knowledge of these acupuncture points has become the foundation upon which modern acupuncture research is built. More recently, acupuncture has been recognized by Western medicine as a scientifically proven means of treating pain and providing relief from many different diseases and conditions.

Traditional acupuncture involves inserting thin stainless-steel disposable needles into points on the surface of the skin, causing an exchange of electrons within the body, similar to the flow of electricity. This transfer sets in motion an elegant interplay of the body's own energies.

According to Western scientific research, acupuncture's effects on the body can be explained by a number of theories. Robert Becker is a researcher in electrophysiology, the study of the relationship of electrical fields to the human body. He was one of the first to use microcurrents to help heal bone fractures. Becker theorized that acupuncture meridians were paths of electrical energy running throughout the body. For electrical energy to flow smoothly, however, there would have to be "amplifiers" along the lines of current. In his book, *The Body Electric*, Becker writes:

> For current measured in nanoamperes and microvolts, the amplifiers would have to be . . . a few inches apart — just like the acupuncture points! — like dark stars sending their electricity along the meridians, an interior galaxy that the Chinese had somehow found and explored. . . . Our readings indicated that the meridians were conducting current. . . . Each point . . . had [an electrical] field surrounding it. . . . If the integrity of health really was maintained by a balanced circulation of invisible energy through this constellation . . . then various patterns of needle placement might indeed bring the currents into harmony. . . .

Another theory addresses the neurological effects of acupuncture. Neural theory holds that inserting needles at acupuncture points stimulates the nervous system, releasing chemicals to either alleviate pain or affect the body's internal regulating system. Acupuncture needles also stimulate specific nerve fibers to carry electrical impulses back to the brain, increasing beta-endorphin concentrations. Higher beta-endorphin concentrations reduce the sympathetic "fight or flight" response in the body and produce a feeling of relaxation and euphoria similar to runner's high. This is one of the reasons people often feel more relaxed after an acupuncture treatment. As one of my patients told me, "At first I was really nervous because I have an aversion to needles, but after my first visit, I found myself looking forward to my next appointment. The needles didn't hurt, and I was incredibly relaxed after the treatment."

Of course, my patients and I are mostly interested in the effects of acupuncture or acupressure on the reproductive and hormonal systems. Pressure exerted by the needle engenders a microelectric current, which causes a release of prostaglandins into the bloodstream. Prostaglandins stimulate the production of a substance in the nerve endings that transmits messages to the hypothalamus, a section at the base of the brain that controls all hormonal activity and is intimately involved with ovulation, menstruation, and pregnancy.

When the hypothalamus receives a message triggered by the stimulation of an acupuncture point, neurotransmitters like dopamine, adrenaline, and serotonin cause the conversion and release of GnRH, which acts on the pituitary gland, which controls the ovary, adrenal, and thyroid glands. The pituitary also produces FSH and LH, both of which are critical elements in a healthy ovulatory cycle. The bottom line is that *acupuncture can stimulate the body's hormonal system to do what it is supposed to: secrete the right hormones at the right time in a woman's cycle.*

Men also can benefit from the pituitary-stimulating effects of acupuncture. *Acupuncture treatments can improve the concentration, volume, and motility of sperm.* One study showed that more than one-third of the men treated with acupuncture showed improved quality of sperm.

If you want to use acupuncture to treat infertility, however, you don't have to subscribe to any of these theories. All you really have to know is that *acupuncture works.* There is scientific proof of its efficacy in treating a wide range of conditions, as well as millions of satisfied patients all over the world.

WORKING WITH THE POINTS THROUGH ACUPUNCTURE

Different acupuncture points have different effects. Some will decrease the sympathetic nervous system response (which becomes important for women who are trying to conceive and are stressed about it). Some points actually cause changes within the cells. Some effect alterations in the brain's chemicals; others can effect chemical changes within the uterine lining. Some improve circulation, and others have mainly local effects.

Points work via feedback. The body is a system of reactions and feedback: something happens with a nerve, which causes something to happen in the brain, which signals neurochemical changes, hormone level

changes, or a million other responses. It's like a chain reaction — for example, when you stimulate a specific acupuncture point, it invigorates the Blood, sending the whole body a message specific to that point and producing blood-thinning chemical reactions. When you stimulate different combinations of points, you can create even greater results and see those results more quickly. But each specific point, as well as each meridian, has a different function, and the art is in orchestrating a combination that achieves the desired effect. Later in this chapter, we'll go over the different points that can be stimulated to help balance a wide range of conditions affecting fertility.

There are several ways to stimulate your acupuncture points. The best known method is the use of acupuncture needles. The metal needle conducts electricity through electron transfer and produces microtrauma and pressure, which are converted into an electrical message transmitted to another part of the body. However, acupuncture needles should be applied only by a licensed and qualified professional.

FINDING AN ACUPUNCTURIST

The National Council for Certification of Acupuncture and Oriental Medicine is the regulatory board responsible for ensuring national compliance with minimum educational and training requirements. Each state also has its own regulatory board, which licenses medical professionals in its state, including doctors, nurses, chiropractors, and acupuncturists. Check with your state medical board to determine local acupuncture licensing requirements.

I also recommend the following guidelines when choosing an acupuncturist to address your fertility issues.

1. Find out your individual state's requirements for certification and go only to a licensed acupuncturist who is steeped in TCM's system of pattern identification and treatment. If you don't, the effects of treatments on your hormonal and reproductive system may be negligible. Western medical training is a plus.

2. Do not rely solely on Internet directories or the Yellow Pages to locate an acupuncturist, as most directories list practitioners who have paid to advertise. Word of mouth is probably the best method of locating an acupuncturist who has been effective in treating infertility. Ask which practitioners have helped others conceive at your local infertility support groups.

3. Call and interview the acupuncturist before you schedule an appointment. Most acupuncturists treat everything, so if you call and ask, "Do you treat infertility?" almost everyone will say yes. But if you ask a more specific question, such as "How many cases of infertility have you been successful in resolving?" the answer will give you more insight into this acupuncturist's level of experience.

4. Make sure you can understand and be understood by the practitioner. Many of the best acupuncturists in the United States come from other countries. Communication is essential in building a relationship with any health care provider. Whenever I have a patient for whom English is a second language, I ask her to bring an interpreter for her first visit so neither of us misses any essential information.

5. Make sure the acupuncturist uses

only disposable needles and cleans the skin with alcohol before needle insertion. (This is standard practice in the United States.) This is especially important if you have a compromised immune system or diabetes.

6. Most important, make sure you feel comfortable and at ease with this particular practitioner. The best doctor in the world may not be the best doctor for you. Find someone with whom you feel you can develop a relationship of trust.

WHEN YOU GO FOR AN ACUPUNCTURE TREATMENT

I make the following suggestions to my own patients for getting the best results from their acupuncture treatments.

1. Make sure you have eaten, but not too recently. It is important not to have your stomach too empty or too full.

2. Try to relax. Acupuncture needles are not hollow like injection needles. They are thin and go in quickly. You rarely even feel a pinprick, and the treatments will make you feel good.

3. Be aware that when you're ovulating or menstruating you may feel more sensitive to your treatments (especially on the hormonal points).

4. Rest after your treatment if you can.

5. Try not to schedule exercises or yoga classes after acupuncture. Exercising or doing yoga before a treatment is fine.

STIMULATING YOUR OWN POINTS

You may also stimulate the acupoints yourself. In order to make Chinese medicine accessible to everyone, I provide a system of acupoint stimulation that you may employ in lieu of acupuncture needles.

Throughout the ages, many other means have been used to stimulate acupuncture points, including stones, bones, plum blossom needles, tacks inserted just barely into the skin, moxibustion, herbal seeds, laser light, liniments, massage, etc. Patients and practitioners have learned that the stimulation is more important than the instrument. And it's actually easy to stimulate many of

the points yourself using *acupressure*. Known as *Tui Na* in China, this form of stimulation energizes specific points with vigorous manual massage.

ACUPRESSURE

Acupoints can be stimulated with the fingertips, thumb, or a small wooden or rubber mallet. You can stimulate many of the points yourself; others (like the ones on the back) will require someone to massage them for you.

Limb and Head Points: With the tip of your finger, apply enough pressure so you feel a slight aching or full sensation at the site. Rub each point vigorously back and forth with your fingertip for a minute or two until you feel the lingering pressure of the massage, every other day.

Abdominal Points: Massage with the fingertip in a deep, clockwise, circular motion for a couple of minutes every other day, before ovulation.

HEAT

Heat packs can also be applied over the points to activate them with warmth. Chinese practitioners use moxibustion (herbal incense that is burned close to the acupoint) to treat patterns of Yang deficiency and cold uterus, especially at those points on the lower abdomen and those tonifying the Kidney Yang. You can also use heat sources like hot water bottles or heating pads over these areas. If your abdomen feels cool below the navel, I recommend warming up the uterus every other day, before ovulation. Heating it up increases the microcirculation and actually stretches the capillaries. We don't want to increase the temperature when an embryo may be implanting, however, so do not apply heat to the lower belly after ovulation.

MAGNETIC STIMULATION

Magnets generate a small magnetic force, creating ongoing electromagnetic stimula-tion that increases circulation through ionic attraction. Magnets may be purchased at some drug, department, and sporting goods stores, and through the Internet at

www.stressreliefproducts.com
www.magnetictherapysales.com
www.magnetemporium.com

Tape the magnets directly to the skin over the acupoints selected for your pattern.

LIGHT THERAPY

Pocket-size laser light pens can be purchased for around $100 and up at alternative medical supply stores or through the Internet at

www.acupuncture.com
www.ycyhealth.com
www.toolsforwellness.com

Light from the red spectrum stimulates acupuncture points in the same manner as needles. The visible red light (660 nanometers) penetrates the tissue and causes changes in the electrical potential and energy of the cell — the same thing acupuncture does but without any microtrauma experienced at the needle site. Light stimulation also causes the release of serotonin, a vasodilator that improves microcirculation. Touch the light directly to the skin of each acupoint for five seconds.

All of these treatments — acupuncture, acupressure, heat, magnets, light therapy —

stimulate the points and produce corresponding reactions in the Organs and systems of the body. The key to success is *precision*: locate the points for your particular condition and stimulate them as indicated. Use the illustrations on pages 123–128 to locate the points as specifically as you can. Don't be afraid of doing harm. Remember, you are stimulating your body to respond in natural ways — in effect, to do what it was meant to do. You may employ these techniques all by yourself or with assistance. The results will range from deep relaxation to improved blood flow and adjustments in your hormonal system.

USING ACUPOINTS TO TREAT YOUR PATTERN/CONDITION

This chapter includes descriptions of each of the points that will either help the energy flow of your entire reproductive system or address the different patterns diagnosed in chapter 4. I also have included points that will help alleviate conditions such as stress, headache, menstrual cramps, excessive uterine bleeding, and grief, as well as those that will assist preparation for IVF treatments or bring on delayed menses. To use this chapter:

1. Locate the symbol or name for your particular pattern.

2. Read the descriptions of the points associated with that pattern.
3. Look at the illustrations on pages 123–128 to locate the points.
4. Stimulate the points as indicated, with acupressure, heat, magnets, or light stimulation (see above).
5. If you believe you have more than one pattern operating, do the same for your other patterns.
6. In almost all cases, you can stimulate the general reproductive points as well.

FOLLOW THE MERIDIANS

To determine which points you should focus on, you need to remember the basics about the Organs and meridian systems from chapter 3, as well as your pattern diagnosis from chapter 4. There are twelve major meridians, or channels, that run throughout the body. Each channel is associated with a specific Organ system. The twelve main channels are usually described in pairs, reflecting the link between energy systems and Organs in TCM. The pairs (and abbreviations) are as follows.

YIN ORGAN	ABBREV.	PAIRED YANG ORGAN	ABBREV.
Lung	Lu	Large Intestine	LI
Spleen	Sp	Stomach	St
Kidney	Ki	Urinary Bladder	UB
Liver	Lv	Gallbladder	GB
Heart	Ht	Small Intestine	SI
Pericardium	Pc	Triple Warmer, or San Jiao	SJ

When you know your diagnosis, you can manipulate the points in your diagnostic categories. For instance, if you have elements of both excess heat (^H) and Heart deficiency (Ht–), you can stimulate points nourishing the Heart and clearing heat. For a Spleen Qi deficiency (Sp–), stimulating Stomach points may be helpful. You may also stimulate other stress-reducing and general reproductive system points.

In TCM, the Pericardium, or the fibrous sac enclosing the heart, is treated as an Organ separate from the Heart itself. In Western medicine the pericardium protects the heart from physical damage. In TCM the Pericardium also shields the heart from emotional stress and strain. Points on the Pericardium meridian are most often associated with psychological states. Remember, in TCM there is no separation between the body, mind, and spirit. Therefore, we stimulate Pericardium points to help us deal with the difficult emotions that may arise around infertility.

The Triple Warmer (San Jiao) is an Organ with no physical counterpart, nor does it have an accompanying function as defined by Western medicine. In TCM, the Triple Warmer is the pathway connecting the Organs in the body that deal with water: Lungs, Spleen, Kidneys, Small Intestine, and the Urinary Bladder. Therefore, stimulating Triple Warmer points can help the Kidneys and Spleen, two Organ systems intimately involved in fertility.

DESCRIBING THE LOCATION OF YOUR ACUPOINTS

The points along each meridian are denoted in two ways: either by an abbreviation of the Organ plus a number (Lv 3 for "Liver channel, point number 3," for example), or by a more poetic name drawn from the point's function (Lv 3 is also known as "Great Rushing" because it promotes the smooth flow of Liver Qi throughout the body). I will use both the abbreviation and the poetic name so you can locate the point easily and understand the physical effects of stimulating the point.

Remember, the meridians linked to these Organ systems run throughout the body. So a Spleen point will be found somewhere on the leg, for instance, and a Heart point on the wrist. Similarly, stimulating a Spleen point will have an effect not just on the Spleen energy but on the entire body. I've provided points by category, with definitions and illustrations.

EXTRAORDINARY MERIDIAN POINTS

In addition to the meridians linking the Organ systems, the body contains four Extraordinary meridians. Some have their own points; others share points with other meridians. The Penetrating meridian (Chong Mai) and the Girdle meridian (Dai Mai) do not have their own points but share them with other meridians. The Governing meridian (Du Mai, abbreviated as Du) and the Conception meridian (Ren Mai, abbreviated as Ren) both have their own points.

As we discussed in chapter 3, a woman's Penetrating meridian originates in the Uterus, and it presides over menstruation, hormones, and psychoneuroendocrinological systems. The Conception and Governing meridians arise from the Penetrating meridian. The Conception meridian is in charge of the body's Yin energy, while the Governing meridian rules the Yang energy.

The Girdle meridian is the only channel in the body that runs horizontally and "holds things in" (e.g., vaginal discharges, fetuses). There are also some points on the face and body not linked to a specific meridian but proven to affect the body's energy.

OTHER POINTS

There is a system of points on the ear and scalp that correspond to the different Organ systems and can easily be stimulated using acupressure. Only those pertaining to the reproductive system are discussed in this book.

THE POINTS

GENERAL REPRODUCTIVE SYSTEM POINTS

These points should be stimulated regardless of the pattern diagnosis. They draw the body's attention to the reproductive system, improve hormonal responsiveness, and increase blood flow, boosting the efficiency of the reproductive organs.

Ear Triangular Fossa. Located in the upper, inner part of the ear, this area contains points that stimulate the Uterus and fallopian tubes, calm the spirit, regulate the sympathetic nervous system, and reduce overall tension and Blood pressure. Massage this area lightly with your fingertip or fingernail once every day or two, and any time you are feeling stressed.

Ear Intertragic Notch. This area, located just above the earlobe in the crevice between the two cartilaginous areas in the lowest point inside the ear, includes endocrine and ovarian points. Massage lightly with your fingernail once every day or two.

Epang II: Scalp Reproductive Points. These points are found above the forehead within the scalp, just inside the upper corner of the hairline above the outside of the eyebrow, or where you feel sensitivity. The area extends from about one half inch below the hairline to one half inch into the hair on the scalp. These scalp points regulate reproductive and pelvic function, including dysmenorrhea. They reinforce the Kidney energies, regulate menstruation, and treat acute urinary dysfunction. Massage gently, especially when tender.

Zigong (Palace of the Child). Located four inches below the navel and three inches lateral to the midline, this point most closely represents the ovaries and is indicated for uterine and menstrual problems, especially infertility. Stimulating Zigong also helps resolve cases of cervical stenosis (a narrowing of the canal between the uterus and the cervical opening). Stimulate with deep, clockwise massage, laser light, or magnets every day or two before ovulation.

Ren 3 (Central Pole of the Conception Meridian). Ren 3 is located on the midline, four inches below the navel. This point represents the center of the body on both a horizontal and vertical plane. It derives its translation, Central Pole, from the Chinese word for "North Star," which is in the center of the sky. It lies over the Uterus on the Conception meridian and regulates menstruation, fortifies the Kidneys, benefits the Urinary Bladder, and removes stagnation and dampness from the pelvis. I use this point to "water the uterus," or subdue toxic heat found in conditions like endometriosis with implantation difficulty and NK cells in the endometrium. Massage with deep, circular motions, but only before ovulation, not after. You may employ heat, light, or magnet therapy as well.

Ren 4 (Origin of the Source of the Conception Meridian). Ren 4 is located on the midline, four inches below the navel. This point represents the source of life, the *Dan Tien*, and the site of the Uterus. It fortifies the original Qi (the life force you inherit from your parents), nourishes Kidney Essence, and assists conception. Massage with deep, circular motions, but only between menstruation and ovulation. You may also use light, heat, or magnet therapy.

St 30 (Rushing Qi). This point is found on the lower abdomen, five inches beneath the navel and two inches lateral to the midline, just above the superior border of the pubic symphysis. This point represents the crossing point of the Penetrating meridian with the ovaries, fallopian tubes, and uterus. It is helpful in treating disorders of menstruation, fertility, and childbirth. It also is said to disperse cold and stagnation in the pelvis. Circular massage, light, and heat are appropriate means of stimulation.

Ki 16 (Vitals Shu). Ki 16 is located one half inch on either side of and level with the umbilicus. This vital point lies where the energy of the Kidneys rises up to the Heart. Ki 16 not only tonifies the Kidney and Heart but also calms the mind. It is also considered a point of transit for the immunologic system and thus removes energetic blockages that have accumulated in the abdomen. Massage with a circular motion, apply heat, or stimulate with light or magnets.

The rest of the points listed in this chapter can be stimulated through acupressure massage, either with your fingers or other massage devices, or with laser light therapy, magnets, or heat (but only if you do not have signs of excess heat).

KI YI– POINTS TO TONIFY THE KIDNEY (YIN)

Ki 3 (Great Ravine). Sometimes an arterial pulsing can be felt at this energetic point, which is located in the depression behind the inner anklebone and in front of the Achilles tendon, just above the heel bone. This "Big Stream," as Ki 3 is also called, nourishes the Essence of the Kidney energies. The Great Ravine clears heat that arises because of a deficiency of Kidney Yin energies.

Ki 6 (Shining Sea). Located in the depression about one inch below the inner anklebone, Ki 6 nourishes Kidney Yin, cools Blood, treats infertility and heat disorders, and is helpful for insomnia and amenorrhea. Together with Lu 7, Ki 6 opens the Conception vessel.

Lu 7 (Broken Sequence). Lu 7 is found above the wrist crease about one and a half inches above the prominent bone on the thumb side of the wrist. This point treats psychoemotional disorders, regulates the Conception meridian, and controls water balance. Along with Ki 6, Lu 7 opens the Conception meridian and is often used to "open the upper canopy" at the end of gestation to allow labor to proceed.

Sp 6 (Joining of the Three Yin). Tucked beneath the calf muscle, Sp 6 is located about three inches above the inner anklebone, just behind the bone. This is the culminating point for all the Yin channels in the leg (Kidney, Spleen, and Liver). In addition to nourishing the Spleen energies, harmonizing the Liver, and tonifying the Kidneys, the Joining of the Three Yin regulates menstruation and treats all reproductive disorders. Sp 6 encourages ovulation and treats menstrual pain. However, because of its strong effect on the Uterus, never stimulate this point during pregnancy.

UB 23 (Back Point of the Kidney). This main point of the Kidney's energies is located in the small of the back at the level of the navel and the second lumbar vertebra. The point is found about one and a half inches from the midline on either side of the spine, where the muscular bulge adjacent to the spine is most prominent. The Back Point of the Kidney tonifies the Kidney energies, both Yin and Yang. In addition to replenishing deficient Kidney energies, stimulating UB 23 can treat irregular menstruation, abnormal vaginal discharge, lower back pain and weakness, and impotence.

UB 52 (Residence of the Will). Located three inches on either side of the second lumbar spine vertebra and one and a half inches lateral to UB 23, on the same level as the navel, UB 52 reinforces the Kidney-tonifying effect of UB 23. It strengthens the lower back, nourishes the Essence in treating impotence and low libido, and treats irregular menstruation. The points on this vertical line of the back also have mental and spiritual significance. The Residence of the Will stimulates determination and lifts the spirit when mental lethargy deprives the will.

Ren 3 (Central Pole of the Conception Vessel). See "General Reproductive System Points."

Ren 4 (Origin of the Source of the Conception Vessel). See "General Reproductive System Points."

KI YAN–/CW POINTS TO TONIFY THE KIDNEY (YANG)

These points help the Kidney Yang and relieve a cold Uterus (**CW**).

Ki 7 (Recover the Current). The seventh point of the Kidney channel is located two inches above the depression behind the inner anklebone, behind the inner leg bone and just on the front border of the Achilles tendon. Ki 7 is the main point of the Kidney meridian that tonifies the Yang of the Kidney. This point also controls whole-body sweating, treats lumbar soreness, resolves dampness in the lower body, and treats Kidney Yang–deficient diarrhea. This point should also be used to address scarred fallopian tubes.

St 36 (Lower Sea of Qi). You find this point by holding your leg straight and measuring three inches below the kneecap at the top of the fleshy musculature, one inch to the outer side of the crest of the upper shinbone. This point strongly tonifies the Qi, giving the patient more vigor after its stimulation. St 36 also fortifies the Spleen, nourishes the Blood and Yin, strengthens resistance, and treats gastrointestinal disorders. Although primarily a Spleen and Stomach point, St 36 also helps the Kidney Yang.

UB 23 (Back Point of the Kidney). See "Points to Tonify the Kidney (Yin)."

Du 4 (Life Gate). This point from the Governing meridian is located on the midline of the lower back at the level of the navel, just beneath the spinal bone protruding from the second lumbar vertebra. This doorway to life is said to reside between the two Kidneys. It affects the womb and is also known as the

"Sea of Blood" and the "Palace of the Essence." Du 4 influences the gate of life — the root of our vitality, or original Qi. Stimulating this point tonifies the Yang of the Kidney, strengthens the source Qi, treats chronic weakness, strengthens the low back and knees, resolves interior cold, warms the gate of life, and treats sexual disorders and impotence.

Ren 6 (Sea of Qi). Ren 6 is located one and a half inches below the navel on the midline of the lower abdomen. This point fosters the original Qi, tonifies the Yang, supplements the Qi, and resolves depression. The Sea of Qi lifts all-encompassing fatigue, when any activity feels like too much effort.

SI 3 (Back Stream). SI 3 is located at the crease between the palm and the back of the hand when you make a fist, just before the pinkie finger knucklebone. This point treats neck pain and night sweating, and calms the spirit. It also opens the Governing meridian with UB 62.

UB 62 (Extending Vessel). UB 62 is found in the depression below the outer anklebone. This point clears excess heat from the head, settles the spirit, and treats insomnia, headache, low back, hip, and leg pain. It also opens the Governing meridian.

SP– POINTS TO SUPPLEMENT THE SPLEEN QI

Sp 6 (Joining of the Three Yin). See "Points to Tonify the Kidney (Yin)."

St 36 (Lower Sea of Qi). See "Points to Tonify the Kidney (Yang)."

Ren 6 (Sea of Qi). See "Points to Tonify the Kidney (Yang)."

Sp 4 (Grandparent Grandchild). Sp 4 is located on the inside of the foot at the base of the bone that makes up the arch of the foot on the same side as the big toe. This point fortifies the Spleen, regulates gynecological disorders, and is used with Pc 6 (see "Other Stress Points") to calm the spirit (in hormonal disorders) and to activate the Penetrating meridian. Sp 4 has a calming effect on the womb and can safely be stimulated during pregnancy.

BL– POINTS TO NOURISH THE BLOOD

Sp 6 (Joining of the Three Yin). See "Points to Tonify the Kidney (Yin)."

St 36 (Lower Sea of Qi). See "Points to Tonify the Kidney (Yang)."

Lv 8 (Curved Spring). Lv 8 is located on the inner side of the leg, toward the back of the knee. When the knee is bent, the Curved

Spring can be found about an inch above the end of the inner knee crease. Lv 8 nourishes the Liver Blood, treats irregular menstruation, and eliminates conditions of dampness in the urinary and reproductive systems.

LV QI X POINTS TO RESOLVE LIVER QI STAGNATION

Lv 2 (Moving Between). Lv 2 is just proximal to the web between the first and second toes. This point subdues patterns of excess heat in the Liver meridian. Its fire-clearing function resolves symptoms like incessant uterine bleeding, early menstruation, eye irritation, migraine headaches, and rage. Moving Between stimulates the Liver to clear excess hormones that can cause symptoms of internal heat.

Lv 3 (Great Rushing). Lv 3 is located about one and a half to two inches proximal to the web between the first and second toes, where the point is tender. This point promotes the smooth flow of Liver Qi, nourishes the Liver Blood, and treats premenstrual breast pain, headache, depression, and mood swings. Lv 3 is often used in conjunction with LI 4 (see "Stress, Tension, and Premenstrual Headaches") to open and activate the body's meridians. (This combination of points is called the Four Gates.) Great Rushing is an important point for regulating menstruation and resolving dysmenorrhea caused by stagnant Liver Qi. This point also has some indications for treating low sperm counts in men with the same pattern.

Lv 14 (Cycle Gate). Located on the same vertical line as the nipple and just below the breast, Cycle Gate can be found on the chest approximately four inches from the midline in the sixth intercostal space, two ribs below the nipple. Cycle Gate is an important point for resolving stagnant Liver Qi, especially when it invades the Stomach, causing gastrointestinal upset. Lv 14 is helpful in resolving premenstrual breast tenderness, breast pain, and menstrual chills and fevers. Lv 14 allows an opening and relaxation for women who have a tense or uneasy aversion to sex. Stimulation of Lv 14 will help a woman become more sexually receptive.

GB 34 (Yang Mound Spring). Behind and just below the crest of the shinbone, Yang Mound Spring is located on the outer side of the upper shin, in the fleshy tissue in front of the head of the fibula. GB 34 promotes the smooth flow of Liver Qi and resolves contractions of the tendons and musculature. This point helps relieve pain, stiffness, cramping, and obstruction anywhere in the body.

LV QI X, HT– STRESS, TENSION, AND PREMENSTRUAL HEADACHES

LI 4 (Joining Valley). LI 4 is found on the muscular area on the back of the hand about one inch inside the web between the base of the thumb and the index finger. LI 4 is often used with Lv 3 (see "Points to Resolve Liver Qi Stagnation") to open up all the channels in the body. Joining Valley alleviates pain and is effective in resolving premenstrual headaches. LI 4 has been found to moderate chemicals responsible for uterine contraction and to calm the uterus prior to implantation. LI 4 should be used only before ovulation. If used during pregnancy, this point might stimulate uterine contractions to help induce labor.

Yintang (Hall of Impression). Located between the eyebrows, Yintang is the closest point to the pituitary gland, and thus regulates its function. The Hall of Impression calms the mind, allays anxiety and agitation, and resolves frontal headaches. This point is often used around the time of implantation and during ART.

Tai Yang (Greater Yang). Tai Yang is found at the temples, in the depression behind the midpoint between the outside of the eye and eyebrow. This point helps resolve temporal stress headaches and TMJ symptoms.

UB 2 (Gathered Bamboo). UB 2 is located just at the inner edge of the eyebrow on the supraorbital notch just above the eye. Together with SI 3 (see "Points to Tonify the Kidney [Yang]"), Gathered Bamboo influences the pituitary gland and is effective in restoring pituitary function. I use this point

when prolactin levels are abnormally elevated. It is also useful when periods don't resume after oral contraceptive use.

OTHER STRESS POINTS

Pc 6 (Inner Pass). Pc 6 is located on the inner wrist, about two inches proximal to the wrist crease in the depression between the two tendons. Inner Pass (often used in conjunction with Sp 4 [see "Points to Supplement the Spleen Qi"] to activate the Penetrating meridian) rectifies the Qi, regulates menstruation, calms the mind, and treats anxiety, insomnia, irritability, and the emotional manifestations of premenstrual tension. Pc 6 is also useful in treating symptoms of chest tightness. Often stimulated prior to IVF transfer, Pc 6 opens the heart.

Ht 7 (Spirit Gate). Ht 7 is located on the inner wrist crease, toward the base of the hand on the side of the little finger. The Spirit Gate calms the mind and regulates the heart. It is useful in addressing symptoms such as heart palpitations, anxiety, agitation, nightmares, depression, mania, insomnia, and restless sleep.

BL X POINTS TO INVIGORATE STAGNANT BLOOD

Sp 6 (Joining of the Three Yin). See "Points to Tonify the Kidney (Yin)."

Sp 8 (Earth Pivot). Sp 8 is located on the inner side of the lower leg on the back side of the tibial bone, one handbreadth below the depression on the inner border of the curved bone below the knee, to the inside of the crest of the shinbone. Earth Pivot resolves Blood stasis in the Uterus and lower abdomen, tonifies the Essence, and treats irregular menstruation and abdominal pain. It also resolves menstrual cramps.

Sp 10 (Sea of Blood). Sp 10 can be found two inches above the upper border of the kneecap toward the inside of the upper thigh. The Sea of Blood is extremely important in treating any menstrual disorder involving Blood stasis. Sp 10 harmonizes menstruation, invigorates (thins) the Blood, and helps resolve abdominal masses as well as Blood stasis conditions often seen in autoimmune disorders. Sp 10 also cools the Blood. The Sea of Blood can alleviate rashes and red-hot allergic conditions. Sp 10 is considered the body's natural heparin (an antiserum factor that prevents clotting) and is often employed in cases of uterine fibroids, endometriosis, and clotty, dark menstrual flow.

UB 17 (Back Point of the Blood and Diaphragm). UB 17 is level with the lower border of the shoulder blade at the same level as the seventh thoracic vertebra, one and a half inches to the sides of the spine, on the most prominent point of the spinal musculature. The Back Point of the Blood treats all diseases of the Blood: it cools hot conditions, resolves Blood stasis, and stops abnormal bleeding.

HT– POINTS TO NOURISH THE HEART

These points also include the ear triangular fossa (see "General Reproductive System Points").

Ht 7 (Spirit Gate). See "Other Stress Points."

Ren 14 (Great Palace). Ren 14 is located two inches below where the ribs join at the center of the upper abdomen and six inches above the navel. This is the front palace of the Heart, where the Heart is cleared of negative influences and obstructions. Ren 14 also calms the mind.

Ren 15 (Dove Tail). Ren 15 is located one inch below the angle where the ribs join, on the midline of the upper abdomen, seven inches above the navel. Dove Tail calms the mind and resolves anxiety, worry, emotional upsets, fears, and obsessions.

UB 15 (Back Point of the Heart). UB 15 is found one and a half inches to the side of the spinal column, on the prominence of the spinal musculature, just to the outside of the vertebral column at the level of the fifth thoracic vertebra, and two inches above the lower border of the shoulder blade. UB 15 nourishes the Heart, regulates the Heart Qi, calms the spirit, resolves Blood stasis, and clears Heart fire. It also calms anxiety and restlessness, and allows sleep.

UB 44 (Spirit Hall). This spirit point is located three inches to either side of the fifth thoracic vertebra, at the level of UB 15 (see above) on the middle inner border of the shoulder blade. The Spirit Hall regulates Qi and drains heat from the Heart. It also tonifies the Qi and nourishes the Essence of the Kidney. Its main indication, however, is to calm the mind (and spirit).

^H COOLING POINTS

Lv 2 (Moving Between). See "Points to Resolve Liver Qi Stagnation."

Sp 10 (Sea of Blood). See "Points to Invigorate Stagnant Blood."

LI 11 (Bent Pond). LI 11 is located on the front (sun-exposed) surface of the arm, level with the elbow. When the arm is bent, LI 11 is found at the end of the crease, midway between the elbow and the bicep tendon. Bent Pond's main function is to clear heat and cool the Blood. It helps resolve symptoms of internal heat such as fever, hypertension, and red, hot skin diseases. It is often used in conjunction with Sp 10 for allergic or autoimmune heat conditions.

UB 40 (Popliteal Center). Located on the back of the leg at the middle of the knee crease, the Popliteal Center clears heat con-

ditions, cools the Blood, and helps resolve acute pain in the sides of the low back. UB 40 is often employed for clearing symptoms of damp heat in the Urinary Bladder that would manifest in conditions like urinary tract infections and cystitis. It can also be used to treat recurrent vaginal and rectal irritation that comes from heat in the Urinary Bladder meridian.

D POINTS TO RESOLVE DAMP CONDITIONS

Sp 9 (Yin Mound Spring). Sp 9 is located in the depression on the inner side of the upper shin, beneath the inner side of the knee to the inside of the crest of the shinbone, where the bone curves. Yin Mound Spring resolves conditions of dampness arising from pathology in the organs in the pelvic region. This includes "damp" diarrhea, vaginal irritation and discharge, urinary tract infections, and the like. It is also employed to treat edema.

St 40 (Abundant Bulge). St 40 is located on the outside of the lower leg, midway between the knee and the ankle, two inches to the outside of the shinbone. Abundant Bulge resolves conditions of accumulated dampness that cause phlegmlike conditions. (In Chinese medicine, obscure obstructive disease mechanisms with unknown causes or cures are often referred to as "phlegm obstruction.") Polycystic ovaries are categorized according to this pattern. When the diagnostic criteria fit, fallopian tube obstruction also involves accumulated dampness in the pelvis.

Ren 12 (Middle Venter). Ren 12 is located on the midline of the stomach, halfway between the navel and the bottom of the sternum, about four inches above the navel. Middle Venter tonifies patterns of deficiency in the Stomach and Spleen, resolving conditions of internal dampness that arise from a weakness in the Spleen/ Stomach. Gently stimulate this point clockwise. Ren 12 is often used in conjunction with St 40 (see above) and Pc 6 (see "Other Stress Points").

Additional points to relieve damp conditions in the reproductive organs (such as uterine and tubal fluid accumulation, and cystitis) include the upper and lower segment of the ear, and the following:

Ren 3 (Central Pole of the Conception Vessel). See "General Reproductive System Points."

Sp 6 (Joining of the Three Yin). See "Points to Tonify the Kidney (Yin)."

UB 66 (Passing Valley). This point resides on the outer edge of the foot, between the base of the little toe and the foot bone, where the sole meets the skin of the upper foot. This point resolves damp heat from the Urinary Bladder channel and is especially useful in cases of cystitis and uterine fluid accumulation.

D POINTS TO DRY ABNORMAL VAGINAL DISCHARGE

SJ 5 (Outer Pass). Located on the back side of the forearm between the two arm bones, two inches above the wrist crease, SJ 5 clears obstructions in the head responsible for headaches, ear problems, and head colds. It addresses various pains in the arm and shoulder, and together with GB 41 (see below) opens the Dai Mai, or Girdle meridian. The Dai Mai governs certain aspects of the menstrual cycle, including infertility associated with abnormal vaginal discharge.

GB 41 (Foot Governor of Tears). GB 41 is located in the depression between the fourth and fifth foot bones, just before the foot tendons extend to the toes. Being a Gallbladder point, GB 41 spreads Liver Qi and, when used with SJ 5 (see above), resolves conditions of abnormal vaginal discharge. Together, these points also treat one-sided headaches associated with the menstrual cycle.

GB 26 (Girdle Vessel). GB 26 is located on the same level as the belly button, just below the free end of the eleventh rib. If you drew an imaginary line from the middle of the armpit down, and one from the umbilicus over to the side, GB 26 would be found at the intersection. This point resolves Liver Qi stagnation, relieves local pain, and treats menstrual and uterine disorders, including abnormal vaginal discharge and infertility.

POINTS TO BRING ON DELAYED MENSES

For primary amenorrhea or complete lack of menstruation, the diagnostic pattern must also be addressed to increase the efficiency of this treatment.

GB 21 (Shoulder Well). This is located at the highest point of the trapezius muscle, located toward the back, between the neck and the shoulder and just above the shoulder blade. Mostly used to treat stiffness of the neck and shoulders, this point also promotes lactation and facilitates difficult labor because of its ability to descend the (uterine) Qi.

NOTE: Do not stimulate this point during pregnancy.

Lv 3 (Great Rushing). See "Points to Resolve Liver Qi Stagnation."

LI 4 (Joining Valley). See "Stress, Tension, and Premenstrual Headaches."

Sp 6 (Joining of the Three Yin). See "Points to Tonify the Kidney (Yin)."

Sp 10 (Sea of Blood). See "Points to Invigorate Stagnant Blood."

POINTS TO ALLEVIATE MENSTRUAL CRAMPS

Use the points on the upper and lower segment of the ear, as well as the following:

LI 4 (Joining Valley). See "Stress, Tension, and Premenstrual Headaches."

Lv 3 (Great Rushing). See "Points to Resolve Liver Qi Stagnation."

Sp 6 (Joining of the Three Yin). See "Points to Tonify the Kidney (Yin)."

Sp 8 (Earth Pivot). See "Points to Invigorate Stagnant Blood."

UB 32 (Second Crevice). Found in the second sacral foramen, this point acts on the uterus via the sacral plexus.

Ren 3 (Central Pole of the Conception Meridian). See "General Reproductive System Points."

POINTS TO STOP UTERINE BLEEDING

Ki 8 (Faith Intersection). Ki 8 is located two inches above the depression behind the inner anklebone, on the rear border of the tibial bone. This point is often used when there is uterine bleeding as a result of Blood stasis. Faith Intersection is also employed to dissolve masses and regulate menstrual problems caused by Blood stasis.

Sp 8 (Earth Pivot). See "Points to Invigorate Stagnant Blood."

Du 20 (Hundred Meetings). Du 20 is at the uppermost aspect of the head, on the same coronal plane as the ears. This is where all the Yang channels meet, and Hundred Meetings is said to lift the Yang Qi. In addition to causing the Qi to ascend, it lifts the Spleen energies, which can stop bleeding that results from Spleen Qi deficiency. Du 20 further lifts the spirit, strengthens the memory, and clears the mind.

POINT TO RESOLVE GRIEF AND CALL TO THE SOUL OF THE UNCONCEIVED CHILD

UB 42 (Door of the Corporeal Soul). Located three inches on both sides of the third thoracic vertebra, UB 42 is found at the midpoint of the shoulder blade, at the level of the bend in its inner edge. The Door of the Corporeal Soul has more spiritual significance in helping to resolve conception difficulties. The corporeal soul is the physical body's connection to its soul. This point, which is related to the Lungs, is especially helpful in resolving the Lungs' emotional pathology, which is sadness and grief. UB 42 has a soothing effect on the spirit and helps replenish its loss of Qi. (Stimulating this point was prescribed by ancient practitioners to "call to the soul of the unborn child.")

POINTS TO IMPROVE BLOOD FLOW TO THE PELVIC ORGANS

Massage the points on the front of the lower abdomen (see "General Reproductive System Points") including Zigong, GB 26, St 30, Ren 3, Ren 4, and Ren 6 (see "Points to Tonify the Kidney [Yang]"); the upper and lower points of the ear; the scalp reproductive points; and the following points:

Sp 6 (Joining of the Three Yin). See "Points to Tonify the Kidney (Yin)."

UB 23 (Back Point of the Kidney). See "Points to Tonify the Kidney (Yin)."

UB 52 (Residence of the Will). See "Points to Tonify the Kidney (Yin)."

UB 31, UB 32, UB 33, UB 34. These four points are found in the holes of the sacrum, where the nerves to the pelvic organs exit. Stimulating these points regulates menstruation, treats lower back and pelvic pain, and resolves impairment to fertility. Studies have shown that electric stimulation of UB 32 (in the second hole of the sacrum) or UB 28 signals the brain that there is too much sympathetic activity at the level of the second lumbar to the second sacral vertebra (the level of the pelvis). The brain then signals the nerves to reduce sympathetic outflow, thereby allowing the blood vessels to dilate and improving blood flow to the pelvic organs.

POINTS TO REGULATE THE HYPOTHALAMIC—PITUITARY—OVARIAN (HPO) AXIS

The HPO axis is involved in almost every aspect of hormonal regulation during the reproductive cycle. The hypothalamus actually "beats," or pulsates, rhythmically about every hour and a half, and acupuncture can speed up the pulsing of gonadotropic hormones, helping with conditions of hormonal deficiency.

Using the Extraordinary meridians, activate points such as Sp 4 + Pc 6 (Penetrating meridian), Lu 7 + Ki 6 (Conception meridian), and UB 62 + SI 3 (Governing meridian), along with points like Sp 6, Ren 3, Ren 4, and Zigong to help regulate the HPO axis.

POINTS TO LOWER ELEVATED PITUITARY HORMONE (PROLACTIN) LEVELS

Yintang + LI 4 + Lv 2 + Lv 3 can help resolve excess prolactin levels — use before ovulation only.

UB 2, located on the inner edge of the eyebrow, along with UB 62 and SI 3, can be used to help harmonize pituitary hormone levels after ovulation.

POINTS TO PREPARE FOR IN VITRO FERTILIZATION (IVF) EMBRYO TRANSFER

Women receiving embryo transfers are generally not in a state of optimum balance. Their hormonal systems have been taxed, their eggs have been surgically extracted, and they feel anything but relaxed. Acupuncture can regulate the endocrine system, improve the uterus's ability to accept an embryo, and calm the state of stress. I could provide hundreds of case histories to illustrate the effectiveness of this treatment.

Stimulate points on the upper and lower segment of the ear, and the following points before embryo transfer:

LI 4 (Joining Valley). See "Stress, Tension, and Premenstrual Headaches." This point keeps the uterus nonreactive. (After implantation, do not stimulate this point.)

Lv 3 (Great Rushing). See "Points to Resolve Liver Qi Stagnation." Together with LI 4, Lv 3 opens the body to make it more receptive.

Pc 6 (Inner Pass). See "Other Stress Points." Pc 6 opens the channel between the Heart and Uterus.

Sp 6 (Joining of the Three Yin). See "Points to Tonify the Kidney (Yin)." Sp 6 opens the Uterus.

Sp 8 (Earth Pivot). See "Points to Invigorate Stagnant Blood." Sp 8 keeps the Blood moving.

Sp 10 (Sea of Blood). See "Points to Invigorate Stagnant Blood."

St 36 (Lower Sea of Qi). See "Points to Tonify the Kidney (Yang)." St 36 tonifies the Spleen Qi.

St 29 (Return). St 29 is found two inches out from the midline, four inches below the navel. This point warms the pelvis, regulates menstruation, and treats fertility impairment, impotence, and pain and swelling in the genital region.

Du 20 (Hundred Meetings). See "Points to Stop Uterine Bleeding." Du 20 lifts the Qi.

If you choose to use acupressure to improve your overall health, remember that it's perfectly fine to stimulate several points in one treatment session if you are experiencing more than one symptom or condition. It's also fine to stimulate all of the points listed as affecting your particular deficiency or excess. Just keep in mind that treatments using TCM are not an instant fix. While you may experience quick relief for some conditions (like headache), other conditions may take several cycles to resolve. You should do everything possible to restore your body to health so it can carry a child, and acupressure is just one way to revitalize yourself.

ACUPOINTS

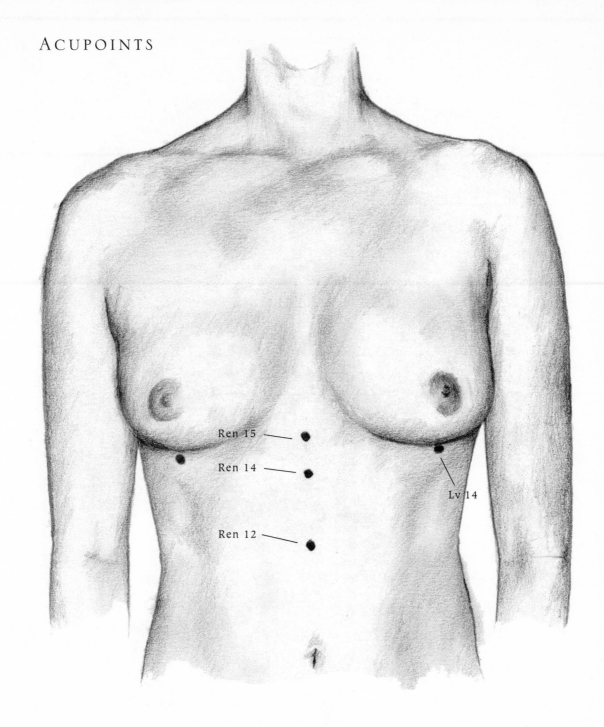

Ren 15

Ren 14

Ren 12

Lv 14

Upper Abdomen

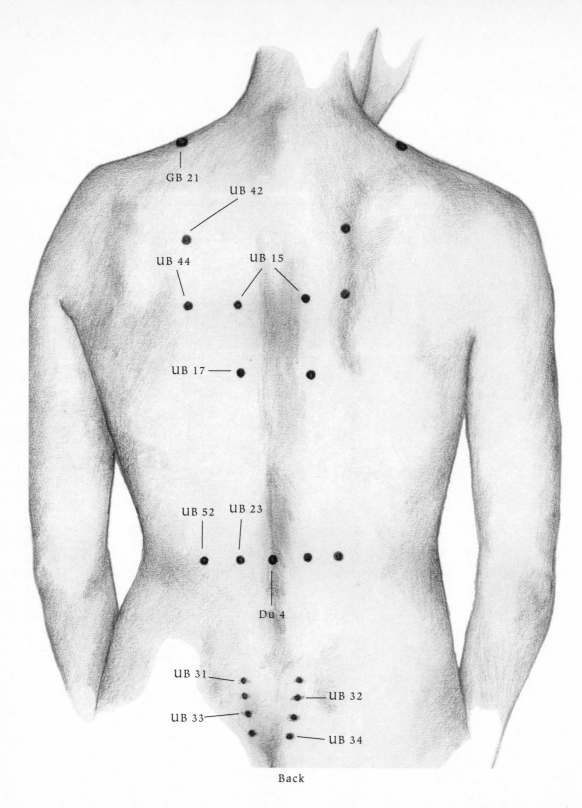

GB 21

UB 42

UB 44

UB 15

UB 17

UB 52

UB 23

Du 4

UB 31

UB 32

UB 33

UB 34

Back

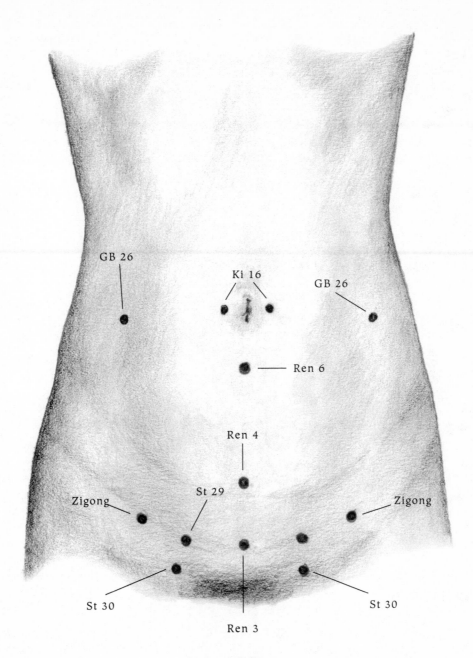

Lower Abdomen

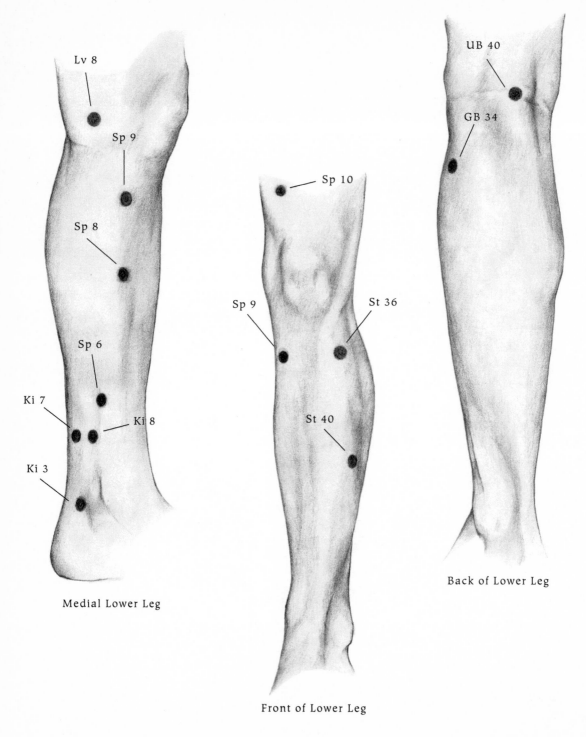

Medial Lower Leg

Lv 8

Sp 9

Sp 8

Sp 6

Ki 7

Ki 8

Ki 3

Front of Lower Leg

Sp 10

Sp 9

St 36

St 40

Back of Lower Leg

UB 40

GB 34

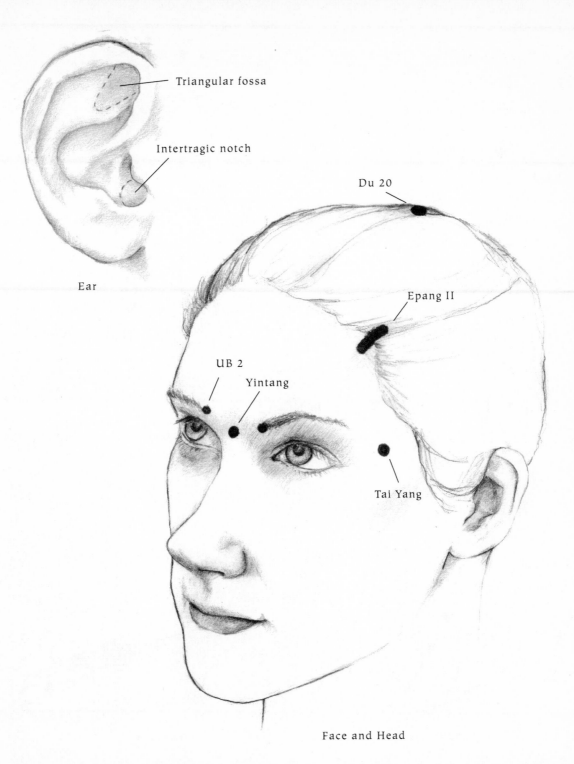

Triangular fossa

Intertragic notch

Ear

Du 20

Epang II

UB 2

Yintang

Tai Yang

Face and Head

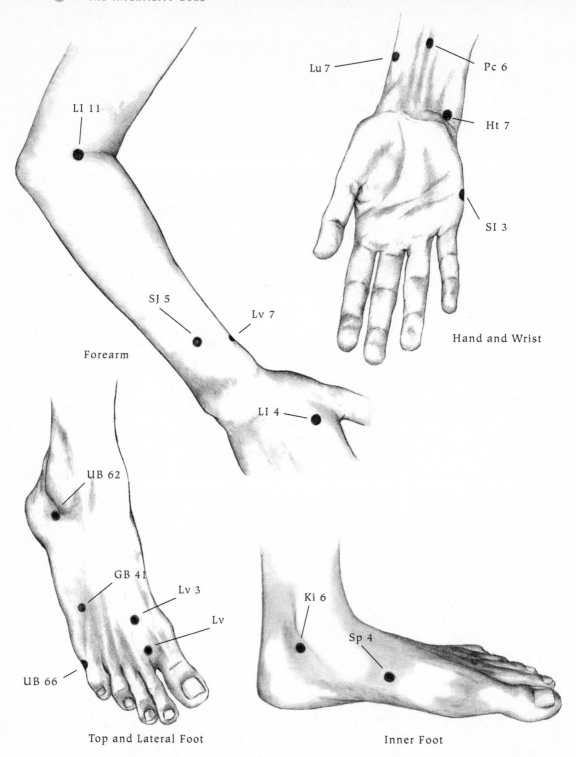

LI 11

SJ 5

Lv 7

Forearm

LI 4

Lu 7

Pc 6

Ht 7

SI 3

Hand and Wrist

UB 62

GB 41

Lv 3

Lv

UB 66

Top and Lateral Foot

Ki 6

Sp 4

Inner Foot

ACUPUNCTURE IN ACTION: VERA

Vera was a vibrant young woman who was cheerful and talked a lot. She was attractive and petite, and epitomized the southern belle. Her unsuccessful attempts to become pregnant seemed to be the only evidence of suffering in Vera's life. She had had laparoscopic surgery because of painful periods and ovulation, but no endometriosis was found. She had undergone the usual hormonal testing (which was normal) and increasingly invasive procedures to get pregnant. Her reproductive endocrinologist put her on Clomid for six months and then did a few cycles of intrauterine insemination and one IVF.

Vera came to me because she said the medical treatments were uncomfortable, she hated being on the hormones, and she wasn't producing many eggs anyway. She described herself as high-strung and somewhat anxious, and said her hands and feet perspired all the time (a condition called hyperhidrosis). Her husband, Lowell, had suggested surgery to correct the excessive perspiration, but Vera said she wanted to get pregnant first. I immediately suspected that her symptoms — painful (but scant) menses and ovulation, poor response to IVF drugs, anxiety, and sweating of the hands and feet — indicated hyperactivity of the sympathetic nervous system, thereby depriving the pelvic organs of blood flow. My diagnosis was confirmed by Vera's pulse, which was tight, weak, and rapid, and her tongue, which was a deep, dark red.

I thought acupuncture twice a week would be the best way to address her disharmony. Many hormonal imbalances respond well to a couple months' administration of herbs to regulate the cycle, but acupuncture immediately addresses energetic disturbances. I regulated Vera's Liver Qi with Lv 2, Lv 3, and LI 4; calmed the spirit with Ht 7 and the ear triangular fossa area (which has a tranquil effect and reduces sympathetic dominance); and harmonized menstruation with Sp 6. I also stimulated Sp 10 to clear excess heat and used electroacupuncture (which stimulates the points more strongly) on her lower back (UB 23, UB 32, UB 52) to override the sympathetic nervous system's control at the level of the pelvic organs' nervous system innervation (second lumbar to second sacral vertebra). I also showed her the femoral massage technique described in chapter 6 so she could perform it on her own.

After beginning treatment, Vera's next menstrual flow was heavier and without any pain. We continued the same regimen during the following follicular phase of her cycle, and she ovulated without pain. During the luteal phase, I used Lv 8, Ht 7, points in ear triangular fossa, Pc 6, and Sp 4 in case she had conceived. Ten days after ovulation, her pulse became rolling and lively. I knew she was pregnant. Months later, Vera gave birth to a healthy baby boy. As far as I know, she no longer needed the surgery to correct her hyperhidrosis.

8

Step Four: Using Herbal Remedies to Promote Vibrant Reproductive Health

The Lord hath created medicines out of the earth; and [s]he that is wise will not abhor them.

— ECCLESIASTICUS 34:4 (APOCRYPHA)

My first experience with Chinese herbs included trying every kind of natural fertility enhancement I could find in my desperate attempt to become pregnant. I consulted a Chinese herbalist, who prescribed different reproductive tonifying herbs. I brewed horrible-smelling concoctions of raw Chinese herbs on the stove, and they tasted no better than their aroma. Three months after I began treatment with TCM, my hormonal problems were resolved, and I became pregnant.

My next experience was when I was in China interning at a TCM hospital, and I was in horrible physical shape. I was breast-feeding my baby, having terribly heavy periods, and feeling constantly fatigued. An internist felt my pulse and reported that I was rather depleted in both Qi and Blood.

The next day, the hospital lunch consisted of mutton soup with the herbs Angelica (Dang Gui) and Astragalus (Huang Qi). Sounds horrible, right? Evidently the doctor had told the hospital pharmacy to give the cook herbs to incorporate into my lunch. I had a bowl of the soup, and although it tasted unusual to my Western palate, after the first cup I began to crave more. I finished the family-size bowl of soup for my meal. And, yes, I started feeling better.

While acupuncture balances the body's energies through the external application of needles, herbs alter the body's internal energies. In both East and West, herbs were the first medicines available. They were used by the ancient Chinese, Greek, and Egyptian civilizations as both fertilizing and postpartum agents. Records of the Chinese pharmacopoeia (the list of herbs and other natural substances used to treat disease and promote health) date back to the third century B.C.E. and have been updated regularly since then. During the second century B.C.E., the Chinese were the first to extract male and female hormones from urine (some modern forms of hormone supplements are still derived from urine). Chinese doctors were also the first to synthesize thyroid hormone from jujube dates to treat goiter. The average Chinese herbalist can compose remedies applying combinations drawn from more than three thousand substances, but most practitioners keep about three hundred herbs for regular use. Of those three hundred, a somewhat smaller number are valuable in promoting fertility.

Chinese herbal medicines differ from Western pharmaceuticals in two important ways. The first is intent. Many Western drugs use a single biologically active compound to treat symptoms: pain relievers for body aches, acid neutralizers for stomach distress, antihistamine creams for itches, decongestants and cough suppressants for a cold, and so on. Even drugs designed to treat underlying problems rarely restore optimum functioning to the body. For instance, cholesterol-lowering medications may keep arteries clear, but they don't teach the body to eliminate excess cholesterol on its own. Asthma medications reduce swelling in the bronchial tubes, but the immune system of the asthmatic still reacts inappropriately to allergens. Traditional Chinese medicine is based on a completely different model. Because TCM endeavors to diagnose and treat the underlying imbalances that are keeping the body from its fullest expression of health, Chinese herbs are prescribed not to mitigate symptoms but to treat their causes.

The second difference is in the medications themselves. If you look at the composition of most Western medications at the molecular level, it's easier to understand some of the problems that can arise when we try to apply these chemical substances in the natural environment of the body. Their potency produces side effects. For example, supplemental estrogen has been used for years in treating menopausal women, as well as those who have undergone hysterectomies or have had their estrogen production inhibited. However, estrogen supplements do not provide the same kind of protection from heart disease as the body's own natural estrogen does. Supplemental estrogen also increases the frequency of breast and uterine cancers. The synthetic supplemental version of estrogen simply does not duplicate the effects of the estrogen produced by a woman's own body.

Herbs contain natural energetic substances whose essence gently corrects underlying deficiencies or removes obstructions. The *synergy* of these substances produces their potent effects. The active ingredients are buffered by the whole plant and blended with other herbs, reducing their side effects. In this case, the whole is definitely more than the sum of its parts.

CATEGORIZING AND UTILIZING CHINESE HERBS

Recall the fundamental premise of Chinese medicine: every condition is a result of excess or deficiency in either an Organ system (like the Kidneys, Spleen, or Liver) or an essential substance (Yin, Yang, Qi, and Blood) or a fluid (Essence and moisture). Herbs are classified by their qualities and by their effects on these different systems.

For example, some herbs are warm; others are cool; still others are neutral (neither warm nor cool). Some herbs stimulate, while others calm the body. Some tonify the Organs; some relax them. Some consolidate energy; others disperse it. Some herbs help purge excess phlegm; others build fluids up. Some herbs help the body's energy rise; others help it descend. Each of these properties can affect the way the body will utilize that particular herb.

The standard of care in Chinese herbal therapy is to use herbs in their raw form. The doctor prescribes a combination of herbal ingredients all bagged together. Outpatients bring their herbs home to make a decoction: they soak each day's herbs in water for up to an hour, then boil the mixture for about forty-five minutes. The herbs are strained, and the remaining "tea" is consumed throughout the day. However, the smell, taste, and amount of effort required to brew these mixtures tend to make Western patients less compliant. I have found that most of my patients prefer to take their herbs in powder or pill form. While this may slightly decrease the herbs' potency, I believe it's better to offer a prescription that the patient will follow.

Here in the United States, herbs are categorized as concentrated food products, and there is little regulatory control over their distribution and usage. But it's important to remember that *these herbs are medicines.* Any substance capable of producing positive physiologic effects is equally capable of creating negative ones. We often hear how this or that herb is responsible for causing untoward side effects, but that is usually because the herbs have been taken improperly — for example, when diuretics are used for weight loss. Drugs, medicines, vitamins, and even benign foods are capable of inducing negative effects if taken in abundance. Therefore, make sure to take only the recommended dosages to treat the specific imbalances for which the herbs have been prescribed, and discontinue the herbs if you experience any negative effects.

USING HERBS TO ENHANCE FERTILITY

The herbal formulas developed by Chinese physicians through the centuries help women enhance their reproductive potential by harmonizing the endocrine system, which regulates the menstrual cycle. The endocrine system operates via feedback. If the body senses an adequate amount of a particular hormone circulating through the bloodstream, the production of that hormone by the body either slows down or ceases altogether. For example, during the first phase of a woman's cycle, estrogen is required for the egg of one follicle in the ovary to mature. If a woman lacks estrogen, her doctor may prescribe estrogen supplementation. However, as soon as the hypothalamus registers that sufficient quantities of estrogen are circulating in the blood, it signals the pituitary gland to quit stimulating the ovary to produce more estrogen. The function of the entire system decreases because an outside source is doing the job instead. It's as if you broke your leg and the doctor put a cast on it and just left it there. Soon the muscles of the leg would atrophy, and eventually the only way you'd be able to walk is with a cast. Similarly, estrogen supplementation can cause the endocrine system to stop triggering the body to produce enough estrogen on its own. In contrast, Chinese herbs act more like a crutch than a cast: they support your reproductive system while it continues to do what it's supposed to.

The effects of these herbs vary. They may act on the ovulatory phase; they may regulate the secretion of mucus; they may stimulate the uterus; or they may assist in the production of adequate progesterone. For instance, many Chinese herbs that produce phytoestrogenic activity (promoting estrogen production) also act on the ovaries, while they impact the central nervous system. They trigger the hypothalamus and pituitary to release hormones that stimulate the timely production of FSH and LH (two necessary elements in preparing for fertilization and implantation of the egg). Because it affects many different parts of the reproductive cycle by triggering the body's own natural processes, herbal medicine is a gentler, more organic response to fertility problems. Many of the ingredients in herbal formulas prescribed for infertility may have little or no direct hormonal actions, but the outcome of the *whole* formula is a substantial increase in hormone levels and the tissues' response to them.

While all Chinese herbal formulas are designed to treat individual patterns, there are some links between the effects of herbal therapies and their Western medical correlations. As you can see from the following table, Chinese herbal medicines can have many of the same results as Western-based fertility treatments, even though they don't have hormones like estrogen and progesterone in them.

TCM Herbal Therapies	Western Correlations
Blood, Essence, and Yin tonics	• Stimulate estrogen production • Increase cervical mucus • Build uterine lining • Strengthen reproductive organs • Lower FSH • In men, help liquefy overly viscous seminal fluid
Blood and Qi tonics	• Increase hemoglobin production • Lower FSH • In men, increase sperm count
Yang and Qi tonics	• Stimulate production of progesterone, testosterone, and thyroid hormones • In men, increase sperm count and motility
Blood invigorators	• Inhibit endometriosis and fibroids • In men, improve sperm morphology
Blood coolers	• Restrain inflammatory processes
Qi regulators	• Lower elevated prolactin levels • Metabolize excess hormones
Dampness drainers	• Lower cholesterol • Control yeast, bacteria, and other pathogens

BEGINNING YOUR OWN HERBAL TREATMENT

The application of Chinese herbal preparations differs from Western herbalism because the concoctions are based and prescribed completely upon pattern discrimination and nothing else. Traditional Chinese medicine practitioners don't prescribe for symptoms, such as "menstrual irregularities," but formulate herbs to address the underlying pattern of imbalance. For example, if menstrual irregularities are caused by Liver Qi stagnation (**Lv Qi X**), they will only respond to herbs found in that category. Taking herbs to build up the Qi without moving it can actually worsen the symptoms. *The treatment must always fit the pattern, not the disease.* And when the proper pattern is identified and treated accordingly, the results will be dramatic.

Here are some guidelines for choosing and using herbs.

1. The herbs you choose should be based on your present symptoms, your BBT chart results, and the patterns you diagnosed in chapter 4, as follows:

net. Other on-line herbal suppliers include www.chineseherbs.com, www.herbalhealer. com, and www.sfherb.com. Patent herbal formulas can be obtained through local Chinese medicine pharmacies located in larger cities, or through a local acupuncturist. You may also order pattern-based herbal formulas through my Web site, www.easternharmony-clinic.com.

2. If you have more than one pattern contributing to your condition, you'll achieve better results if you treat each pattern concurrently. Recognize that a change in one kind of energy requires adjustments in the other. For instance, say you find yourself defi-

Abbreviation	Pattern	Herbal Treatment
Ki Yi–	Kidney Yin deficiency	Kidney Yin tonics
Ki–	Kidney Yin and Yang deficiency	Kidney Essence tonics
Ki Yan–	Kidney Yang deficiency	Kidney Yang tonics
Sp–	Spleen Qi deficiency	Spleen Qi supplements
Bl–	Blood deficiency	Blood builders
Sp–/Bl–	Combined Spleen Qi deficiency and Blood deficiency	Qi and Blood supplements
Ht–	Heart deficiency	Heart supplements
Bl X	Blood stasis	Blood movers
Lv Qi X	Liver Qi stagnation	Qi movers
^H	Excess heat	Heat clearers
D	Dampness	Damp drainers
DH	Damp heat	Damp heat resolvers

You can acquire your herbs from almost any natural foods store. Some co-ops and larger grocers also carry organic products and herbs. East Earth Trade Winds (www. eastearthtrade.com) sells both individual Chinese herbs and patent formulas via the Inter-

cient in the Spleen Qi energies (**Sp–**), but you are also experiencing some Liver Qi stagnation (**Lv Qi X**). If you focus on strongly tonifying the Spleen without resolving the Liver stagnation, it will be like putting too much air in a tire. There will be more energy than space to hold it, generating increased pressure, which will then produce negative side effects (too much pressure in a confined space produces heat).

3. Side effects are caused by overdosage or improper pattern diagnosis. Too much Yin tonification can potentially cause dampness; strongly clearing dampness can produce dryness; overinvigorating the Blood can cause bleeding; and so on. Take a look at your overall pattern diagnosis and choose the herbs in each category that address your patterns. Then adjust your formula based on the effects you notice and keep fine-tuning until you have the results you want. You may then discontinue the herbs.

4. Consistency, accuracy, and patience are important. But if you forget to take your herbs, resume the same dosage when you remember. Take what's prescribed in the recommended dosage; be consistent and accurate. Almost anything can be harmful if used in the wrong way or in too great a quantity.

Also, be patient. While you may see improvements in your symptoms quickly, bringing the body back into harmony takes time.

5. It is important to keep your reproductive medical health team abreast of the complementary measures you are employing concurrently with their procedures. Western health care practitioners are becoming wary of patients who take self-prescribed herbal preparations because of the potential for side effects and interaction with Western treatments. For example, invigorating herbs may prolong bleeding time during surgery; certain herbs have the potential to alter the metabolism of hormones or the effects of anesthesia. Unless you have your doctor's blessing, you should not take over-the-counter herbal preparations during hormonal stimulation, as there is potential for adverse interactions. Communication between you and your physician will allow you to trust that everything you are doing for yourself will only enhance the medical protocol.

❧ HERBAL THERAPIES FOR YOUR CYCLE PHASE AND SPECIFIC CONDITION

Whether you are preparing your body for pregnancy or trying to get pregnant, there are herbs for every stage of your cycle. Beginning on page 139, I have listed each herb by its Chinese name and its common name. (Western herbal reproductive therapies, often easier to obtain than some of the Chinese herbs, are also included here, but I adhere to the patterns of TCM in their application.) Each herb is described in terms of its functions and when to use it. Although I have chosen herbs that have the fewest interactions, if there are any potential risks or side effects, you will be forewarned under

"Cautions." "Dosage" indicates the average daily dosage of loose herbs in grams.

Different herbs are grouped according to the underlying pattern of imbalance. Always address your underlying pattern of imbalance first. Some herbs are harder to find than others, but I have listed several herbs in each category. If you can't find one, move on to the next. If you fall within multiple diagnostic categories, treat them together in addition to using the following guiding principles for choosing the herbs for the phases of your monthly cycle.

- *During Phase I (follicular phase):* Nourish Yin and Blood.
- *During Phase II (ovulation):* Ensure both Qi and Blood are adequate and unobstructed; move Qi and Blood.
- *During Phase III (luteal phase):* Tonify Qi and Yang.
- *During Phase IV (premenstrual phase):* Move (stagnant Liver) Qi.
- *During Phase V (menstruation):* Take nothing unless there are problems with severe pain or bleeding. Menstruation is considered a hormonal zero point and we should allow the body to rest during the time of bleeding. If, however, there is severe Blood stasis causing clotty, painful menstruation, the Blood or Qi may need to be moved, or heat may need to be cleared during this time. If the bleeding is too heavy, we may need to tonify the Qi, clear heat, or resolve stasis — whichever pattern(s) fits.

HOW TO TAKE YOUR HERBS

Herbs come in many different preparations: premade tablets, granulated concentrates, tinctures, or in raw form. Each manufacturer will provide daily dosage recommendations. Here are some general guidelines:

1. If you prefer herbs in capsule or tablet form, take the manufacturers' recommended number of pills per day. You can combine different herbs — say, 1-gram capsules of Kidney Yin tonic at three times a day, 1-gram capsules of Blood supplement three times a day, and 1-gram capsules of Heart tonic at three times a day for a daily total of nine capsules per day. If you are addressing a single pattern like Spleen Qi deficiency, you can combine different herbs from a single category in the same manner, taking three different Spleen tonic pills, three times per day.

2. Some suppliers sell powdered concentrates. Granulated powders vary in concentration, but generally 1 teaspoon = 3 grams. These can be mixed together and put into capsules (one capsule = 1 gram; empty capsules are available at herbal suppliers), or can be dissolved in water and consumed as a tea (the powder will dissolve, so there is no need to strain). Stir one-third of your daily dosage into a cup of hot water and drink three cups per day. For example, 9 grams of a kidney supplement would translate to: 1 teaspoon (3 grams) per cup of hot water. Drink 3 cups of tea per day.

3. If you take herbs in tincture form, the dosages will be much smaller. Watch for

alcohol content; many tinctures now come in water-based preparations, which are preferable. Place the number of drops the manufacturer recommends under your tongue.

4. If you prefer to take raw herbs obtained through a Chinese pharmacy, the herbs will be packaged in daily dosages. Different herbs can be brewed together. Raw herbs are sometimes prescribed by the ounce — one-fourth of an ounce = 8 grams. Cover the herbs with about 4 cups of water and let soak for at least one hour, then boil and simmer for forty-five minutes. Drain the liquid from the herbs; keep the liquid and discard the herbs. Drink the liquid (about 3 cups) throughout the day.

5. Stop taking the herbs immediately if you experience any of the effects listed under "Cautions." Side effects usually are caused by overdosage, sensitivity to a particular herb, or improper pattern diagnosis. Even when you're taking the right herbs for your condition, overcorrecting the problem can produce negative symptoms. Too much Yin tonification can potentially cause dampness, which can result in abnormal vaginal discharge or an overall sluggish feeling; strongly clearing dampness can produce dryness, which can cause thirst and vaginal dryness; overinvigorating the Blood can cause uterine bleeding; strongly tonifying Qi without clearing the Liver Qi can produce stomach upset, headaches, and so on. Take a look at your overall pattern diagnosis and choose the herbs in each category that address your patterns. Then adjust your formula based on the effects you notice, and keep fine-tuning until you have the results you want (a restoration of health and balance to your body).

If after adjusting the formula you continue to notice any side effects, such as nausea, headaches, sleeplessness, anxiety, digestive upset, and so on, the dosage of these particular herbs may be more than your body can handle. In such cases I generally suggest that patients decrease the amounts of herbs they are taking, and when the symptoms go away, stay at the lower dose. If symptoms continue, it's possible you are reacting to a particular herb, and you may need to change to a different herb in that category. Luckily, most patterns and conditions have a variety of herbal treatments.

Sometimes side effects are due to incorrect pattern diagnosis, causing the treatment to be incorrect as well. Check your symptoms and conditions against the lists in chapter 4 and see if there may be another pattern that is contributing to your particular problem.

Most of all, be alert to the changes in your body produced by *any* kind of treatment, Eastern or Western. You're the only one who truly knows how your body feels and whether the treatments you are using are having positive or negative effects. Certainly, treatment is a process, and you can't expect instant results (especially with TCM), but learning to listen to and heed your body's innate sense of what's working and what's not is a vital step in any fertility treatment.

KI YI– KIDNEY YIN TONICS

Yin-tonifying herbs nurture and moisten. They are generally classified as being sweet and cool in nature. They should be used with caution in persons with Spleen Qi deficiency (**Sp–**). The cloying nature of Yin tonics, if used in overabundance, can cause dampness if the Spleen Qi is not tonified concurrently.

Kidney Yin deficiency manifestations include weakness or soreness of the lower back and the knees, warm palms and soles, low-grade sensation of heat, night sweats, dry mouth or eyes, vaginal dryness, and diminished sexual function.

Although these herbs can help with glucose metabolism and estrogen production, they do not contain hormones. However, they often contain hormonal precursors (the chemical building blocks of hormones), which, when the body is in balance, allow the body to produce its own adequate amounts of hormone. Since the follicular phase is dominated by Yin energies, these herbs are especially helpful from the end of menstruation until ovulation.

TIAN MEN DONG (asparagus root)

Functions: nourishes the Yin of the Kidney and Lung, generates fluid, and moistens the intestines.

Treats: thirst; irritated, scanty, or frequent urination; backache; and impotence. Often used by diabetics to lower blood sugar. Inhibits many bacteria; has an anticancer effect in leukemic cells, preventing the conversion of normal cells into malignant ones.

Cautions: should not be used in abundance in patients with acute rheumatism or gout because its high purine content may aggravate these conditions. Avoid use during an acute urinary tract infection. Also should be avoided during the third trimester of pregnancy.

Dosage: 12 grams

MAI MEN DONG (Ophiopogon root)

Functions: moistens the Lungs; augments Stomach Yin and generates fluids; clears the Heart; moistens the intestines.

Treats: irritability, constipation, elevated serum glucose levels.

Dosage: 12 grams

HAN LIAN CAO (Eclipta)

Functions: nourishes the Yin of the Liver and Kidneys, cools the Blood.

Treats: dizziness, vertigo, blurred vision, bleeding caused by Blood heat.

Dosage: 12 grams

NU ZHEN ZI (Ligustrum, privet fruit)

Functions: nourishes the Liver and Kidney Yin.

Treats: dizziness, ringing in the ears, blurred vision.

Dosage: 10 grams

HE SHOU WU (Solomon's seal root, fleeceflower root)

Functions: tonifies Kidneys and Liver, Blood and Essence, moistens Intestines.

Treats: low back pain and weakness, insomnia, excessive vaginal discharge, constipation, restores color to prematurely gray hair.

Cautions: Overdosages can cause nausea, diarrhea, and gastric complaints.

Dosage: 15 grams

SANG JI SHENG (Loranthus, mulberry, mistletoe)

Functions: tonifies the Liver and Kidneys, nourishes Blood, relaxes the Uterus during pregnancy, and strengthens the bones and tendons.

Treats: joint problems in the lower back and knees; dry, scaly skin. Prevents miscarriage. Has been found to have a diuretic effect and lower blood pressure.

Cautions: Do not use if you have been diagnosed with low blood pressure or if you frequently get light-headed when you stand up fast.

Dosage: 15 grams

CHINESE MEDICAL PATENT FORMULAS TO TONIFY KIDNEY YIN

(All the Chinese patent formulas listed in this chapter are available only through Chinese herbal pharmacies.)

Liu Wei Di Huang Wan (Six Flavor Rehmannia Pill) to tonify the Kidney Yin — contains Cornus fruit (Shan Zhu Yu), cooked Rehmannia root (Shu Di Huang), Dioscorea root (Shan Yao), Poria cocos (Fu Ling), moutan (Mu Dan Pi), and Alisma (Ze Xie).

Zhi Bai Di Huang Wan (Anemarrhena, Phellodendron, and Rehmannia Pill) — consists of the above formula, which tonifies the Kidney Yin, with added Anemarrhena rhizome (Zhi Mu) and Phellodendron bark (Huang Bai), which cool deficiency heat. I prescribe this formula for women who have perimenopausal heat symptoms like night sweating, or who ovulate too early.

KI– KIDNEY ESSENCE TONICS (TO STABILIZE KIDNEY ESSENCE AND RAISE THE REPRODUCTIVE QI)

HELONIAS (false unicorn root)

Functions: retains the Essence (both Yin and Yang) of the Kidneys, nourishes the reproductive Qi.

Treats: low fertility, irregular menstruation, low progesterone levels, excessive vaginal discharge, menstrual pain, and threatened miscarriage.

Cautions: Since this is a "dry" herb, care should be taken when using this herb alone in conditions of severe Yin deficiency where there is scant fertile cervical mucus.

Dosage: 7 grams

FU PEN ZI (Rubus, Chinese raspberry)

Functions: stabilizes the Kidneys, preserves the Essence, and assists the Yang energies.

Treats: excessive urine, nocturnal emission, and excessive vaginal discharge.

Cautions: Use carefully in cases of Yin deficiency with heat signs.

Dosage: 7 grams

SHAN ZHU YU (Cornus, Asian Cornelian cherry fruit)

Functions: stabilizes the Kidneys to preserve the Essence (hold on to its reproductive function), tonifies Yang.

Treats: incontinence, excessive menstruation, and low sperm motility.

Dosage: 7 grams

KI YAN– KIDNEY YANG TONICS

The Kidney Yang energies are warm; therefore, tonifying Yang adds more heat to the system. If your menstrual cycles are short and you have signs of heat or Yin deficiency, use Yang supplements cautiously. Many people assume that if they have short cycles, they do not have enough progesterone, which is Yang. However, if they have heat signs, tonifying with warm, Yang herbs can actually worsen or shorten an already brief luteal phase.

However, if you have profuse or frequent, clear urination, long menstrual cycles, feel cold (especially cold feet at night), have low libido, and lower back pain, then Yang supplements can be therapeutic, especially during the luteal phase. Some Yang supplements can regulate the function of the adrenal cortex, promote sexual function, strengthen immune resistance, and invigorate metabolism. Yang supplements provide the natural triggers to increase production of thyroid hormone and progesterone (two temperature-raising hormones) if they are deficient.

MAN JING ZI (chaste tree berry, Vitex fruit)

Functions: acts on the hypothalamus, which then signals the pituitary to increase the production of LH while it mildly inhibits FSH release, resulting in an indirect increase in levels of progesterone in proportion to estrogen. Lowers the release of prolactin, which inhibits ovulation.

Treats: low progesterone, breast milk leakage, some PMS complaints.

Cautions: can interfere with hormone therapy, oral contraceptives, and dopamine-blocking drugs. Man Jing Zi should not be used in conditions of short menstrual cycles as a result of heat, as it will tend to cause even earlier menstruation. May cause (heat) rashes. Man Jing Zi should not be used during pregnancy.

Dosage: 300 milligrams per day in capsule or tablet form, or 35 milligrams of aqueous-alcohol extracts

DAMIANA, MEXICAN WILD YAM

Functions: tonifies the reproductive Qi, fortifies the Yang.

Treats: impotence, frigidity, incontinence, low testosterone production, vaginal discharge, and urinary leakage. Because of the relationship of the Kidney system to the brain, Damiana nourishes the nervous system to restore mental clarity.

Cautions: Should be applied with care in patients with irritable bowel syndrome or an otherwise hyperfunctioning sympathetic nervous system.

Dosage: 6 grams infusion, 2 milliliters tincture

SAW PALMETTO

Functions: nourishes the reproductive Qi, fortifies the Kidney Yang and Spleen Qi, enhances pituitary function via its hormonal influence on the endocrine glands, including the ovary, testicle, thyroid gland, and breasts.

Treats: impotence, amenorrhea, long menstrual cycles, and lack of sexual desire.

Cautions: Because it is oily, avoid usage in conditions of dampness with loose stools.

Dosage: 6 grams dry; 2 milliliters in tincture form

BA JI TIAN (Morinda root)

Functions: tonifies the Kidneys and fortifies the Yang, strengthens and warms the reproductive system.

Treats: infertility, joint pain.

Dosage: 12 grams

YIN YANG HUO (Epimedium, goatweed)

Functions: tonifies deficient Kidney Yang.

Treats: low libido, painfully cold lower back and knees, frequent urination, long menstrual cycles, impotence, premature ejaculation.

Dosage: 9 grams

XIAN MAO (immortal grass, goldeneye grass, Curculigo)

Functions: warms and tonifies the Kidney Yang.

Treats: Cold Uterus (CW) causes of infertility, luteal phase defect, impotence, arthritis.

Cautions: for short term use only; take Xian Mao for only one menstrual cycle at a time.

Dosage: 6 grams

DU ZHONG (Eucommia bark)

Functions: tonifies the Liver and Kidneys, treats cold-deficient Yang patterns, promotes circulation.

Treats: lower back pain and weakness, frequent urination, high blood pressure, threatened miscarriage with back pain.

Dosage: 12 grams

XU DUAN (Japanese teasel root, Dipsacus)

Function: tonifies the Liver and Kidneys and strengthens the tendons and bones (because of the Kidneys' relationship with the bones).

Treats: soreness, pain, and trauma; poor circulation; threatened miscarriage with cramping and bleeding.

Dosage: 15 grams

ROU CONG RONG (Broomrape stem, Cistanches)

Functions: tonifies the Kidney Yang and "moistens" the Intestines.

Treats: constipation, cold Uterus, impotence.

Cautions: Rou Cong Rong should not be used if there is diarrhea as a result of Spleen Qi deficiency.

Dosage: 15 grams

PATENT CHINESE HERBAL FORMULAS TO TONIFY THE KIDNEY YANG:

Eight Ingredient Pill with Rehmannia (Ba Wei Di Huang Wan) or **Kidney Qi Pill from the Golden Cabinet** (Jin Gui Shen Qi Wan) — contains the same ingredients as Liu Wei Di Huang Wan, with added aconite (Fu Zi) and cinnamon twig (Gui Zhi) to warm the Kidneys. Found in one study to lower elevated prolactin levels in both men and women.

Two Immortals Decoction (Er Xian Tang) — includes Curculigo (Xian Mao), Epimedium (Yin Yang Huo), Morinda (Ba Ji Tian), Angelica (Dang Gui), Phellodendron (Huang Bai), and Anemarrhena root (Zhi Mu). Especially important in addressing menopausal symptoms.

SP– SPLEEN QI SUPPLEMENTS

When the Qi is weak, all systems suffer. Weakened Spleen Qi can result in fatigue and emaciation, and the body's defenses may also be compromised. Spleen Qi deficiency is characterized by lethargy, weak extremities, lack of appetite, and digestive complaints like loose stools and abdominal pain.

Qi supplements are generally sweet and somewhat heavy or stodgy in nature. Sometimes when a patient with Qi deficiency starts to take Qi supplements, she may experience digestive disturbances such as abdominal bloating and nausea because these rich herbs are difficult for the weakened digestive system to absorb. Start slowly or combine with herbs like Chen Pi to moderate their richness.

Spleen Qi supplements strengthen the body's immunologic functions, or "defensive Qi." They are useful in treating certain Blood disorders, including anemia.

REN SHEN (ginseng root)

Functions: used by ancient Chinese emperors as a potent stimulant for physical and mental stamina, strongly tonifies the source Qi and strengthens the Spleen, boosts immunity.

Treats: fatigue, low testosterone, low sperm counts. Regulates immunologic disorders and helps the body adapt to environmental stressors.

Cautions: Because ginseng stimulates the central and peripheral nervous systems, anyone with symptoms of severe Qi stagnation or a hypersympathetic nervous system should choose a milder Qi tonic. Avoid in cases of Yin deficiency with heat signs, or with high blood pressure. Overdosage may lead to insomnia, palpitations, headaches, and a rise in blood pressure.

🍃 NOTE: Korean ginseng is stronger than Chinese ginseng.

Dosage: 6 grams

AMERICAN GINSENG

Functions: weaker than Chinese ginseng, used for concurrent Qi and Yang deficiency. Tonifies the digestive Qi, enhances immunity.

Treats: fatigue; poor endocrine, immune, and nervous system functions.

Dosage: 6 grams

SIBERIAN GINSENG

Functions: protects and regulates the immune system, and especially affects the adrenal glands.

Treats: low energy, poor capacity to handle stress.

Dosage: 3 grams

DANG SHEN (Codonopsis root)

Functions: not as strong as ginseng but has the same ability to augment the Qi.

Dosage: 15 grams

HUANG QI (Astragalus root)

Functions: tonifies the Spleen Qi, raises Yang Qi, and augments protective Qi.

Treats: weakened immunity, as in immunologic infertility factors. Astragalus helps the body mend broken parts (e.g., the fallopian tubes, tissue after surgery, etc.). Astragalus, like ginseng, helps the body adapt to stress.

Cautions: Astragalus can impair the effects of some immunosuppressive drugs and can increase the effects of immune-stimulating drugs.

Dosage: 15 grams

SHAN YAO (Chinese yam, Dioscorea root)

Functions: tonifies the Spleen energies as it nourishes, stabilizes, and preserves Kidney function.

Treats: fatigue, frequent urination. Used in many deficient conditions, including diabetes.

Cautions: Use with care when there is any excess condition of dampness, stasis, or stagnant obstruction.

Dosage: 15 grams

BAI ZHU (Atractylodes)

Functions: tonifies the Spleen Qi while drying dampness

Treats: fatigue, day sweats, miscarriage as a result of Spleen deficiency.

Cautions: Use carefully when Yin-deficient heat is present. Has a diuretic effect and has been found to lower plasma glucose levels. Prolongs the presence of prothrombin (a factor involved in blood clotting), significant when someone has a bleeding condition or is planning to have surgery.

Dosage: 6 grams

PATENT CHINESE HERBAL FORMULAS TO SUPPLEMENT SPLEEN QI

Tonify the Middle and Augment Qi Decoction (Bu Zhong Yi Qi Tang) — contains Astragalus (Huang Qi), ginseng (Ren Shen), Atractylodes (Bai Zhu), baked Glycyrrhiza (Zhi Gan Cao), Angelica (Dang Gui), dried tangerine peel (Chen Pi), black cohosh (Sheng Ma), and Bupleurum (Chai Hu). Tonifies and raises the Qi.

Four Gentlemen Decoction (Si Jun Zi Tang) — consists of ginseng (Ren Shen), Atractylodes (Bai Zhu), Poria cocos (Fu Ling), and baked Glycyrrhiza (Zhi Gan Cao). Tonifies the Spleen Qi.

BL— BLOOD BUILDERS

Blood deficiency is commonly characterized by scant menstrual flow, dry skin, dry hair, hair loss, and similar signs of blood not reaching tissues for proper nourishment. Like Kidney Yin tonics, Blood builders help tissues respond to estrogen. In Blood-deficient patterns, Blood builders help improve uterine lining and ovarian response.

DANG GUI, DONG QUAI (Angelica)

Functions: nourishes and invigorates the Blood.

Treats: irregular menstruation, amenorrhea, perimenopausal symptoms like hot flashes and night sweats, and menstrual difficulties such as painful menstruation. Possesses mild estrogenic qualities and has a regulatory effect in the uterus, hence its ability to normalize contractions in dysmenorrhea.

Cautions: Angelica can cause excess bleeding in people who are already taking blood-thinning medications. In rare cases, it may cause heart palpitations.

Dosage: 9 grams

SHU DI HUANG (cooked Rehmannia, Chinese foxglove root)

Functions: tonifies the Blood and Essence and nourishes the Kidney Yin.

Treats: menstrual problems due to Blood deficiency.

SHENG DI HUANG (fresh Rehmannia, Chinese foxglove root)

Functions: nourishes the Yin, generates fluid, cools the Blood.

Treats: elevated blood sugar levels, Liver disharmony. Used to control heat conditions that cause rheumatoid arthritis symptoms and skin conditions like eczema.

Cautions: Rich and cloying, Rehmannia should be used with care when Spleen deficiency with dampness is present.

Dosage: 15 grams

BAI SHAO (white peony)

Functions: nourishes the Blood, softens the Liver, and regulates menses.

Treats: symptoms of Liver Qi stagnation resulting from improperly nourished Liver Blood: PMS, night sweats, pain, and spasms.

Dosage: 12 grams

NETTLES

Functions: nourishes the Blood and restores deficient Liver Blood and Yin, drains urinary dampness.

Treats: relieves scanty lactation, nourishes dry hair, clears damp reproductive symptoms, and detoxifies.

Dosage: 15 grams, or 5-milliliter tincture

GOU QI ZI (Chinese wolfberry fruit, Lycium)

Functions: nourishes the Blood, tonifies the Liver and Kidneys, and benefits the Essence.

Treats: poor vision, dry eyes, impotence, lower body weakness. Gou Qi Zi is one of the "five seeds," which are said to "nourish the ancestral Qi," or strengthen the genetic constitution. The other four seeds are: Tu Si Zi (Cuscuta), a Yang supplement; Fu Pen Zi (Rubus), which stabilizes the Kidneys and boosts the Yang; Wu Wei Zi (Schisandra), which tonifies the Kidneys and restrains the Essence; and Che Qian Zi (Plantago seed), a dampness-draining herb.

Dosage: 12 grams

PATENT CHINESE HERBAL FORMULA TO BUILD THE BLOOD

Four Substances Decoction (Si Wu Tang) — cooked Rehmannia (Shu Di Huang), white peony (Bai Shao), Angelica (Dang Gui), Ligusticum (Chuan Xiong). Tonifies the Blood.

QI–/BL– HERBS TO SUPPLEMENT QI AND BLOOD

The Qi and Blood are closely related in TCM because the Qi travels with the Blood. A deficiency of one most always leads to a relative deficiency of the other. Therefore, many nourishing preparations tonify both the Qi and the Blood. Although we might think low hemoglobin concentrations in anemia would intuitively seem to be a blood deficiency, this situation will actually respond better to Qi supplements rather than Blood builders.

AVENA SATIVA, OAT BERRY AND STRAW, AVENA FATUA

Functions: provides nourishment to the endocrine, nervous, and immune systems and tonifies Qi, Blood, and Essence.

Treats: infertility, impotence, endocrine deficiencies, insomnia, and PMS caused by Liver and Kidney depletion.

Dosage: 20 grams or 30 drops of tincture

PATENT CHINESE HERBAL FORMULAS TO SUPPLEMENT QI AND BLOOD

Eight Treasure Decoction (Ba Zhen Tang) — a blend of the ingredients found in Four Gentlemen and Four Substances. Tonifies Qi and Blood. Adding Kidney supplements such as Cuscuta (Tu Si Zi), Psoralea fruit (Bu Gu Zhi), and Eucommia (Du Zhong) has been found to lower FSH in women with Qi, Blood, and Kidney Yang deficiency.

Restore the Spleen Decoction (Gui Pi Tang) — tonifies the Spleen Qi as it nourishes Heart Blood. Contains Four Gentlemen plus Zizyphus (Suan Zao Ren), longan (Long Yan Rou), Aucklandia (Mu Xiang), and Polygonatum root (Yuan Zhi).

LV QI X LIVER QI MOVERS

These herbs "get things moving," energetically speaking. Qi is an expression of the body tissues' functional activities. When the Liver Qi is stagnant, the organ function or tissue health will become stifled. Qi-moving herbs remove energy blockages. Since the Liver metabolizes hormones, some of the herbs that clear the Liver can help metabolize excess hormones. Excess estradiol, for example, can result in depression, irritability, menstrual irregularities, swollen and tender breasts, and precancerous conditions — all signs of Liver Qi stagnation. The treatment calls for Liver Qi movers. Most of these herbs are aromatic and drying in nature and also disperse the Qi, so they must be used cautiously in conditions of Qi and Yin deficiency.

CHAI HU (Bupleurum root, hare's-ear)

Functions: resolves Liver Qi stagnation by lifting and up-bearing sunken Qi; vents toxins through the pores.

Treats: emotional instabilities, depression, menstrual irregularities, headaches, chest tightness, gastric upset, and irritability.

Cautions: This herb can be somewhat dry-

ing, so it should be used with caution in cases of Yin deficiency, or else combined with Yin- or Blood-nourishing herbs. Chai Hu can increase the effects of some sedatives.

Dosage: 7 grams

SHENG MA (black cohosh, Cimicifuga)

Functions: raises the Yang Qi, meaning it has an energetic lifting effect. Vents the body of hot influences.

Treats: infertility, prolapse, PMS

Cautions: Because of its upward and outward energetic, Sheng Ma can have a drying effect and, therefore, should be used with care in cases of Yin deficiency. Paradoxically, this herb also resolves menopausal hot flashes and irritability. Since Sheng Ma dilates blood vessels, it should be avoided if you are taking anticoagulants like heparin.

Dosage: 6 grams

CHEN PI (dried tangerine peel)

Functions: regulates the Spleen Qi and prevents all types of stagnation — Liver Qi, dampness, and phlegm obstruction.

Treats: stomach upset; used in conjunction with heavy, cloying herbs to stimulate their digestion.

Dosage: 6 grams

XIANG FU (Cyperus, nut-grass rhizome)

Functions: spreads and regulates the Liver Qi.

Treats: irregular menstruation, menstrual pain. The volatile oils of Cyperus have been found to have an estrogenlike effect.

Dosage: 9 grams

MILK-THISTLE SEED

Functions: softens, detoxifies, and decongests the Liver; purifies the Blood; stimulates the Uterus.

Treats: hepatitis. Helps the Liver metabolize excess hormones, drugs, and environmental toxins.

Dosage: 600 milligrams per day

PATENT CHINESE HERBAL
FORMULAS TO MOVE LIVER QI

Frigid Extremities Powder (Si Ni San) — contains Bupleurum (Chai Hu), immature bitter orange (Zhi Shi), white peony (Bai Shao), and baked Glycyrrhiza (licorice, Zhi Gan Cao). Resolves stagnant (stuck) Liver Qi.

Rambling Powder (Xiao Yao San) — Bupleurum (Chai Hu), Angelica (Dang Gui), white peony (Bai Shao), Atractylodes (Bai Zhu), Poria (Fu Ling), baked Glycyrrhiza (Zhi Gan Cao), roasted ginger (Wei Jiang), mint (Bo

He). Resolves Liver Qi stagnation with Spleen Qi and Blood deficiency. Commonly used in treating menstrual irregularities and PMS.

BL X B L O O D   M O V E R S

We rarely find Blood stasis by itself. It is frequently associated with Blood or Kidney deficiency, and sometimes with Liver Qi stagnation (indicated by lots of PMS symptoms) and Spleen Qi deficiency (indicated by symptoms of fatigue, low blood pressure, and varicose veins). When a woman comes to my clinic with stagnant uterine Blood (which produces fibroids, endometriosis, or just dark, clotty, brown, or sticky menstrual blood), one of my first goals will be to "cleanse the Uterus" with the use of one or several of these Blood invigorators. After she takes the herbs for a while, her menstrual flow should become a fresh red in color.

Herbs that invigorate the Blood also help establish or promote menstruation in cases of amenorrhea or delayed menstruation as long as all other deficiency causes have been resolved first. For instance, I won't try to establish a menstrual cycle in an anorexic woman with amenorrhea until her Qi and Blood have been adequately tonified. Then Blood invigorators may restore regular menstruation.

Blood-invigorating herbs are blood thinners and should be utilized with care, especially if you have surgery scheduled. They also should be consumed cautiously if you are already taking aspirin or other blood thinners like heparin, because they function in somewhat the same manner.

YI MU CAO (Leonurus, Chinese motherwort)

Functions: invigorates the Blood of the Heart, Liver, and Urinary Bladder, and regulates the menses.

Treats: gynecological disorders involving Blood stasis, pelvic masses, and infertility. Because it stimulates the uterus, it should not be used during pregnancy. It may be used, however, to help the uterus contract after delivery.

Dosage: 30 grams

The seed of this herb, Leonurus (Chong Wei Zi), has more of a tonifying quality than its mother herb. I use it to build the uterine lining and to promote ovulation when Blood stasis is present (indicated by sharp, stabbing ovulatory pain).

Dosage: 6 grams

TAO REN (Persica, peach kernel)

Functions: breaks up Blood stasis to resolve menstrual disorders, moistens the bowels.

Treats: lack of menstruation, menstrual pain, constipation.

Cautions: This herb should not be used during pregnancy or after ovulation. A knowledgeable practitioner, however, may prescribe this anticoagulant herb to treat disorders that can prevent implantation or cause miscarriages (where the body "clots off" blood flow to the uterus), just as baby aspirin is often employed to thin the blood to improve blood flow to the uterus.

Dosage: 6 grams

HONG HUA (Carthamus, safflower)

Functions: invigorates Liver and Heart Blood, unblocks menstruation, alleviates pain.

Treats: amenorrhea, abdominal pain.

Cautions: stimulates the Uterus and should be avoided during pregnancy.

Dosage: 6 grams

BLUE COHOSH ROOT

Functions: raises estrogen levels, moderates and warms the Uterus, and promotes menstruation.

Treats: menopausal symptoms. Alleviates false labor pains yet enhances true uterine contractions. Conversely, it can be used to treat painful menstruation by relaxing the uterus. The relaxant effect is also used to treat ovulation pains and irritable bowel syndrome. Promotes urination and sweating to balance excess fluids.

Dosage: 6 grams; tincture 2 milliliters

PATENT CHINESE HERBAL FORMULAS TO MOVE THE BLOOD

Four Substances Decoction with Safflower and Peach Pit (Tao Hong Si Wu Tang) — Four Substances with Tao Ren and Hong Hua. Treats Blood deficiency and Blood stasis.

Warm the Menses Decoction (Wen Jing Tang) — Evodia fruit (Wu Zhu Yu), cinnamon twig (Gui Zhi), Angelica (Dang Gui), Ligusticum (Chuan Xiong), red/white peony (Chi or Bai Shao), gelatin (E Jiao), Ophiopogon (Mai Men Dong), moutan (Mu Dan Pi), ginseng (Ren Shen), fresh ginger (Sheng Jiang), Pinellia (Ban Xia), Glycyrrhiza (Zhi Gan Cao). Warms the Uterus to resolve Blood stasis. Treats the cold Uterus (CW) pattern. A study in 1989 showed an increase in response to Clomid when combined with Wen Jing Tang. If women didn't ovulate after three cycles of Clomid, they were given Wen Jing Tang along with the Clomid, which then made them ovulate.

Cinnamon Twig and Poria Decoction (Gui Zhi Fu Ling Wan) — cinnamon twig (Gui Zhi), Poria (Fu Ling), moutan (Mu Dan Pi), peach kernel (Tao Ren), red peony (Chi Shao). Invigorates the Blood, warms the menses, and, during pregnancy, treats Blood stasis in the womb that may deprive the fetus of nourishment. I use this decoction with many women who have endometriosis or fibroids and are attempting to conceive.

HT– HEART SUPPLEMENTS

Spirit-calming medicinals usually (but not always) enter the Heart channel because the Heart is where the spirit is said to reside. These herbs are generally heavy, and some have a high mineral content. They settle insomnia, anxiety, and restlessness. In Chinese medicine, the Heart is the Organ that sends the Blood to the Uterus. Therefore, the Heart must be calm, nourished, and unobstructed for conception to occur.

SUAN ZAO REN (Zizyphus, sour jujube seed)

Functions: nourishes the Yin of the Heart, augments Liver Blood, and quiets the spirit.

Treats: irritability, night sweats, and spontaneous sweating. It is somewhat of a sedative and lowers body temperature and blood pressure.

Dosage: 15 grams

MU LI (oystershell)

Functions: settles and calms a restless spirit.

Treats: palpitations, anxiety, restlessness, and insomnia.

Dosage: 20 grams

VALERIAN ROOT

Functions: calms and sedates.

Treats: insomnia, cramping and spasms of the uterus, intestines, and muscles. Considered a "nervine," or stress reducer, it allows deeper levels of sleep.

Dosage: 500 milligrams per day, usually taken before bed

PATENT CHINESE HERBAL
FORMULAS TO TONIFY THE HEART

Sour Jujube Decoction (Suan Zao Ren Tang) — Zizyphus (Suan Zao Ren), Ligusticum (Chuan Xiong), Poria (Fu Ling or Fu Shen), Anemarrhena (Zhi Mu), licorice (Gan Cao). Nourishes the Heart, calms the spirit, and supplements Liver Blood.

Heavenly Emperor's Special Pill to Tonify the Heart (Tian Wang Bu Xin Dang) — fresh Rehmannia (Sheng Di Huang), ginseng (Ren Shen), asparagus root (Tian Men Dong), Ophiopogon (Mai Men Dong), Scrophularia (Xuan Shen), Salvia root (Dan Shen), Poria (Fu Ling), Angelica (Dang Gui), Polygonatum root (Yuan Zhi), Schisandra (Wu Wei Zi), Stemona root (Bai Bu), Biota seed (Bai Zi Ren), Zizyphus seed (Suan Zao Ren), Platycodon (Jie Geng), licorice (Gan Cao). Harmonizes the relationship between the Heart and Kidneys.

^H HEAT-CLEARING HERBS

Some herbs in the heat-clearing category have excellent anti-inflammatory, antibacterial, antiviral, and antitumor effects. They also can eliminate rashes and other forms of internal heat. The heat-clearing herbs I describe are those I utilize primarily in treating infertility caused by heat conditions. Short cycles are often a result of heat, as are certain autoimmune conditions and miscarriage presentations.

DI GU PI (Chinese wolfberry root bark)

Functions: clears heat from Yin deficiency.

Treats: night sweats, hot flashes, and genital itching.

Dosage: 10 grams

CHI SHAO (red peony)

Functions: clears heat, cools and invigorates the Blood.

Treats: early menstruation, premenstrual headaches, rashes, and Blood stasis (fibroids; endometriosis; and dark, clotty, painful menses).

Dosage: 6 grams

MU DAN PI (moutan, peony root bark)

Functions: clears heat, cools the Blood, and invigorates static Blood.

Treats: gynecological disorders, early menstruation.

Cautions: Mu Dan Pi should not be used during pregnancy or excessive menstruation.

Dosage: 9 grams

DH HERBS TO DRAIN DAMP HEAT

These herbs are bitter and cold, and are thus used to treat disorders of damp heat. The *Chinese Herbal Medicine: Materia Medica* says, "From a modern biomedical perspective, they seem to have antimicrobial, antipyretic, and anti-inflammatory effects." They are often used in excess conditions (such as Liver Qi stagnation or Blood stasis) in combination with herbs that clear heat. Because of their bitter and cold nature, they should be used with discretion in cases of Spleen and Yang deficiency.

HUANG QIN (Scutellaria, skullcap root)

Functions: clears heat and drains damp heat from the upper part of the body.

Treats: premenstrual acne around the mouth and chin area caused by heat arising from Liver Qi stagnation. Clears other damp heat skin conditions like eczema, fevers, headaches, irritability, and red eyes from excess Yang. Stops bleeding caused by excess heat, forestalls threatened miscarriage during patterns of Liver Qi stagnation with heat. Because it inhibits the release of enzymes from mast (immune) cells, Huang Qin has been found to have an anti-immune effect and can act as a diuretic or antibiotic, as well as lower cholesterol, fevers, and blood pressure.

Dosage: 6 grams

HUANG LIAN (Coptis)

Functions: strongly clears heat and damp heat from the middle part of the body.

Treats: irritability and manic episodes; resolves skin problems caused by damp heat; and can defeat antimicrobial, antiviral, and antifungal pathogens. Can be applied topically to treat Trichomonas vaginitis. It has been found to lower blood pressure and has antiadrenaline and anti-inflammatory effects.

Dosage: 4.5 grams

HUANG BAI (Phellodendron bark, Amur cork bark)

Functions: drains damp heat from the lower part of the body.

Treats: vaginitis with abnormal vaginal discharges, cystitis, Trichomonas vaginitis, and cervical inflammation.

Dosage: 7 grams

PATENT CHINESE HERBAL FORMULAS
TO DRAIN DAMP HEAT

Eight Herb Powder for Rectification (Ba
Zheng San) — Clematis (Mu Tong), Dian-
thus (Qu Mai), Polygonum (Bian Xu), Plantago seed (Che Qian Zi), licorice (Gan Cao),
gardenia fuit (Zhi Zi), rhubarb (Da Huang),
sassafras medulla (Deng Xin Cao), talcum
(Hua Shi).

D DAMP DRAINERS

Some herbs categorized as "draining dampness" in Chinese medicine are found to
lower cholesterol and triglyceride levels.
Some inhibit yeast overgrowth, and others
can act as diuretics.

FU LING (Poria cocos)

Functions: strengthens the Spleen and promotes urination, transforms dampness and
phlegm, calms the spirit, and relaxes smooth
muscles and the nervous system.

Treats: fatigue, sluggishness, diarrhea, urinary difficulty. Reduces blood sugar levels.

Dosage: 12 grams

KUN BU (kelp)

Functions: reduces phlegm conditions and
promotes urination.

Treats: thyroid abnormalities caused by
lack of iodine and goiter. Treats fibrocystic
breasts and restores endocrine and immune
system functions.

Cautions: avoid in conditions of hyperthyroid.

Dosage: 10 grams

HAI ZAO (seaweed, sargasso)

Functions: clears heat and reduces phlegm,
promotes urination, and reduces edema.

Treats: both hypo- and hyperthyroid disorders, fibrocystic breasts, high cholesterol,
clotting (has an anticoagulant effect).

Dosage: 10 grams

ZAO JIAO CI (Gleditsia fruit)

Functions: dispels abscesses caused by
damp obstruction, revives the spirit, and dis-
sipates phlegm.

Treats: PCOS; dissolves the waxy coating
found around polycystic ovaries and induces ovulation.

Cautions: slightly toxic; take in small
amounts prior to ovulation only. Contraindicated during pregnancy.

Dosage: 1 gram

PATENT CHINESE HERBAL FORMULAS TO DRAIN DAMPNESS

Six Gentlemen Decoction (Liu Jun Zi Tang) — contains the same ingredients as Four Gentlemen, with added dried tangerine peel (Chen Pi) and Pinellia (Ban Xia). Tonifies the Spleen Qi and dries dampness.

Two Cured Decoction (Er Chen Tang) — contains Pinellia (Ban Xia), dried tangerine peel (Chen Pi), Poria (Fu Ling), and baked licorice (Gan Cao). Dries dampness, transforms phlegm, and regulates Qi.

"CALM THE FETUS" TO PREVENT MISCARRIAGE

Although there is not a Chinese herbal category for miscarriage prevention, many herbs have the inherent effect of "calming the fetus" (or relaxing the uterus) to prevent miscarriage. Some of them tonify the Kidneys or Liver, supplement Blood or Qi, stop bleeding, or clear heat. However, the premises of Chinese pattern differentiation still hold true: we must treat the underlying pattern responsible for the threatened miscarriage. These herbs are often added to other Chinese formulas.

Atractylodes *Bai Zhu* — tonifies Qi.

Gelatin *E Jiao* — tonifies Blood, stops bleeding.

Dipsacus *Xu Duan* — tonifies Liver and Kidneys.

Sangjisheng *Sang Ji Sheng* — tonifies Liver and Kidneys.

Scutellaria *Huang Qin* — clears damp heat.

Eucommia *Du Zhong* — tonifies Kidney Yang.

Perilla fruit *Zi Su Ye* — warms and harmonizes the Spleen and Stomach to treat cold conditions.

Amomum *Sha Ren* — aromatic, Sha Ren clears dampness, strengthens the Spleen and Stomach.

Cuscuta *Tu Si Zi* — tonifies Kidney Yang.

Artemisia *Ai Ye* — warms the womb to stop bleeding, treats cold Uterus (CW) conditions, and in so doing, helps build up thin uterine linings.

Astragalus *Huang Qi* — tonifies Spleen Qi.

HERBS TO HELP THE FALLOPIAN TUBES

Don't rely on herbal medicine alone to treat blocked fallopian tubes. However, if the blockage is partial or the tubes are "sluggish," these herbs can help. I have seen many women whose tubes were at least partially obstructed and who became pregnant after treatment with acupuncture, massage and exercises, and herbal therapy.

Platycodon *Jie Geng* — a phlegm-resolving medicinal, assists cilia movement, responsible for getting the egg to the uterus in fallopian tubes.

Tribulus *Bai Ji Li* — decreases swelling to help heal tissue.

Astragalus *Huang Qi* — helps heal tissue.

HERBS TO STOP BLEEDING

Herbs that stop uterine bleeding can be used in cases of bleeding during the luteal phase, or where menstrual bleeding does not stop when it should. Of course, the underlying cause of the bleeding must be determined and treated as well. When there is Blood loss, usually the Blood and Yin must be tonified.

Bulrush, cattail pollen *Pu Huang* — invigorates static Blood to stop bleeding.

Agrimonia *Xian He Cao* — restrains bleeding. May be used with bleeding caused by heat, cold, excess, or deficiency.

Pseudoginseng *San Qi* — invigorates static Blood to stop bleeding.

Japonicus, Japanese thistle *Da Ji* — cools the Blood to stop bleeding.

Artemisia *Ai Ye* — warms the womb to stop bleeding.

HERBS TO BUILD UP THE UTERINE LINING

When the uterine lining is shown to be less than 7 millimeters on ultrasound, the endometrium is considered too thin for implantation to occur. At least eight millimeters or more with a triple layer (trilaminar) pattern is ideal. If you have not had an ultrasound and don't know if your lining is thick enough, I consider scant menstrual blood with light flow occurring for less than three days indicative of a thin uterine lining.

Artemisia *Ai Ye* — warms the Uterus and stops bleeding.

Leonurus *Yi Mu Cao* — invigorates uterine Blood.

Placenta *Zi He Che* — tonifies Kidney Yang.

Four Substances Decoction (*Si Wu Tang*) — patent herbal formula used to tonify the Blood.

Red raspberry leaf — Steep in water and drink daily as a tea to tonify the uterus.

HERBS IN ACTION: SOPHIE

Sophie came to see me after three years of marriage. She and James had been trying to conceive for two and a half of those years. They were from England, where they had begun their fertility workups and treatment. Although Sophie's hormone tests were all within normal limits, she spotted light-colored blood every month a few days before her period came, bled heavily during her period, and spotted for a few days afterward. She experienced a heavy, downward cramping sensation with the onset of menses. Sophie was usually fatigued and had a history of low blood pressure and hemorrhoids.

By now you should identify that Sophie was deficient in her Spleen energies. James had a borderline low sperm count as well. I asked James to take nutritional supplements, including two amino acids and relatively high dosages of antioxidants and ginseng. Sophie came for acupuncture treatments every other week, during which I tonified her Spleen. I put her on the formula Bu Zhong Yi Qi Tang to supplement and lift the Spleen Qi, which she took for two months. After the first month, she did not have any more premenstrual spotting, and her period lasted five days and then stopped. The next cycle, during her second monthly visit, her pulse had the characteristic rapid, slippery quality that told me she was pregnant. Both Sophie and James came for her following appointment to confirm that they were expecting their first child.

SUMMARY

Diet and lifestyle changes, blood flow and meditative exercises, herbal supplementation, and acupoint stimulation are the most effective elements of TCM for improving your fertility status. Yet, for individual reasons, not everybody can apply all of these modifications. Come up with a program with which you are comfortable and to which you can adhere for perhaps months. Any of these methods alone will help; the combination of all, however, usually provides the best results.

PART III

FERTILITY IN SPECIAL CIRCUMSTANCES: HOW TO HELP WESTERN-DIAGNOSED OBSTACLES TO FERTILITY

If we remain obsessed with seeds and eggs, we are married to the fertile reproductive valley of the Mysterious Mother, but not to her immeasurable heart and all-knowing mind.

— HUA HU CHING (TRANSLATED BY BRIAN WALKER)

The women who come to see me are usually highly informed about their particular medical problems. They can give me details on their FSH levels, autoimmune issues, polycystic ovaries and fallopian tube blockages, lack of pituitary function, or insufficient ovarian response to hormonal medications. Having been trained in both Western and Eastern medicine, I not only understand what their fertility conditions mean but can apply what I know from both medical disciplines to diagnose and eventually correct the real issues of energetic and Organ system imbalances. In this way, I have been able to build a bridge between Western science and Eastern treatment, resulting in greater reproductive health for my patients.

The therapies I recommend for Western-diagnosed conditions like luteal phase defect, advanced maternal age, PCOS, endometriosis, immunological issues, and so on, are not based simply on ancient Chinese traditional remedies but also founded on scientific research and clinical results. Yes, the acupuncture, herbs, and dietary recommendations will balance your Qi or decrease heat or tonify your Kidney Essence. But the *effects* of these remedies will be normalization of your hormone levels, or the shrinking of your endometriosis, or the enlivening of your ovaries. Your menstrual cycle will follow a more regular schedule — and yes, you will be more likely to conceive.

Western medicine has done wonders for many women and men who wish to have children. However, for millions of others, each month is yet another disappointment and another unsuccessful treatment. Some conditions — like unexplained infertility, poor ovarian response, and uterine lining issues — are only occasionally addressed with success by Western medicine. And sometimes the remedies can be worse than the problem itself.

In many cases, men and women who have not responded to Western prescriptions find their answers in the health-restoring practices of TCM. Of course, I'm not saying TCM can guarantee everyone will be able to have a child, but it can provide a new approach that is capable of doing what Western medicine is not. And with its focus on healing the reproductive system by restoring health to the entire body, you are far more likely to gain greater health and well-being along the way.

9

Luteal Phase Defect: Strengthening the Kidneys and Spleen

Progesterone is the fuel for the body's incubator.

— ANONYMOUS

None of the phases of reproduction is an isolated event. As with all other physiologic processes, each one depends on the proper working of the entire system. This is especially true when it comes to the luteal phase of the reproductive cycle.

Problems with the luteal phase concern not just the egg itself or its production, or even its journey from the ovary through the fallopian tube to the uterus. Luteal phase defect (LPD) affects the body's "incubator," hampering the production and response of the endometrial lining of the uterus, where a fertilized egg should implant.

LUTEAL PHASE DEFECT: DIAGNOSIS AND EFFECTS

Most infertility specialists consider LPD an insufficiency of progesterone production. Yet, administering progesterone does not cure it, so we know this is not the only factor. Some studies have demonstrated that there is impaired follicle development in women with LPD. Other studies have implicated impairment of the levels of FSH or LH as causative. All these factors may play a role in this condition.

Luteal phase defect also can mean that the events signaling endometrial development are out of sync with the rest of the hormonal cycle. For pregnancy to occur, the endometrium must be ready to receive the fertilized egg between four and eight days after ovulation. If the endometrium is ready any earlier or later, the blastocyst will find it unreceptive for implantation and pass through undetected. If the embryo finds the endometrium receptive to initial implantation, then the mucinous glands, which are necessary for the embryo's continued growth in the uterus, must continue to develop in response to progesterone stimulation. When this process does not occur smoothly, the body's own immune system is often to blame for not allowing the pregnancy to continue.

If your Western medical doctor suspects LPD, you may be asked to undergo any or all of the following tests:

1. *Plasma progesterone level measurement* — to see if you've ovulated. A normal midluteal range would be 10 nanograms per milliliter or more.
2. *Other hormone tests* — to measure levels of prolactin (excess prolactin can interfere with normal ovulation) and androgen (high levels of androgen indicate PCOS, hypothalamic and / or pituitary dysfunction).
3. *Endometrial biopsy* or *endometrial function test* — to see how well your uterine lining is prepared for the implantation of a fertilized egg. If your endometrial development is more than two days off the normal curve, this indicates luteal phase defect.
4. *Vaginal ultrasound* — to document thickness and patterns of endometrial development, and to determine whether the dominant follicle has ruptured.

Several signs may make your doctor suspect LPD, including a luteal phase of less than twelve days long, menopausal symptoms, low serum progesterone levels (less than 6 nanograms per milliliter) midway through the luteal phase, and spotting before menstruation.

Basal body temperature also can be considered. It is generally agreed that progesterone has a heating effect and raises the BBT at least four-tenths of a degree to one full degree after ovulation. A slow or low rise in body temperature after ovulation might indicate a lack of progesterone production. Progesterone levels and basal temperatures should remain elevated for fourteen days after ovulation. Progesterone levels peak during the middle of the luteal phase, about a week after ovulation. If the corpus luteum is not producing adequate quantities of progesterone, or if the uterine lining is not properly primed to respond, spotting may occur, the BBT may drop, or the period may come early.

Treatment of LPD may include using medications to stimulate follicular growth and the corpus luteum, or medications that act directly on the endometrium. Clomiphene (Clomid), FSH, or human menopausal gonadotropin (hMG) can be used to stimulate follicle growth in different phases of the reproductive cycle. Clomiphene is often used to treat LPD because it increases production of follicles and corpus lutea and, in turn, progesterone, which can improve the quality of the uterine lining and/or lengthen the luteal phase of the cycle. (However, as I said earlier, in some cases this drug can actually *increase* a woman's chances of implantation problems by thinning her uterine lining.) A series of injections of hCG after ovulation also can help support the corpus luteum and uterine lining.

Progesterone treatment is used to mature a properly primed endometrium and is usually started two to three days after ovulation. Progesterone can be given in pill form, by vaginal suppository or gel, or by intramuscular injection. However, in some women, synthetic progesterone is metabolized into a dopaminelike chemical, which makes them feel tired, woozy, and disoriented.

❧ THE EASTERN VIEW

The Eastern view of the luteal phase takes into account the interrelation of the other four phases of the reproductive cycle. You may recall from chapter 5 that Phase I is the follicular, estrogen-dominated Yin stage, in which a dominant follicle in the ovary is encouraged to grow and prepare its egg for release. Then, during ovulation (Phase II), Yin reaches its apogee and transforms into Yang, but *only* if Qi, Blood, Yin, and Yang are functioning optimally. Phase III is the luteal phase, governed by the Yang hormone progesterone. The warming Yang energy prepares the endometrium to accept the fertilized egg. This phase can thrive only if the Yin of Phase I has been transformed into

Yang during ovulation (Phase II). Phase IV is the premenstrual phase, governed by the Liver Qi, which transforms the Yang energy back into Yin, and Phase V is the menstrual, Blood, or zero (hormonal-resting) stage, when Yin and Yang are balanced.

Most cases of LPD include a condition of low progesterone, the harmone governed by Kidney Yang and Spleen Qi. Therefore, these two elements almost always need supplementation in cases of LPD. In addition, the other phases also must be in harmony for progesterone to be released. Adequate hormonal precursors (chemical building blocks of hormones) need to be present in Phase I and during ovulation, and no obstruction — mechanical, anatomical, or energetic — can be present if the luteal phase is to be in sync.

According to TCM there can be many reasons for luteal phase insufficiency. These include:

◆ not enough Yin in Phase I to transform into Yang (**Ki Yi–**)
◆ obstructed Blood (**Bl X**)
◆ Liver Qi stagnation (**Lv Qi X**)
◆ not enough Kidney Yang or Spleen Qi to promote or hold the luteal phase (**Ki Yan–/Sp–**)
◆ cold Uterus (**CW**)

Each of these reasons will require different kinds of treatment to balance the body's energies. This is where correct pattern discrimination can make the difference in treatment outcome.

A woman's BBT graph can reveal disharmony during the luteal phase. For instance, in one form of LPD the temperatures go along normally during the follicular phase, the fertile cervical fluid appears, and the fertility monitor says ovulation has occurred. However, the BBT does not rise as dramatically as it should after ovulation. If the BBT graph rises, lowers, and rises again (fig. 9.1), this horseshoe-shaped curve points to problems with corpus luteum functioning.

In TCM, this pattern often indicates Kidney Yang (**Ki Yan–**) or Spleen Qi (**Sp–**) deficiency. Sometimes this pattern also appears with Blood stasis (**Bl X**) or damp heat (**DH**) obstruction, especially in the presence of endometriosis.

SP– SPLEEN QI DEFICIENCY

Spleen Qi deficiency is almost always involved at some level with LPD. A woman might find she is particularly fatigued around ovulation. She may sweat spontaneously during the luteal phase. She may be prone to abdominal cramping and diarrhea. She may have a history of low blood pressure. She can always tell that her period is coming because her stools become loose. During menstruation, she bleeds heavily, but the blood is somewhat thin and watery, and appears almost pink in color. Her energy is especially low during her period. Going back to the diagnostic checklists in chapter 4, this woman fits the category of Spleen Qi deficiency: there is an insuffi-

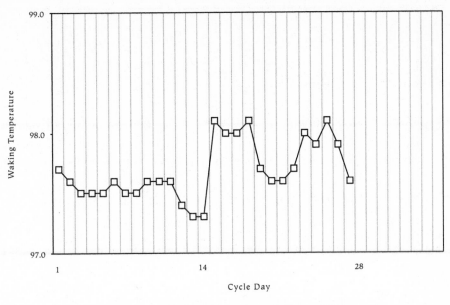

Figure 9.1: BBT Graph — Luteal Phase Defect

ciency of Spleen Qi to support the Yang of the Kidney. This is what is creating the LPD.

Adding progesterone to this woman's system using either Western or Eastern means would not get to the root of her problem. We could give her progesterone supplements, or use herbs like Angelica to invigorate the Blood, and she would get no response. The only way to correct her deficiency is to supplement Spleen Qi. This woman should take herbs such as ginseng (Ren Shen), Atractylodes (Bai Zhu), Dioscorea (Shan Yao), and Astragalus (Huang Qi), which build up Spleen Qi. There are also dietary changes she could make: avoiding cold, raw foods and eliminating sweets and refined carbohydrates. In addition, she may wish to use acupressure to stimulate Spleen Qi

points like St 36 (Lower Sea of Qi) and Ren 6 (Sea of Qi). Using these dietary recommendations, adding the herbs, and stimulating the Spleen Qi points should allow the luteal phase to correct itself, making it possible for the woman to conceive.

KI YAN– KIDNEY YANG DEFICIENCY

Kidney Yang deficiency also is common in cases of LPD. With Kidney Yang deficiency, the BBT stays low during the follicular phase, as it should. In fact, the problem is that the temperature *doesn't* go up — because there's not enough Yang to make it rise (see fig. 9.2).

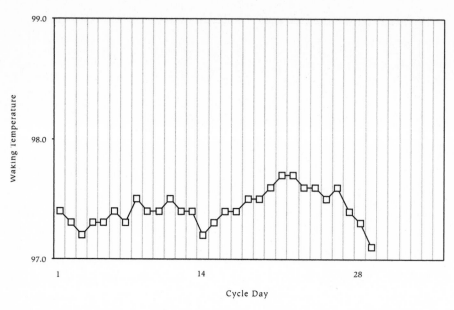

Figure 9.2: BBT Graph — Luteal Phase Defect Caused by
Kidney Yang Deficiency (**Ki Yan–**)

A woman with Kidney Yang deficiency always feels cold; her feet are especially cold at night. Midcycle vaginal discharge appears on schedule and may even be profuse in amount. Ovulation occurs, but she has almost no sexual desire, so intercourse feels like a chore. Her BBT never rises very much — the pre- and postovulatory baselines may differ only by about two- or three-tenths of a degree. This woman's back is almost always weak and sometimes feels sore. She sleeps well but has to wake up to urinate at least one or two times per night. Sometimes she spots about a week before her period is due. She can usually tell she is not pregnant and her period is coming because her back aches more than usual. Her bowel movements become somewhat loose on the morning she starts bleeding.

Going back to the diagnostic checklists, this woman most closely resembles the Kidney Yang deficiency scenario. (She also has some symptoms of Spleen Qi deficiency, but when the Kidney Yang is depleted it will sometimes "borrow" from the Spleen energies. Overlapping symptoms are common.) Kidney Yang deficiency can be helped by diminishing activities that tax the Kidney system. Traditional Chinese medicine would recommend that this woman reduce her consumption of caffeine and other stimulants, including alcohol, cigarettes, or herbal "pick-me-ups" like Ephedra (Ma Huang). (Nicotine is a serious fertility killer. Women who wish to get pregnant shouldn't consume any type of nicotine, including gum and patches. And secondhand smoke impairs fertility almost as much as smoking cigarettes yourself.) It's also important for a woman with Kidney Yang deficiency to avoid overexercise and overwork, and to get enough sleep.

Dietary choices also can help increase Kidney Yang. This woman should choose foods that tonify the Kidney system, like black beans, legumes, kelp, parsley, tofu, raspberries, walnuts, wild rice, spirulina, wheat germ, and wheatgrass. Many of these foods are rich in vitamin B6, which is helpful in cases of LPD because it boosts progesterone and lowers elevated prolactin levels. String beans, mulberry, millet, and non–hormonally treated organ meats are helpful, as well as black sesame seeds, Lycium fruit, adzuki beans, gelatin, chestnuts, and corn. Supplementing the diet with extra vitamin B6 and L-arginine may be indicated, and some women with low libido find DHEA helpful. Although fresh pineapple is not considered a Yang food, eating it can assist in implantation.

Beneficial herbs include Eucommia (Du Zhong), Epimedium (Yin Yang Huo), Dipsacus (Xu Duan), Cuscuta (Tu Si Zi), Morinda (Ba Ji Tian), and Psoralea (Bu Gu Zhi). Black cohosh (Sheng Ma) raises the Yang Qi during the luteal phase as well. Psoralea tonifies the Yang when there is a concomitant Spleen Qi deficiency. Helonias root (false unicorn root) is considered a uterine restorative, which stimulates hormonal precursors to trigger progesterone release. It also improves progesterone production and moderates menstruation. Acupoints Ki 7 and Ren 4 should be stimulated.

CW COLD UTERUS

The condition termed "cold womb" basically means that the uterus is not responding to the heating effect of progesterone. I find women with this condition usually have Kidney Yang deficiency (**Ki Yan–**), which is often accompanied by Blood stasis (**Bl X**). They often experience a sensation about a week after ovulation telling them their period will be coming this month. It may be a fluttering feeling or a cramp in the area where they think their uterus is. In addition, their temperature may go down at this time. Their lower abdomen, below the belly button, may feel cooler to the touch than the rest of the body.

If the Uterus is cold, the solution is to warm it up. You can improve Blood flow to the Uterus with femoral massage (see page 88) and with Qi Gong breathing techniques (see page 89). Apply a hot water bottle or heating pad over the lower abdomen before ovulation. It's also good to eat warm foods. You can stimulate all the acupuncture points in the lower abdomen (Ren 3, Ren 4, Ren 6, St 29, St 30, and Zigong), as well as Ki 7, to tonify Kidney Yang, and Sp 8, to resolve Blood stasis.

TREATING OTHER FACTORS INVOLVED IN LPD

As mentioned previously, there are other endocrine factors affecting the luteal phase. If there is not enough Yin in the follicular phase, for instance, the Yin will not reach the apogee required for transformation into Yang. (In Western medical terminology, there is not enough estrogen to prepare the cervix, trigger ovulation, or thicken the endometrium for implantation.) In this case, there will be signs of Yin deficiency, and the woman's cycle most often will be prolonged. This will be evident in the BBT graph pattern of consistently low temperatures, with possible sawtooth variations indicating Liver and /or Heart fire (see fig. 9.3).

Chinese medicine seeks to resolve the underlying imbalance responsible for the body's inherent lack of progesterone production. If you fall into the category of luteal phase defect or think you may have a deficiency in progesterone production, I also advise the use of natural United States Certified Potency (U.S.P.) progesterone cream, to be taken topically (applied to the skin) twice per day after ovulation, as recommended by the manufacturer. (Topical creams containing other herbal blends do not seem to be as effective.) My patients usually apply the progesterone cream during the luteal phase *only* for three successive cycles, and then take one month off.

WHEN PROGESTERONE AND CLOMIPHENE ARE NOT THE ANSWER

Some modern "infertility diets" recommend the consumption of yams during the first half of the menstrual cycle to help improve progesterone during the second half. Yams are said to act like a natural form of clomiphene citrate (which is both estrogenic and antiestrogenic at different stages of a woman's cycle), giving more stimulation to the ovary so more follicles are produced. Chinese yam (Dioscorea [Shan Yao]) is categorized as a Qi supplement and is often used to treat gynecological disorders. Women who are diagnosed with Kidney Yang (**Ki Yan–**) or Spleen Qi (**Sp–**) deficiency will tend to respond more favorably to the administration of clomiphene, just as they will respond favorably to Chinese yams. However, those who fall into a different category of imbalance will *not* respond favorably to either clomiphene or yams. In fact, the administration of either may potentially do more harm than good.

For example, women diagnosed with Liver Qi stagnation (**Lv Qi X**) with heat will not become pregnant with clomiphene. Their systems are already under too much stress, and clomiphene further invigorates the Yang Qi, basically creating more internal pressure. The body cannot handle the intensification of Qi in a confined space. This increased force produces a toxic environment unfavorable to implantation, regardless of the level of progesterone. Their temperatures tend to jump around madly (see fig. 9.4); anyone can see that this is not a harmonized pattern. It is a stagnant Liver Qi pattern to which too much Yang was added.

If women with Liver Qi stagnation and heat from the internal pressure take

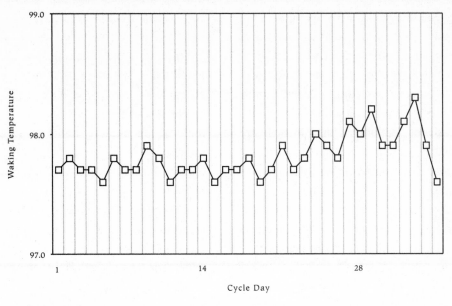

Figure 9.3: BBT Graph — Luteal Phase Defect Caused by Kidney Yin
Deficiency (**Ki Yi–**) and Liver and Heart Fire

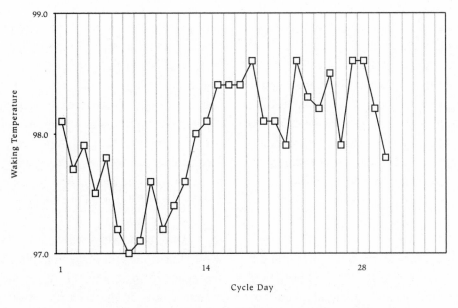

Figure 9.4: BBT Graph — Effect of Clomid on a Woman Diagnosed
with Liver Qi Stagnation (**Lv Qi X**) with Heat (**^H**)

clomiphene, they often will experience only its negative side effects, such as headache, heat sensation, sweating, and irritability. What's worse is that they are much less likely to become pregnant. Women with severe premenstrual symptoms also should not be given clomiphene; they most likely already have adequate production of progesterone. If a woman fitting this category is nonetheless prescribed clomiphene, we would use TCM to rectify the Qi to reduce internal pressure and give the clomiphene a chance to succeed. The acupuncture prescription might include Lv 2, Lv 3, LI 4, LI 11, and Sp 10, stimulated only during clomiphene administration *before* ovulation, not after. Some of these points, like LI 4, are not to be used during pregnancy.

On the other hand, women with Kidney Yin deficiency (**Ki Yi–**) will tend to experience more of the antiestrogenic properties of clomiphene administration, such as night sweats, reduced cervical fluid, and thin uterine lining. In this case we would use acupuncture points like Sp 6 and Ki 3 to nourish Yin and Sp 10 and LI 11 to clear heat, and/or herbs like Anemarrhena, Phellodendron, and Rehmannia Pill (Zhi Bai Di Huang Wan) to supplement the Yin and clear heat.

TCM IN ACTION: STEPHANIE'S STORY

Stephanie came to my clinic after trying to conceive for nine years. She had been diagnosed with unexplained infertility and possible LPD. She had previously taken clomiphene for eight months without suc-cess. Then she and her husband had done four cycles of ovulation induction with intrauterine inseminations — all failures. Finally, they gathered up their savings and attempted one IVF procedure. She had a fair response to the medication and produced quite a few mature follicles. Three were transferred into her uterus, but no pregnancy resulted. Eventually, Stephanie and her husband adopted a child.

After hearing one of my lectures, Stephanie reluctantly called my clinic just to see if I thought there was any chance she might conceive (she was quite convinced there wasn't). She did not want to get her hopes up and didn't even tell her husband she was coming for a consultation. Her diagnostic questionnaire revealed a pattern of poor eating habits and bouts of abdominal cramping and diarrhea, which had been diagnosed as irritable bowel syndrome. She was tired most of the time but blamed it on having a small child at home. She admitted she couldn't remember ever feeling energetic, though. Stephanie's history included symptoms of bruising easily, hemorrhoids, and premenstrual loose stools. Her menses were characterized as light in amount and watery in consistency. She had low blood pressure and became light-headed when she stood up fast.

During my examination, I noted that her pulse was fine and soggy in quality, and her tongue was pale and slightly swollen, with teeth marks on the sides and a slimy coating. I asked her to monitor her BBT for a couple of months, and at her next visit, she

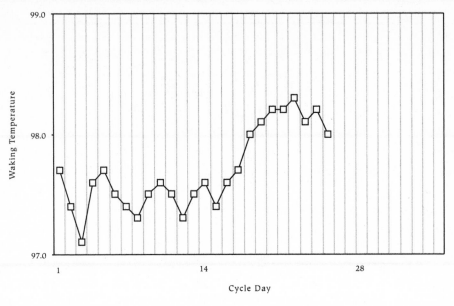

Figure 9.5: Stephanie's BBT Graph — Luteal Phase Defect

brought me graphs she had kept several years earlier (fig. 9.5).

Based upon her medical history, her current physical signs, and her previous BBT graphs, Stephanie was diagnosed with a luteal phase defect caused by Spleen Qi deficiency. I suggested she clean up her diet by not eating so many refined junk foods and avoiding carbonated sodas as a first step. I also suggested she supplement her diet with vitamin B6.

To boost her Spleen Qi, I gave Stephanie an herbal formula including ginseng root (Ren Shen), Astragalus (Huang Qi), Poria cocos (Fu Ling), and Atractylodes (Bai Zhu). I also gave her acupuncture treatments twice a month, one before and one right after ovulation, to boost her Qi and focus it on the reproductive system dur-

ing the time when it would be most effective. I directed her treatments mostly to the Conception meridian and the Spleen/Stomach channels, stimulating St 36, Ren 6, Sp 6, and Ki 7.

Upon starting treatment, Stephanie's symptoms improved almost immediately. She felt more energetic, her digestion improved, and her menstrual blood became redder and more profuse. Her BBT graph showed changes as well (fig. 9.6). Within two months of starting treatment, Stephanie became pregnant. Her BBT graph showed the typical pattern of pregnancy (fig. 9.7). (This is the temperature pattern you are looking for if you wish to become pregnant.) Stephanie gave birth to a healthy baby girl nine months later.

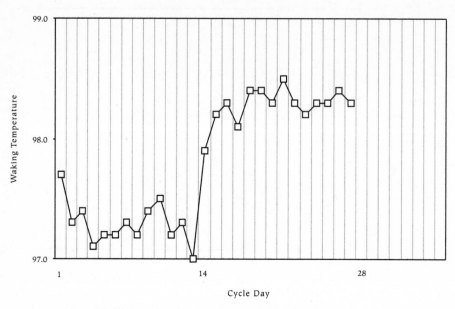

Figure 9.6: Stephanie's BBT Graph — Luteal Phase Defect Improved

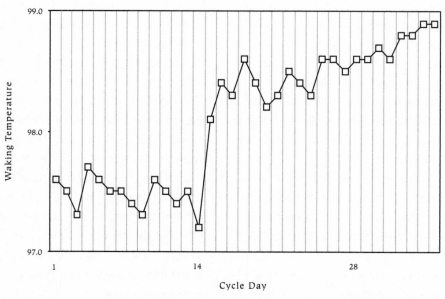

Figure 9.7: Stephanie's BBT Graph — Typical Pregnancy Pattern

10

Advanced Maternal Age (If You're over Thirty-Five, Please Read)

I remember sitting in the clinic waiting room . . . and a woman — she was in her mid-forties and had tried everything to get pregnant — told me that one of the doctors had glanced at her chart and said, "What are you doing here? You are wasting your time." It was so cruel. She was holding out for that one last glimpse of hope. How horrible was it to shoot that hope down?

NANCY GIBBS, "MAKING TIME FOR A BABY," *TIME*, APRIL 15, 2002

The *Nei Jing* recounts a dialogue between the Yellow Emperor and an old Taoist teacher named Chi-Po. The Yellow Emperor asks, "Why does medicine exist?" Chi-Po answers, "Because people have severed themselves from their roots (the Tao)." Chi-Po might very well have answered that medicine exists to help us live longer. Most forms of medicine throughout history have sought to improve longevity. The Chinese believe longevity is deeply connected with one's inner harmony, allowing us to live full, healthy lives. When harmony is disturbed in any way, the result is disease and a shorter life span.

The same is true of our reproductive life span, which is somewhat shorter than our chronological one. For women, the reproductive years are marked by two rites of passage: the first and last menstrual period. In between, however, as every woman will tell you, the menstrual cycle is constantly changing. It is like the ocean, in which every wave is different, its shape determined by a hundred separate factors. A woman's monthly cycle is influenced by physiological, emotional, mental, and spiritual factors. Conventional Western medicine treats her physical body but does very little to restore her overall balance. That is where Chinese medicine provides far more well-being, especially as the "waves" of a woman's reproductive "tides" ebb and she moves closer to menopause.

Many in the Western reproductive medical community believe age is the only factor determining ovarian health. Medical studies conclude that our ovaries start to produce fewer and fewer healthy eggs when we reach our thirties. By age forty, they tell us, we have scant chance of producing an undamaged, healthy egg that can be fertilized. Like the woman Nancy Gibbs describes at the beginning of this chapter, most women in their mid-forties are told they are wasting their time if they seek to become pregnant. But believing these assertions about age-related fertility decline is like believing the only thing influencing the creation of a wave is the amount of water it contains. Certainly, the natural process of aging in every human being brings with it some decrease in fertility. But there are many factors that can help us maintain our fertility regardless of our

age. The ocean of our fertility doesn't dry up; it just becomes still. And with help, it can flow once more.

I liken Western medicine's current view of fertility and aging to the view it used to hold about exercise and aging. Twenty years ago, we were told it was natural for our muscles to get weaker, our bones to shrink, our reflexes to decline, and our faculties to diminish with age. But then researchers discovered that senior citizens who kept doing cardiovascular and weight-training exercises were able to maintain greater levels of strength, bone mass, and agility. They also found that seniors who ate healthy diets and had active social lives were sharper and healthier, and retained their faculties at the levels of much-younger people. Now doctors recognize that the physical decline they had associated with aging has much less to do with biology and more to do with lack of physical activity, poor diet, and lack of mental stimulation.

In the same way, a woman's fertility is influenced by many factors, no matter what her age. Understanding which energies decline with maturation can help restore youthful energetics and, in essence, turn back the reproductive clock. With a little help, we should be able to prolong our reproductive health and longevity.

❧ THE TRUTH ABOUT OUR EGGS

Our ovaries and the millions of eggs residing in them are present before we are born. The number of eggs dwindles to hundreds of thousands by the time we reach puberty. In the perimenopausal period (defined as the period ten years or so before menstruation stops), there are still thousands of eggs remaining in the ovaries. Why is it, then, that our fertility gets lower and the chance of defective eggs higher as we age?

Certainly the DNA contained within our eggs becomes less stable as we get older, and a woman's eggs are usually "healthier" when she's thirty-two than when she's forty. But contrary to what Western medicine would lead us to believe, a woman's eggs do not have an "expiration date." They respond to their surroundings just as the rest of our bodily systems do. This news is a double-edged sword — our ovaries and eggs respond negatively to poor diet, drugs, toxins, and stress hormones, but they also respond positively to a healthy diet and pure lifestyle.

Ultimately, what makes our eggs less responsive is not age but *hormonal fluctuations*. These fluctuations begin in the hypothalamus, the brain's "hormone central." The hypothalamus controls levels of GnRH, which in turn triggers the pituitary to release FSH, which then stimulates our ovaries to develop the follicles, ripen the eggs, release the eggs, produce progesterone, and so on. As we approach middle age, however, our hormonal makeup wavers. The HPO axis —

the invisible network of hormonal relationships governing our reproductive status — becomes less stable. The body pays more attention to maintaining its other systems and less attention to the reproductive system. As a result, the ovaries starve and become less predictable. The eggs contained within them quit responding so well to FSH. More and more of the eggs cycle through the ovary and go to their "resting" state, or atresia, where they no longer respond to hormonal messages. But let me stress that *the ovaries are still well endowed with follicles while these neuroendocrine changes take place.*

Follicle-stimulating hormone is only one of the many hormones and neurochemicals needed to produce healthy eggs. Most women know how long it takes for an egg to develop in the ovary, be released (ovulation), travel to the uterus, and then either be fertilized or be sloughed off in the process of menstruation. This cycle takes anywhere from twenty-five to thirty-one days in most women; its rhythm is the basis of our lives for more than thirty years. But in truth, for an egg to grow from a follicle in its resting state into a full-blown egg ready to be released takes up to *150* days.

Indeed, follicles are selected from the pool of resting follicles almost a year before ovulation, when they are recruited to become biologically active. Then, about five months before ovulation, the 0.03-millimeter follicle is chosen from the pool to double in size (to about 0.06 millimeter) and become a primary follicle. Approximately 120 days before ovulation, it again doubles in size as it reaches its secondary stage. The follicle then cycles through stages called the preantral and antral phases, during which it takes on the appearance of a circular chamber, growing from about 0.12 millimeter to about 1 millimeter in approximately 65 days. Over the course of five months, the follicle has quadrupled in size and has gone through many stages of proliferation.

During this period (before the follicle is signaled by FSH from the pituitary), the follicle responds to hormone-regulating factors within the ovary itself. One important factor that emerges to influence ovarian health is called insulinlike growth factor, which is also the precursor to human growth hormone (hGH), the youth hormone secreted by the thymus gland. Other hormonal factors in the ovaries have names such as insulinlike growth factor binding protein, interleukin, tumor necrosis factor, inhibin, vascular endothelial growth factor, and activin. These ovarian growth factors help determine the eventual fertility potential of the egg. During the time in which a follicle is developing its residing egg, these regulator proteins prepare it to be healthy and responsive.

Only during the last two to three weeks of its cycle through the ovary does the follicle become dominant. During the selection phase, which lasts approximately ten days, the follicle activates mechanisms to make itself responsive to FSH. Now the follicle grows to twice its previous size, rises to the surface of the ovary, and becomes an estrogen-producing follicle. Then it fulfills its major purpose and releases its egg, which leaves the ovary and travels down the fallopian tube, seeking its chance to become fertilized. The follicle ends its life cycle by becoming its own endocrine gland, called the corpus luteum, which secretes the progesterone needed to maintain a pregnancy should the egg be fertilized.

Imagine the potential energy required for these great follicular achievements! It's not surprising that even a small disturbance in this intricate chain of hormonal and physiological events can have a detrimental effect on our fertility. And age is only one of the factors that can disturb this delicate balance.

THE EFFECTS OF AGING ON OUR FERTILITY

A woman in her forties often will be turned away from any chance at Western medicine's ART because of her age and the "poor" state of her ovaries. She may indeed fail to respond as favorably as her younger counterpart to the hormones provided by ARTs because her eggs have become less receptive to hormonal stimulation. She may produce fewer eggs, and their outer capsule may be tougher, diminishing their potential for fertilization. Eggs that do become fertilized may have more inclusions (waste products put out by the mitochondria) during early embryologic development. Fewer fertilized eggs make it to the blastocyst (five-day) stage, even fewer are capable of implantation, and fewer still make it through full embryonic development. That is why a woman over age forty is statistically less likely to give birth and is encouraged to find alternative ways of becoming a mother. Her reproductive endocrinologist will tell her she has poor-quality eggs and then strongly suggest she consider using the eggs of a younger donor. This technique does make her chances of having a baby (and thus her doctor's success rate) much higher. But even with donor eggs, older women have less of a chance of conceiving. The problem with all ART isn't just the quality of the eggs an older woman produces: the real problem is that the only portion of the hormonal process ART addresses is the last few weeks of an egg's journey from initial follicle to released egg.

True, as a woman ages, the many-month process of follicular development becomes susceptible to breakdown. However, this has three very specific and measurable causes. First, if we don't take good care of our bodies in general, no reproductive therapy will make up for our lack of health. For the seed to be planted, the field as well as the seed must possess the conditions of fertility. If women wish to become pregnant, they had better be eating well, exercising, and reducing the stress levels in their life.

Second, as our bodies age, the blood flow to the ovaries begins to decline precipitously. As we approach menopause, the ovarian blood flow is around five times less than when we were in our reproductive prime. The follicular fluid contains rising levels of vascular endothelial growth factor, the same chemical found in a damaged heart. It signals the body that the follicular tissue is being starved of blood flow. (Better circulation to any organ improves its function, and this is also true of the ovaries and their residing eggs. Acupuncture and acupressure are the only known methods to improve the blood flow to the ovaries.)

Third, as I explained earlier, a woman's hormone levels fluctuate more as she ages. The lack of communication between the brain, the pituitary gland, and the ovaries makes the follicles resistant, and they quit paying attention to FSH — not surprising, since the poor ovaries are undernourished by lack of blood flow. And trying to trigger the undernourished follicles to develop into eggs is like trying to whip a starving ox into working harder. He doesn't need more lashes; he needs more food! Unfortunately, the FSH-producing chemicals used in ART aren't going to produce any better response than a woman's own FSH.

It seems logical to assume that if we could encourage a woman's body to return to more youthful levels of hormonal balance and blood flow, then the ovaries would produce and release eggs in the same way they did when we were younger. This assumption was confirmed in a recent scientific study in which the ovaries of older rats that had stopped ovulating were transplanted into hormonally youthful rats' bodies. Once the older rats' ovaries were placed in the hormonally youthful environment of the younger rats, the old ovaries became capable of ovulating again.

If women want to become pregnant in their forties, they need to provide more hormonal fuel and blood flow to their remaining thousands of eggs. Western medicine has attempted to do this with injections of hormones designed to hyperstimulate our ovaries. However, this approach does not address the root causes of age-related infertility: imbalances within the HPO axis, reduction of blood flow to the ovaries, and the internal environment, which affects follicular development over the months prior to ovulation. Luckily, the techniques of Chinese medicine have been proven to restore communication to the HPO axis and nourish the ovaries. The result is plentiful hormone production and proper follicular response.

How do we give the HPO axis the attention it needs to express its full reproductive vigor? Fortunately, the steps involved in turning back the reproductive clock are all natural. Unfortunately, rejuvenating the reproductive system takes time. With a little effort, however, older women can give the entire reproductive-psychoneuroendocrinologic system the attention that a young woman's body provides effortlessly. Through TCM, we can help direct the body's attention to the midbrain, pituitary, ovaries, and uterus, as well as create the spiritual, mental, and emotional health required to produce healthy eggs, provide appropriate conditions for their fertilization, and foster a welcoming environment in the uterus so the egg may be implanted, grow into a fetus, and be carried to term.

❦ THE CHINESE VIEW OF AGING

Turn your attention back to three of the Extraordinary meridians covered in chapter 3 — the Penetrating, Conception, and Governing. In TCM, these three meridians are the equivalent of the HPO axis. The energies flowing through these meridians become fulfilled when a girl reaches menarche and depleted when a woman enters menopause. (Statistically, the earlier a young woman first menstruates, the later her entrance into menopause will be.) A woman's reproductive age span is primarily a function of her underlying congenital source Qi, the lifetime Essence of the Kidney, which we have at birth and which can be supplemented by Spleen Qi throughout life.

The Penetrating meridian originates in the Uterus, presides over the function of menstruation, and governs the hormonal cycles. The energies of the Conception and Governing meridians — the Yin and the Yang of the endocrine system — arise from the Penetrating meridian. The inherent functions of these meridians are the basic forces of our internal nature that determine genetic health, cellular division, continued development, maturity, and decline. According to the *Nei Jing,* as a woman approaches the age of seven times seven (forty-nine), her Kidney Essence declines, her menses cease, and *then* she is incapable of bearing children. We all have been programmed with a certain reproductive energetic potential controlling hormonal fluctuations and eventual

regression. But even the *Nei Jing* concedes that our reproductive potential is not fixed but subject to certain environmental and internal factors that can stave off or accelerate the decline of our fertility.

The usual process of reproductive transition from a fertile to a nonfertile state spans many years. Ideally, it should be a smooth evolution from an energetic focus on self (prepuberty) to an energetic focus on reproduction (menarche) to an eventual outward energetic shift toward wisdom (menopause). This transition is physiological, psychological, and spiritual. The physical ramifications of these shifting energies begin when a girl enters menarche, when the hormonal system is effulgent and the Penetrating meridian brims over. After this, the menses arrive like a tide as the Uterus fills and empties from one full moon to the next. When a woman's reproductive life span nears completion, the energies are transferred from the Uterus to the Heart via the Penetrating and Conception meridians. A woman moves from a state of procreation (represented by the Kidney system) to a state of wisdom (represented by the Heart). This is seen as a literal shifting of energies.

If our bodies are resistant to this energetic transition from the Uterus upward to the Heart, these rising energies, under pressure, will produce heat signs like hot flashes and night sweats. Irritability will result from the obstructed flow of Qi. The Kidney system will become depleted and will no longer be able to support bone growth, leading to osteoporosis. When we treat menopause with TCM, we make this transition smooth and complete. When we treat age-related fertility factors, we interrupt and stall this transition, regulating the hormones and making them function as if they were young again.

Two specific areas are affected by the aging of a woman's reproductive system: the Kidney and the Spleen. Treat these with acupuncture, diet and lifestyle, and herbs, and you can often turn back the clock and restore higher levels of fertility.

THE KIDNEY SYSTEM

In Chinese medicine, the Kidney system is the seat of our genetic constitution and underlies all other metabolic processes. The Kidneys dictate growth and development. They are responsible for bone and teeth formation and overall brain function. They control water balance and elimination. The Kidney system supports and links the reproductive system, the skeletal system, the neurological system, and the endocrine system. The Kidneys provide Essence for the Uterus and menstruation. When the Kidney Essence becomes depleted, women go into menopause. The Extraordinary meridians governing endocrine relationships cannot be separated from the Kidney system. The signs and symptoms of declining Kidney function parallel an actual decline in hormone levels.

When the Kidney system begins to decline as a woman ages, she will manifest symptoms that include signs of Kidney Yin deficiency (**Ki Yi–**), Kidney Yang deficiency (**Ki Yan–**), or both. As you may remember from chapter 4, signs and symptoms of Kidney Yin deficiency (**Ki Yi–**) include:

- low levels of estrogen
- night sweats
- hot flashes
- vaginal dryness
- low back weakness, soreness, or pain
- knee problems
- ringing in the ears
- dizziness
- scanty fertile cervical mucus
- excessive fear
- dark circles around the eyes
- scanty menstruation
- a tongue lacking in coating and appearing shiny or peeled

Symptoms of Kidney Yang deficiency (**Ki Yan–**) include:

- a sore or weak lower back that tends to feel worse premenstrually
- cold feet at night
- feeling cold in general
- low libido
- frequent, diluted, or nighttime urination
- excessive fear
- early morning loose, urgent stools
- profuse vaginal discharge
- dull menstrual blood
- menstrual cramps that respond to a heating pad
- a moist, pale tongue

TCM IN ACTION: CHARLOTTE'S STORY

Charlotte was forty-one when she first came to see me. She was a dietician who had recently married a gynecologist, and they had just failed their tenth cycle of hormonally stimulated IUIs. She didn't feel she was getting satisfactory results from her reproductive endocrinologist and came to see me because her friend had become pregnant through my clinic. Even so, Charlotte was skeptical about my ability to improve her situation. Her husband humored her for seeking alternatives but did not support her decision.

Charlotte had been diagnosed with cervical stenosis (a narrowed or constricted cervix) and advanced maternal age, hence the hormonal stimulation and IUIs. Her greatest concern, however, was her "aging" eggs, which she imagined (and her doctor confirmed) were responsible for her failure to conceive. She ovulated every month, but she had no fertile cervical mucus and no cervical response to the hormonal stimulation. The inseminations were always painful (as well as unsuccessful) because her cervix was closed at ovulation.

Charlotte had all the signs and symptoms of both Kidney Yin and Kidney Yang deficiency: sore low back premenstrually, weak knees, nighttime urination, low libido, lack of cervical fluid, etc. Her cervix was not responding to the hormonal stimulation because she didn't have the endocrine balance required to orchestrate the many series of physiologic changes for successful ovula-

tion, fertilization, implantation, and pregnancy. I began treating her with acupuncture and herbs to nourish the Kidney system. She took variants of the herbal formulas Six Flavor Pill with Rehmannia (Liu Wei Di Huang Wan), Eight Ingredient Pill with Rehmannia (Ba Wei Di Huang Wan), and Four Substances Decoction with Curculigo (Si Wu Tang with Xian Mao), along with Epimedium (Yin Yang Huo) and the five seeds — Rubus (Fu Pen Zi), Lycium (Gou Qi Zi), Plantago (Che Qian Zi), Cuscuta (Tu Si Zi), and Schisandra (Wu Wei Zi). I stimulated acupoints Ki 3, Ki 7, Ren 3, Ren 4, Ren 6, Zigong, St 30, and the intertragic notch of the ear. Charlotte had been a vegetarian for most of her adult life, aggravating the Yang aspect of her Kidney deficiency (and, therefore, affecting the Essence and Yin), so I urged her to eat more Yang-tonifying foods like walnuts.

After two months of tonifying her Kidney system, Charlotte was producing cervical mucus, and after three months, when an insemination was performed, her cervix was wide open. She conceived that same month. Her pulse changed dramatically upon conception, and we knew she was pregnant well before she saw the double line on the urine pregnancy test.

Western medical treatments had merely addressed the manifestation of her problem rather than its cause. When we addressed and corrected the root of the imbalance, Charlotte became pregnant. (Even Charlotte's gynecologist husband conceded that the acupuncture and herbal treatments were what finally made the difference.) They have since had a second child, this time without any hormonal stimulation or inseminations.

SP– SPLEEN QI DEFICIENCY

The Spleen energies weaken with age right along with the Kidneys', and often precede the Kidneys' decline. Since the Spleen supplements Kidney Essence, both organ systems must be maintained for optimum reproductive health. The first clue that Spleen function is waning is fatigue. We just seem to require more energy to get the same amount of work done than we did a few years ago. To combat our fatigue, many of us turn to caffeine, which artificially stimulates the brain and allows us to function with a little more energy. However, caffeine itself provides no additional energy to the body. It merely borrows it from — you guessed it — the Kidneys. When the Kidneys are taxed by caffeine and other stressors and still have to

preside over menstruation, hormonal functioning, the skeletal system, the neurological system, and the endocrine system, guess what suffers? Reproduction — a process that is unnecessary for the body's survival.

Another sign of waning Spleen energies is when things start to "fall." Our skin begins to sag, our breasts fall, veins appear on the surface of our skin, we get hemorrhoids, and our uterus falls into our bladder. We have to pee more often. Our blood pressure fluctuates. Our digestion and elimination become more sensitive. Progesterone levels drop off during the luteal phase. Periods come earlier and are often accompanied by loose stools. Our metabolism changes. Even our protective mechanisms start to falter. We react more to our environment and catch cold more often. Sounds like a pretty accurate description of the aging process for women, doesn't it? Luckily, strengthening our Spleen energies can help reverse these uncomfortable signs of aging.

TREATMENT FOR AGE-RELATED FERTILITY DECLINE

To improve our chances of getting pregnant after age forty, we first need to make sure our bodies are maintained at peak efficiency and health. We know our overall capacity for cell repair and resistance can be affected by improving our environment; exercising; reducing stressors; eating a more organic,

whole-foods diet; and taking appropriate nutritional and herbal supplements. Therefore, correct dietary practices and exercise routines are the first things you should adopt to raise your fertility quotient and maintain reproductive vigor.

Even Western medicine recognizes the

importance of these two factors in reproductive health. In *Definition & Character of Reproductive Aging & Senescence*, R. G. Godsen and C. E. Finch state, "Dietary and endocrine manipulations can also slow the pace of ovarian aging." A study in *Biological Reproduction* (Nelsen, Godsen, and Felicio, 1985) reported that feeding a low-calorie diet to rodents slowed the disappearance of ovarian follicles. Whole foods that nourish the Spleen, the Kidneys, and the Blood (see specific dietary recommendations below, as well as in chapter 6) will help restore vitality, as will avoiding alcohol, caffeine, and nicotine. Any form of stimulant will age us prematurely. In fact, even moderate tobacco use has been estimated to advance the onset of menopause by up to three years and increase the rate of follicular atresia (causing more eggs to go into the resting phase rather than be released) by 7 percent. Moderate exercise at least three times per week helps improve the circulation to the internal organs and boosts skin and musculoskeletal tone.

In addition to increasing the fundamental health of our cells, we should also employ methods to tonify the energies of both the Spleen and the Kidney. Below are several suggestions to help you support your reproductive system as well as your Spleen, Kidney, and Penetrating meridian. Along with these steps, however, you must make sure your overall health is supported. Exercise regularly. Get enough sleep. Maintain a positive attitude. Connect with your inner source. Feel yourself in tune with a beneficent nature. You are doing everything you can to allow conception to happen naturally. Let nature take its course while you restore your body's natural state of health and fertility.

DIET AND SUPPLEMENTS

DIET

- Avoid junk food, caffeine, tobacco, sodas, sweeteners, and refined carbohydrates.
- Whenever possible, avoid dairy products, raw vegetables, and cold foods.
- Do not eat any meat or animal products treated with growth hormone. This includes most of the meat, eggs, milk products, and cheese found at the supermarket. You can find hormone-free dairy and meat products at many health-food stores.
- Eat the foods recommended to tonify the Kidney and Spleen (see chapter 6). Supplement your diet with royal jelly, blue-green algae, wheatgrass, and chlorella.

SUPPLEMENTS

- *Coenzyme Q-10 (co Q-10)* — this is a supplement commonly used for cardiovascular disorders. Co Q-10 helps support and improve mitochondrial function, which is the powerhouse of the cell. One of the hallmarks of aging is damage to mitochondrial DNA caused by oxygen metabolism and the presence of free radicals in the system. This damage has also been shown to contribute to age-related decline in egg quality. A way to improve cellular function is to supplement your diet with enzymes like co Q-10. Antioxidants (vitamins C, E, A, zinc, and selenium) and superantioxidants (pycnogenol) also help prevent free-radical damage to cell mitochondria.

- *Human growth hormone (hGH)* — many women are taking hGH analogues such as insulinlike growth factor (a precursor to growth hormone that naturally declines with age) to improve the quality and quantity of their egg production. However, this method has not been proven effective scientifically. Some companies are manufacturing products touted to encourage your pituitary gland to produce more hGH using amino acids like L-arginine, glycine, L-ornithine HCl, L-glutamine, L-lysine, and bovine colostrum. Human growth hormone is not available as a dietary supplement because the molecule cannot be utilized orally. In the United States, hGH is available by prescribed injection as Somatropin.
- *Dehydroepiandrosterone (DHEA)* — some studies have shown that DHEA (a hormonal building block) can be used instead of growth hormone to help ovarian response. A study published in *Human Reproduction* (2000) reported that taking 80 milligrams per day of DHEA for two months improved response to ovarian stimulation in each woman in the study. The ovaries of the women who took DHEA responded better to the gonadotropic drugs.

❧ NOTE: Women who have elevated levels of male hormones should not supplement with DHEA.

- *L-arginine* — a study published in *Human Reproduction* (1999) found increased ovarian response, endometrial receptivity, and pregnancy rates in IVF patients who supplemented daily with large doses (16 grams) of oral L-arginine, an amino acid. These studies have not been reproduced in women who are experiencing a natural cycle, but the response remains the same: increased blood flow to the ovaries. I generally recommend that women take no more than 4 grams per day of L-arginine.

BALANCING ENERGIES
USING ACUPUNCTURE,
ACUPRESSURE, AND MASSAGE

- Perform the femoral massage technique described in chapter 6 to direct more blood flow to the ovaries and uterus.
- Perform daily acupressure, magnet, or light therapy on the uterus and ovary points on the lower abdomen.
- Massage the endocrine (intertragic notch) and reproductive organ (triangular fossa) points on the ear each day.
- Stimulate the acupressure points to tonify the Kidney and Spleen every other day (see chapter 7).

HERBAL THERAPIES

The following herbs help nourish the Blood, Qi, and Kidneys. In addition, when they are taken for the correctly diagnosed pattern (see above and chapter 4), they can help lower FSH levels. See chapter 8 for more information on the specific properties of these herbs.

Astragalus (Huang Qi)
ginseng (Ren Shen)
chaste tree berry (Vitex)
false unicorn (Helonias)
Angelica (Dang Gui)
Epimedium (Yin Yang Huo)
Dipsacus (Xu Duan)
Atractylodes (Bai Zhu)
Dioscorea (Shan Yao)
Eucommia (Du Zhong)
Codonopsis (Dang Shen)
Rubus (Fu Pen Zi)
Cuscuta (Tu Si Zi)
Cornus (Shan Zhu Yu)

Here are three specific herbal formulas prescribed in TCM for age-related reproductive decline.

Two Immortals Decoction — indicated for perimenopausal symptoms including amenorrhea, hot flashes, night sweats, fatigue, depression, insomnia, irritability, and hypertension, and other symptoms of Kidney Yin and Yang deficiency (**Ki Yi–, Ki Yan–**) with deficiency heat. Two Immortals contains Curculigo (Xian Mao), Epimedium (Yin Yang Huo), Morinda (Ba Ji Tian), Phellodendron (Huang Bai), Anemarrhena (Zhi Mu), and Angelica (Dang Gui).

Special Pill to Aid Fertility — treats symptoms of Kidney Yang deficiency (**Ki Yan–**), Qi and Blood deficiency (**Qi–/Bl–**). In addition to aching and weakness of the lower back, symptoms of fatigue and listlessness would be common in this presentation. The mixture contains aconite (Fu Zi), cinnamon bark (Rou Gui), Cistanches (Rou Cong Rong), Morinda (Ba Ji Tian), Epimedium (Yin Yang Huo), Cnidium (She Chuang Zi), Curculigo (Xian Mao), Cornus (Shan Zhu Yu), Eucommia (Du Zhong), cooked Rehmannia (Shu Di Huang), Angelica (Dang Gui), Lycium (Gou Qi Zi), and Atractylodes (Bai Zhu).

Er Si Wu He Ji — puts the emphasis on the Kidney Essence, Yang, and Blood. It is very commonly used for treating fertility problems in China. It contains Curculigo (Xian Mao), Epimedium (Yin Yang Huo), white peony (Bai Shao), Ligusticum (Chuan Xiong), cooked Rehmannia (Shu Di Huang), Schisandra (Wu Wei Zi), Cuscuta (Tu Si Zi), Rubus (Fu Pen Zi), Lycium (Gou Qi Zi), and Plantago (Che Qian Zi).

Here is the conundrum for a woman with age-related infertility: it takes a minimum of three months to maximize the health of the developing follicle and its residing egg. Yet with each month of natural treatment, we are losing precious time. We feel we don't *have* three or six months to wait. This process requires an extraordinary level of patience. The good news is that with the natural treatments provided by TCM, we can extend our fertility past the age when many Western medical doctors tell us it is impossible for us to get pregnant. And, as you'll see from the following story, TCM can make it not only possible but natural for us to conceive and bear a healthy child.

TCM in Action: Barbara's Baby

When she first consulted me, Barbara was forty-two years and eight months old. She was single and had her own business, which took her out of the country each month. Although she didn't have a partner, she knew she wanted a child, and her age was not going to provide her the luxury of finding the right father. She had been having IUIs with frozen sperm purchased from a sperm bank every month, but she would start to spot about a week after ovulation. She had been diagnosed by her Western medical doctors with a thyroid imbalance and was currently taking synthetic thyroid hormone (Synthroid). The reproductive clinic also prescribed progesterone suppositories for her to take after the inseminations, but this did not curtail the bleeding. She had previously done three cycles of Clomid stimulation, but her response had not changed.

Barbara put herself in my care with complete trust. Her diet was already healthy — she had been reading about nutrition and consulted a nutritionist for supplementation.

She was tired most of the time, was beginning to get varicose veins, bruised easily, and had low blood pressure. Her menstrual flow started out light pink in color and was rather watery in consistency. Then the flow became quite heavy and lasted about seven days. I diagnosed her with a Spleen Qi deficiency. We began weekly treatments of acupuncture, and she took herbal formulas religiously to supplement her Spleen Qi. She decided not to resume inseminations until she could hold a luteal phase. She also began monitoring her BBT so we could assess her hormonal status.

Barbara's chart proved somewhat erratic. In her first month, she ovulated later than usual and had a short luteal phase with a chaotic pattern. After about two months on the herbs, her luteal phase lengthened, but she was still spotting. She also reported that she got a nosebleed each month just before her period. Once again this confirmed the diagnosis of deficient Spleen Qi, which was unable to hold the blood in its proper place.

Barbara began to feel as if the Synthroid was doing her more harm than good, and after consulting her internist, she quit taking it. She continued with the herbs I'd prescribed to supplement her Spleen Qi (which, coincidentally, affects thyroid imbalances as well), and within six weeks, her thyroid levels were within normal limits. Her energy was much better than it had been previously, and her menstrual blood became less profuse.

By this time, Barbara had turned forty-three and was becoming anxious about her biological clock. She began the monthly inseminations again, even though her spotting and nosebleeds were still present. Meanwhile, her BBT graphs were improving. They showed she was ovulating on day 15 or 16, and was having 29- to 30-day cycles. The luteal phase was adequate in length, but her temperature would still dip when she spotted. I counseled patience. After three more (agonizing) months of acupuncture and herbs, the nosebleeds and spotting were gone.

The next month was the magical one. About twelve days after Barbara's insemination, she came in for her regular appointment and told me she knew she wasn't pregnant because her breasts weren't tender, and she just didn't feel like it had been successful. But when I felt her pulse, it had taken on the lively, vibrant quality of pregnancy. I assured her she had succeeded. Barbara carried her baby to term and gave birth soon after she turned forty-four. Mother and daughter make a great team.

TCM IN ACTION: EDITH'S IVF

Edith, a nurse practitioner, came to my clinic after years of trying to become pregnant naturally and almost two years of back-to-back IVF cycles. She had married late in life, at age thirty-eight, and she and her new husband had tried to start a family immediately. But month after month, she failed to conceive. Edith was not emotionally prepared for the disappointment. She gave up her profession to focus on becoming a mother. She went to numerous infertility specialists and reproductive endocrinolo-gists. She had her fallopian tubes evaluated and her hormone levels checked; she took (and passed) Clomid challenge tests; she had her uterus inspected hysteroscopically and had uterine biopsies and ultrasounds. She had no history of abnormal menstrual bleeding, ovarian cysts, endometriosis, fibroids, or any other menstrual disorder. Still she couldn't conceive, and even with all the tests, her doctors could come no closer to explaining why she was unable to become pregnant. The only possible reason, they told her, was her age.

The doctors started Edith on a course of hormonally stimulated IUIs, and when those were not successful, IVF procedures. Although Edith's response to the IVF drugs was adequate, no pregnancy resulted. Until she turned forty-two, she was always encouraged by her physicians to keep trying; it was just a matter of beating the odds. However, by the time Edith was forty-four (nine IVFs later), she had still not achieved a pregnancy. Now her previous fertility specialists wouldn't treat her anymore because she was just "too old."

Edith called me very close to her forty-fifth birthday. When I answered the phone, she demanded answers. She wanted to know my experience with age-related infertility, my background and training, my success rates, and, lastly, if I believed I could help her. She had obviously come to the point of mistrusting her health care providers. Although I answered all of her questions to her satisfaction, quite frankly I did not know if she had any remaining potential. I told her she may have called too late. She insisted on coming in for an evaluation, and I agreed. (While I am brutally frank with my patients, I always give them a chance.)

I saw Edith twice a week (at her urging) for about five months. She was strong, had normal menstrual cycles, ovulated mid-cycle, had a fourteen-day luteal phase, and was otherwise very healthy. She had a slight Spleen Qi deficiency that manifested as urinary problems, including cystitis. She never thought this problem was related to her inability to conceive, but I did. I used acupuncture and herbal techniques to strengthen the Spleen, lift the Qi, and resolve the damp heat condition I had diagnosed. I also supplemented her Kidneys, assuming that they were involved because of her age.

After five months of treatment, Edith told me she had found a reproductive endocrinologist in another state who would treat women over forty-three. She wanted to go through one more IVF procedure and asked me to "gear her up." I did. We stimulated her ovaries with acupuncture treatments to flood them with more energy and Blood. She continued to take herbs to tonify the Spleen, lift the Qi, nourish the Uterus, and supplement the Kidneys.

After her egg retrieval, Edith called me, absolutely ecstatic. She reported that she had had her best cycle ever: eight eggs had been retrieved, and all of them were successfully fertilized. She became pregnant with twins, but lost one of the babies shortly after implantation. After Edith's forty-sixth birthday, she gave birth to her son. She is probably the proudest mother I have ever met.

While Barbara's and Edith's stories are inspirational, and enhancing our natural reproductive capacity will usually maximize the possibility of conceiving a child, we cannot wait too long and override nature. According to an old Chinese proverb "The Yangtze never runs backwards . . . man recaptures not his youth." It is important for women of all ages to realize that there is much that can be done to preserve, enhance, and increase our fertility at almost every stage of life. However, life's other stages are just as important — and rewarding — as our childbearing years. The time of childhood before sexual maturity is one of incredible physical, mental, and emotional growth. The time of wisdom, when our fertile years are over, can be equally fulfilling. Our energies move from our reproductive center to the heart. We become nurturers in a different sense. There is much we can do to extend our childbearing years if needed, but we also must learn to celebrate the stages of our lives as they occur and to maintain our health at its highest level no matter what our age.

11

"Unexplained Infertility": Overcoming the Most Frustrating Diagnosis

Let [her] who seeks, not cease seeking until [s]he finds.

— THE GOSPEL ACCORDING TO SAINT THOMAS

"We don't know why you're not getting pregnant." These are some of the most frustrating words a woman can hear from her doctor. Usually, by the time she hears that sentence, she has undergone an extensive array of tests. If none of these tests pinpoint her problem, her doctor will likely recommend some kind of surgical procedure to evaluate the health of her reproductive organs. Finally, if the doctor suspects that male as well as female factors are causing the problem (as is true in one of every four infertile couples), the woman's partner will undergo his own series of tests, measurements, and even surgeries.

Even with all these tests and all this information, unexplained infertility is still an all-too-common diagnosis. According to RESOLVE, a national nonprofit infertility network, up to 30 percent of all cases of infertility in women and 25 percent in men are the result of idiopathic (unexplained) causes. Multitudes of women diagnosed with infertility will never know the cause of their condition.

"Unexplained infertility" means that there is no medical reason the doctors can find within the realm of modern scientific understanding to explain why conception is not occurring. Many women with irregular menstrual cycles who are unable to conceive are given the diagnosis of unexplained infertility because their laboratory blood analyses show hormonal levels within the "normal" range. Couples with unexplained infertility are either told to go home and keep trying, or they are subjected to different clinical procedures in the hope that one of the solutions offered by Western medicine will work. Often these couples are pointed toward ART procedures, the theory being that putting sperm directly into the uterus (as is done during an IUI), or fertilizing her eggs outside the body and then providing a chemically enhanced environment

for their implantation, might bypass their mysterious fertility problems.

There are many steps in the journey of fertility, and even a small misstep can make the difference between a happy mother and a woman faced with unexplained infertility. One hormone produced at the wrong time in the menstrual cycle, a tiny change in the pH of cervical mucus, or a millimeter less depth in the endometrial lining can be the deciding factor between a pregnancy and yet another period. Western medicine may be very good at measuring such differences when they reach critical levels; but what of subclinical — i.e., too small to be measured — problems that may still be significant enough to keep a woman from getting pregnant?

THE EASTERN APPROACH TO UNEXPLAINED INFERTILITY

Luckily, TCM is particularly effective in treating women (and men) with this frustrating diagnosis. In Eastern medicine, "unexplained infertility" translates simply to "impaired reproductive functioning," and reproductive functioning can be healed and supported by bringing the entire body back into balance.

The first step is always to address the manifestation of the problem and determine the underlying pattern. In most cases of unexplained infertility, there is some sort of indication of where the problem lies —

whether it be in symptoms involving the menstrual cycle, or feelings of hot or cold, lethargy or nervousness, and so on. As you remember from chapter 4, when you are diagnosed using the principles of TCM, all these objective and subjective symptoms are taken into account. In addition, TCM uses the diagnostic tools of pulse reading and examination of the tongue to unveil imbalances in your particular system. And when these imbalances are addressed, the reproductive system can begin to function normally.

The Western approach is like trying to

return a lake to purity once it's been contaminated by toxic waste. You could try to treat the lake by finding out exactly what the contaminants in the water are, then using different chemicals to neutralize their effects — but all you'd end up with is water with even more chemicals in it. The Eastern way to purify the water isn't to add more chemicals but to put more clean water into the lake. You can do that by making sure that the streams feeding the lake are clean, healthy, and flowing as freely as possible, and that the old, toxic water can flow out as new water flows in. Once the ecological balance of the water is restored, the entire lake will return to health, and the fish and animals living in and around the lake will thrive. That's what TCM does for a woman's body: it allows clean, pure, healthy energy to flow in while allowing old, toxic energy to be eliminated. With balanced energy, the body restores its natural condition of health. The organs and different systems of the body, including the reproductive system, function as they were designed to do. And the resulting conditions are far more conducive for conception.

MENSTRUAL FLOW IRREGULARITIES

One of the first places we can look to diagnose unexplained infertility is the menstrual flow itself. Many women have told me, "I've always thought my period was abnormal, but my doctor told me it didn't matter." If the menstrual blood is unusual in amount, color, and consistency, this usually indicates a problem within the uterine lining. If the blood flow is scanty and all other signs lead to Blood deficiency (**Bl–**), then you should tonify the Blood by following the Spleen-fortifying diet, which helps the Spleen produce more Blood during the follicular phase. You also can take herbs like Angelica (Dang Gui), red raspberry, and white peony (Bai Shao). Once the Blood is rectified, the blood flow will increase, and the endometrial lining will thicken.

If the menstrual blood is scant, black or very dark, and accompanied by stabbing pain, this indicates a condition of Blood stasis (**Bl X**). You should supplement the diet with seaweed, evening primrose oil, and safflower. Local application of warm castor-oil packs may resolve the Blood stasis and its associated toxic residue. This allows the uterine lining to respond with fresh, healthy endometrial tissue — the type of environment embryos prefer when searching for a home.

Another manifestation of the failure of the uterine lining to respond appropriately to the warming hormone (progesterone) is known as cold Uterus, or cold Womb (**CW**). Cold Uterus causes the vessels supplying blood to the uterus to constrict as a result of the "cold" response. Women with this diagnosis often have a combination of Kidney Yang deficiency (**Ki Yan–**) and Blood stasis (**Bl X**). They usually will have premenstrual lower back pain, cramps that respond to heating pads, and clotty menstrual blood. I prescribe warming herbs like Vitex, Damiana, and Morinda, and Blood-invigorating supplements like fish oil and OPC/pycnogenol, as well as peach kernel (Tao Ren). The acupoints SP 10 and UB 17 also invigorate the blood. The Chinese herbal formula Wen Jing Tang (Warm the Menses Decoction) warms the Yang and invigorates the Blood. It's also helpful to warm the lower abdomen with heat packs or a water bottle before ovulation.

USING BBT MONITORING TO DIAGNOSE YOUR PATTERN

Monitoring BBT can give you lots of information regarding any imbalances in your cycle. Relatively low temperatures (around 97 degrees Fahrenheit) that do not exhibit a biphasic pattern at all and are accompanied by cold signs like feeling cold; having cold feet, especially at night; and clear, profuse urination reveal a diagnostic pattern of Kidney Yang deficiency (**Ki Yan–**). When Kidney Yang is supplemented, a biphasic ovulatory pattern will begin to emerge, and reproductive hormones will respond accordingly. On the other hand, a single-phase pattern of high temperatures accompanied by heat signs like feeling too hot; red skin; red, irritated eyes; and sweating will respond to Yin supplementation and clearing of heat. You can supplement Yin and clear heat with the Chinese herbal formula Anemarrhena, Phellodendron, and Rehmannia Pill (Zhi Bai Di Huang Wan) and acupoints like Ki 3, Sp 6, Sp 10, and LI 11.

WHAT ABOUT STRESS?

I believe that one of the most underdiagnosed contributing factors to unexplained infertility is stress. The body knows we should not be pregnant when we are under tremendous stress: after all, the body's first priority is keeping us out of danger, and taking care of a fetus when we are experiencing a precarious or tense situation is an overwhelming strain. Indeed, our hormonal response to stress is actually antagonistic to our fertility. For instance, the hormone adrenaline is released by the adrenal glands during conditions of stress. Although adrenaline helps us to escape from danger, it also inhibits our ability to utilize progesterone, thus impeding our fertility. Another hormone, prolactin, is usually released by the pituitary gland to stimulate lactation in preparation for nursing. Prolactin also inhibits a woman's fertility so she won't become pregnant again while she is nursing. However, in times of stress, the pituitary gland emits higher levels of prolactin. It's as if our bodies don't want us pregnant during times of high stress. (High prolactin levels also tell me the Qi is obstructed and needs to be circulated.)

Liver Qi stagnation (**Lv Qi X**) occurs as a result of our poor adaptation to stress. Liver Qi stagnation is often indicated by a sawtoothed, erratic temperature pattern on the BBT graph, showing there is not enough hormonal regulation to normalize the cycle. In addition, women who exhibit no pattern at all to their menstrual cycles often have Liver Qi stagnation. One month, the cycle may last thirty-five days, and the next month, it is twenty-six days. There are severe premenstrual signs some months, and other months there are almost none. The problem most assuredly lies in the Liver Qi and is caused by stress and its associated endocrine effects. The remedy will be to soften the Liver and rectify the Qi with meditation, deep-breathing exercises, and stimulation of acupoints Lv 3, Lv 8, and Lv 14.

When we are under stress, the sympathetic nervous system (the part that accelerates heart rate, constricts blood vessels, and raises blood pressure) can become hyperstimulated, flooding the muscles with blood and telling us to either fight or flee from danger. However, a hyperstimulated nervous system sends *less* blood to the uterus and ovaries, thereby impairing their optimal functioning. If you tend to sweat more than normal; have cold, sweaty, or clammy hands and/or feet, especially under stress; have consistently dilated pupils or sweat when you feel anxious; grind your teeth or have tension headaches, you probably have a hyperstimu-

lated nervous system. This translates into excess heat, which is either caused by Liver Qi stagnation (**Lv Qi X**) or heat from a Heart deficiency (**Ht–**). To calm and supplement the sympathetic nervous system, you might supplement with calcium and magnesium, and take herbs like unripened· wheat grain (Fu Xiao Mai) and Ephedra root (Ma Huang Gen), which are usually prescribed to stop abnormal sweating.

🐦 NOTE: Ma Huang Gen is the root of the Ephedra plant and is not to be mistaken for Ma Huang, the stem, which has a stimulant effect. The two herbs are *not* interchangeable.

Much of the stress we experience in modern times has nothing to do with the "life or death" response that triggers adrenaline, prolactin, and sympathetic nervous system hyperstimulation. Most of our stress has more to do with perception rather than real danger. Indeed, one of the biggest stresses for women is the failure to conceive and a diagnosis of infertility, often compounded when the diagnosis is unexplained infertility.

When the stressor is only one of perception, or when you are responding inappropriately to stress with nervous tension, you must retrain your body and let it know you are not in immediate danger regardless of your environmental situation. You can help the body overcome the stress response in a number of ways. First, get rid of as many external stressors in your life as you are able to control. If your job is causing you a lot of stress, change it. If certain people are causing you stress, you may wish to avoid them for a while. If you're one of those women who do too much and are stressed about it, figure out ways to cut back on the number of demands being placed on you from outside.

Then turn attention to yourself. Following are some simple suggestions for reducing the amount of stress in your life.

◆ Exercise.
◆ Meditate.
◆ Employ meditative breathing techniques whenever possible.
◆ Sit down when you eat.
◆ Eat frequent, small meals to keep the blood sugar level more stable and inhibit the release of adrenaline.
◆ Chew your food sufficiently, mixing enough saliva with the food to make digestion easier.
◆ Drink a lot of water, but not during a meal.
◆ Do not drink alcohol or caffeine, or smoke cigarettes.
◆ Incorporate the Spleen Qi deficiency dietary principles described in chapter 6.
◆ Use herbs that move the Qi, like peppermint, rosemary, spearmint, turmeric, and thyme.
◆ Supplement with herbs that resolve Liver Qi stagnation (see chapter 8).
◆ If your prolactin levels are high, take malt barley sprout (Mai Ya).
◆ Perform the acupressure techniques described in chapter 7 to rectify the Liver Qi.

Stress is not the only factor causing unexplained infertility. Many subtle endocrine and hormonal factors also affect our ability to conceive. But finding and treating the underlying pattern will resolve the hormonal imbalance, no matter how slight. Take a look at your symptoms and use the diagnostic guidelines in chapter 4 to discover your pattern of imbalance. Then use diet, lifestyle, acupressure or acupuncture, and herbs to restore your body to health and balance.

Subclinical infertility often responds quickly to small changes in the body's overall functioning. Of course, nothing is certain, but with a greater level of health it's likely you will stand a greater chance of conceiving.

TCM IN ACTION: SONJA'S STORY

Sonja was a thirty-two-year-old secretary married to a schoolteacher. They had been trying to conceive for two years, and the doctors were unable to find a mechanical cause or laboratory abnormality to account for their infertility. She was not ready for hormonal stimulation and did not want to pursue ART. When she came to my office, she was pleasant and upbeat, and had no outward signs of angst. Therefore, I was somewhat surprised when she said she had a psychiatric history of depression, for which she was being treated with three different medications. She spoke of the fear of her depression more than the depression itself.

Most of Sonja's symptoms revealed themselves in the mood category. Her men-

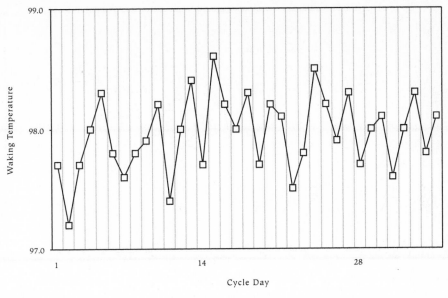

Figure 11.1: Sonja's BBT Graph — Anovulation Caused By Liver Qi Stagnation (**Lv Qi X**)

strual cycles were about thirty-two days in length, and the blood flow lasted about five days. She didn't notice any signs of increased fertile vaginal discharge midcycle but said she felt pains in her ovaries during the middle of the month. She had some menstrual discomfort and breast distension, but no significant symptoms of premenstrual syndrome. However, she said she felt tense and irritable all the time, and she didn't sleep well. She was often constipated, but she blamed this on her medication.

When she started to monitor her BBT, we saw it was monophasic and sawtoothed (fig. 11.1). She wasn't ovulating at all.

I diagnosed Liver Qi stagnation. Sonja came for acupuncture once a week, but we did not use any herbs because she was afraid they would interfere with her anti-depressant regimen. I taught her Qi Gong breathing for the purpose of regulating her hormonal cycles and relaxing her, and she started doing it every time she got upset. She also used the breathing techniques while sitting at her desk or talking on the phone, as well as every night to help her sleep. Her patterns began to stabilize, and within four months we could tell from her BBT that she had ovulated (fig. 11.2).

Sonja talked to her psychiatrist about reducing her antidepressant medication because she had started to feel better. By the time she ovulated, she was off two of the drugs she had been relying on for most of her adult life. She still took one selective serotonin reuptake inhibitor (SSRI) that was

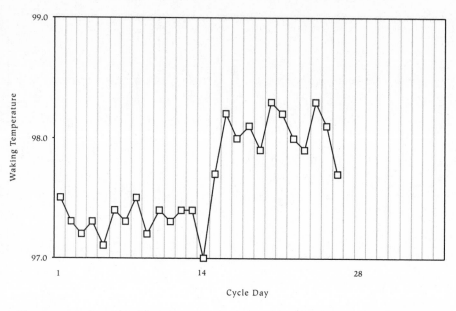

Figure 11.2: Sonja's BBT Graph — Liver Qi Stagnation (**Lv Qi X**) Improved

safe even during pregnancy. She conceived shortly thereafter and had an uncomplicated pregnancy. She did experience some postpartum depression, but the last I heard, she had not gone back on the other antidepressant medicines.

TCM IN ACTION: CINDY'S JOURNEY TO HEALTH

Cindy was an attractive, thirty-six-year-old professional woman married to Mark, who appeared very angry and cold. During their initial interview at my clinic, Mark would often answer the questions I asked Cindy, but he would look away when I talked to him. They had married when Cindy was twenty-eight. She always had had very heavy menstrual cycles, and when she was thirty,

doctors discovered three fibroids in her uterus and moderate endometriosis in her pelvic cavity, of all which were surgically excised. Cindy said her menstrual cycles had been normal for the last six years, although they varied in length. Her shortest cycles were thirty days; longer cycles lasted up to thirty-eight days. She and Mark had tried to conceive every month for the last eight years, but even though all their laboratory tests were normal, she had not become pregnant. She had tried Clomid for six cycles and had good egg production and a thick uterine lining, but she still had not conceived. She said the Clomid made her very anxious and gave her severe headaches and acne.

It was clear that Cindy was not comfortable answering questions regarding her menstrual cycles in Mark's presence, but she did report that the blood flow was normal in amount and that there was very little pain, premenstrual syndrome, or breast tenderness. She listed no other symptoms and said she had no difficulty with circulation, digestion, elimination, sleeping patterns, or moods. I decided not to press the questioning further and got right to her pulse, which had a fine but taut quality. Her tongue (which she scraped daily) had a slightly grayish hue.

In the month after our initial conversation, Cindy monitored her BBT. When she showed me her chart, I saw the pattern was extremely erratic (fig 11.3).

I diagnosed Liver Qi stagnation and treated her accordingly. I stimulated acupoints LI 4 and Lv 3 to open up the Liver channels and resolve stagnant Qi. I needled the spirit point within the ear triangular fossa and the point between the eyebrows, Yintang, to calm the spirit. I also prescribed an herbal formula to nourish the spirit and resolve Liver Qi stagnation.

Over the next couple of months, Cindy began to open up and admitted that she had not disclosed some of her symptoms at her initial visit. She reported that her periods were becoming much less painful, she was sleeping better, and she was feeling less "crazy" premenstrually. I made dietary and lifestyle recommendations to support the acupuncture treatments, and she incorporated every suggestion I made. She started walking every day during her lunch break. She did breathing exercises every day at work. She changed her (and Mark's) diet.

Within four months, Cindy said she was happier. She made a few comments about Mark and said she didn't let him "get to her"

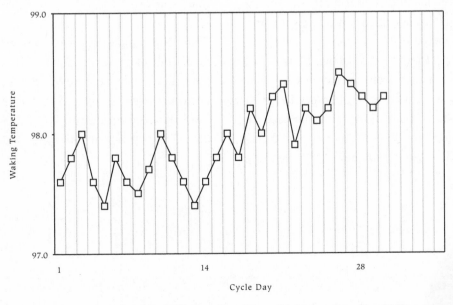

Figure 11.3: Cindy's BBT Graph — Liver Qi Stagnation (**Lv Qi X**)

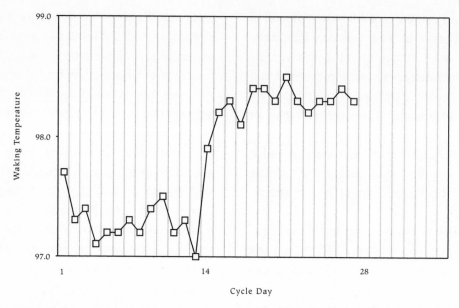

Figure 11.4: Cindy's BBT Graph — Liver Qi Stagnation (**Lv Qi X**) Improved

anymore. She quit grinding her teeth at night. She rearranged her bedroom so she felt more comfortable in it. Each month, her cycle stabilized a little more as we got closer to the source of her disharmony. Her BBT graphs reflected the change (fig. 11.4).

As I incorporated medicinals to clear Liver and Heart heat — Biota seed (Bai Zi Ren), gambir (Gou Teng), and mimosa tree bark (He Huan Pi) — Cindy responded dramatically. Within six months of starting treatment, she was pregnant. Mark, Cindy, and their baby, Ethan, came to visit later to thank me.

Both Sonja's and Cindy's hormones were definitely out of whack, but the cause of their problem was not clear to Western medicine. Restoring their systems to balance using TCM provided an elegant and simple solution, giving them healthy, happy children.

12

Immunologic Reaction and Recurrent Miscarriage: Bringing Your Body into Harmony with Itself

The wrong done oneself is born of oneself, is produced in oneself.

— *The Dhammapada*

The immune system functions to define or recognize "self" and to destroy "nonself." If this complex system loses its ability to recognize and regulate which is which, it will begin to destroy certain "self" components. Autoimmune disorders are abnormal reactions to parts of our own bodies. In such disorders, the immune system loses its ability to discriminate between what is "safe" and what is "harmful."

Pregnancy creates conditions in which immunologic reactions can be triggered, yet reproductive medicine has focused precious little on treating its immunologic components. By definition, when a woman becomes pregnant her body is being invaded by something foreign. In some cases, the woman actually produces antisperm cells, which attack the sperm as it enters the vagina in the same way T cells attack germs in the bloodstream. For any woman to conceive and carry a fetus to term, there must be a natural suppression of her T-helper immune response. However, overriding this suppression can cause the embryo or fetus to abort.

In other cases, when a woman's egg becomes fertilized, certain immune components cause clotting at the placental attachment site, starving the embryo and causing it to abort. Markers of other potential immunological fertility factors include antinuclear antibodies and premature elevations of FSH, natural killer (NK) cells, lupus anticoagulant, and other clotting factors. Some of these represent a reaction to the man's "nonself" tissue interacting with the woman's "self" tissue, thereby causing an overly sensitive immune response. A woman may even have antibodies to her own hormones and neurotransmitters. In some cases, a woman's cells produce a kind of cytokine protein that literally will kill the developing embryo.

Other hormonal disturbances can create immune reactions leading to conditions like premature ovarian failure (POF). One such hormonal disturbance of the thyroid is diagnosed by the presence of antithyroid antibodies in a woman's bloodstream. According to RESOLVE, approximately 23 to 35 percent of women with recurrent miscarriage have antithyroid antibodies, compared with 10 to 17 percent of women who carry children to term. Antithyroid antibodies can be indicative of hypothyroidism, which may contribute to a woman's tendency to miscarry.

Another version of improper immunologic reproductive response is endometrial glandular developmental arrest, when the glands of the uterine lining fail to respond adequately to the signals of rising progesterone. Autoimmune issues also can cause vascular and blood flow abnormalities. Women with these problems often demonstrate characteristic groups of symptoms and conditions. For example, migraine headaches and endometriosis occurring together can indicate an autoimmune reaction within the blood vessels. (Countries in Asia and Europe have recognized endometriosis as an autoimmune disease for many years.)

The usual treatment for autoimmune fertility disorders is to suppress or override the immune system so implantation may occur. A woman who is suspected of having a blood-clotting component to her infertility or habitual miscarriage is given daily doses of aspirin to "thin the blood" and inhibit the clotting pathway. If this is not effective, heparin (a stronger blood thinner) is employed. Because of the side effects of heparin therapy, however, it is not chosen as the first course of action in treating immunologic infertility. Blood products that bind up immune cells through intravenous infusions to prepare a patient for transplants are used by some physicians to address severe autoimmune conditions, and steroids like prednisone are also used to suppress overactive immune systems.

These procedures are not only severe, but also can be unpleasant, with long-term side effects. Perhaps there is a better way, one that doesn't involve suppressing the immune system but retraining it.

❧ THE EASTERN VIEW

While Western reproductive endocrinology has recognized the impact of immunologic factors for only a decade or so, TCM has been treating autoimmune infertility for thousands of years. According to the Eastern medical paradigm, it is not so important what the autoantibody is, be it antinuclear antibody (ANA), anticardiolipin antibody (ACA), antiphospholipid antibody (APA), or lupus anticoagulant. It doesn't matter if T cells are low or if NK cells are high. What matters is the process initially causing the immune system to go awry. When we treat the root problem, the immunologic markers correct themselves. Many women with previously diagnosed "unexplained infertility" or autoimmune fertility factors have been treated effectively with TCM's prescriptions of diet, herbal therapy, and acupuncture.

In the view of TCM, immunologic factors hostile to pregnancy may be caused by imbalances in levels of heat and/or damp; in Blood flow (stagnation or overabundance); in the levels of Yin or Yang; or in the level of Qi energy. As with all TCM treatments, however, a proper diagnostic pattern must be established before treatment will be effective. The key is to use the symptoms presented by the patient to diagnose her particular deficiencies and excesses, and to prescribe treatment to bring her back to balance.

For instance, many women in my clinic typically report that around the time of implantation they experience a strange sensation in their uterus (a fluttering, tugging, or burning), often accompanied by systemic changes like whole-body rashes or hives, a feverish sensation, cold sweats, and the like. Their symptoms tell me that these women are having a reaction to implantation, and the body and Uterus need to be quieted. This often involves clearing heat from the Blood (with acupoints Sp 10 and LI 11) and damp heat from the Uterus (using points Sp 9, Sp 6, and Lv 8). Before implantation, I will sedate Ren 3, bringing the Yin energies to "water" the Uterus to put out its toxic state of fire (which produces NK cells).

When Our Body Becomes a Battleground

One must still have chaos in oneself
to be able to give birth
to a dancing star.

— NIETZSCHE

We may view the immune system as our body's defense against invaders. The soldiers of the army that make up the immune system are formed primarily in the bone marrow (B cells — humoral immunity), and the thymus gland (T cells — cellular immunity). To tonify our defensive forces, we should strengthen these four components:

1. Origin — ensure a strong foundation by choosing the best soldiers.
2. Circulation — allow transit of these troops via safe passages.
3. Sustenance — provide adequate nourishment to keep the forces healthy.
4. Mobilization — don't allow the regiment to stagnate or revolt.

Origin Our immune system, as with almost every other system, originates in the Kidney (and Liver). Therefore, basic tonification of the immune system must begin with the Kidneys. Stimulate points Ki 3, Ki 7, Lv 14, UB 23, UB 52, and Du 4.

Circulation Elements of the immune system circulate through the Penetrating meridian. To activate the immune cells, stimulate points St 30, Sp 4, and Pc 6.

Sustenance The Spleen nourishes the immune system. Stimulate points St 36, Ren 6, Ren 12.

Mobilization When the soldiers gather and become idle, there is a risk of mutiny. Say the defensive forces that have been trained to "fight" offensive influences find endometrial cells that have invaded the pelvic cavity. Their job is to protect their territory and destroy invaders. When their opponent is immobilized, they move on and find a multitude of enemies in the Uterus, where they assemble. They have been trained to fight, and they have found a battleground rife with foes. Yet when the adversaries are gone, the troops stagnate, become bored, and may turn against their host. These immune cells must be neutralized and moved out so the Uterus may resume its function of receiving an embryo. To remove these energetic blockages, stimulate points UB 23, Ki 16, and St 30.

And, of course, always treat the pattern that is present.

In ancient Chinese literature, a combination of the herbs Angelica (Dang Gui) and Ligusticum (Chuan Xiong) was given to women (the emperor's concubines) whose periods were late. These herbs would help bring on the menses if a woman wasn't pregnant; if she had conceived, they would have no effect, and the pregnancy would go on. Both Angelica and Ligusticum invigorate the Blood. They have the same blood-thinning effects as aspirin and heparin, but are a more natural and harmless approach. Thus, women who are suspected of having an immunologic reaction to the conception process might be treated with Angelica and Ligusticum if symptoms indicate there is Blood stasis (**Bl X**) in the Uterus in early pregnancy. These signs and symptoms might include uterine cramping; a history of dark, clotty menstrual flow; and a pulse whose quality is not smooth and whose strength seems to come and go in one or both wrists around the time of implantation and into early pregnancy.

OTHER AUTOIMMUNE REACTIONS AND PATTERNS

Serotonin is one of the chemicals involved in preparing the Uterus for pregnancy. Some women are found to make antibodies to the serotonin circulating in their blood. Reproductive immunology has recognized a group of common symptoms in women with this condition. They include:

◆ body aches
◆ increasing depression, irritability, and premenstrual symptoms
◆ early morning insomnia

◆ night sweats, especially over the breastbone area
◆ panic attacks
◆ thin uterine lining (less than 8 millimeters on days 13 or 14)
◆ poor response to high levels of follicle-stimulating hormone
◆ hormone levels crashing in the middle of the cycle

In TCM, these symptoms correspond to a pattern of Liver Qi stagnation (**Lv Qi X**) and Yin deficiency, with heat in the Heart and Liver. These symptoms are likely to be accompanied by irregular menstrual cycles and a sawtoothed, erratic BBT graph. Women with this presentation should follow the dietary, lifestyle, acupressure, herbal, and meditative practices listed for these patterns in chapters 6, 7, and 8.

When pituitary and ovarian functions are imbalanced, the Heart should be suspect, and if accompanied by other signs of Heart disharmony, like restlessness, heart palpitations, and insomnia, they too should be addressed. Herbs to calm the Heart and Liver (see chapter 8) are very effective in resolving this scenario and can be incorporated into other prescriptions.

BALANCING SPLEEN QI

Any immunologic issue, regardless of the physical or symptomatic manifestation, requires supplementation of the Spleen Qi. Chinese medicine ascribes all immunologic functions to an energetic aspect called "protective Qi." Protective Qi incorporates some of the functions of the Spleen and Lung systems. Herbs that strengthen protective Qi include Astragalus (Huang Qi), Atractylodes (Bai Zhu), Codonopsis (Dang Shen), and Dioscorea (Shan Yao). Since Chinese medicine recognizes no separation of mind, body, and spirit, the mental processes of overconcern and worry also are said to damage the function of the Spleen. Meditative techniques like the Qi Gong breathing in chapter 6 can assist women in managing the concerns of everyday life and protecting the Spleen energy.

Dietary management is probably the most essential element in ensuring proper functioning of the Spleen Qi. Women whose Spleen Qi is deficient are advised not to eat cold foods (anything straight out of the refrigerator or freezer), to avoid too many raw fruits and vegetables, to consume no fruit juices, and to avoid too many dairy products, fats, oils, or sweets. An overabundance of wheat can also dampen and impair Spleen functioning.

TREATMENTS BASED UPON PATTERN DISCRIMINATION

A *Clinical Handbook of Chinese Medicine Gynecology* by Shen Shong-li describes four patterns associated with allergic and autoimmune causes of infertility and recommends treatment methods to resolve them. I have modified some of the herbal formulas listed below to include herbs that are easier to obtain and have added some acupoints and dietary suggestions.

PHLEGM OBSTRUCTION

Main symptoms: Inability to conceive after one year of unprotected intercourse. The woman may or may not be overweight, but she usually is suffering from fatigue, lack of strength, lower back pain, heavy lower legs, and a heavy, dragging feeling. There is often profuse vaginal discharge, which is sticky and thick in consistency. Indeed, there may be no clinical symptoms except for this vaginal discharge and positive sperm (Blood, Essence) antibodies. The tongue has a thin, white coating; the pulse is fine but feels "slippery" or viscous, as if there are ball bearings moving through it.

Pattern diagnosis: Spleen Qi deficiency (**Sp–**) and dampness (**D**). Phlegm is considered condensed dampness.

Treatment methods: Supplement the Spleen, dry dampness, and transform phlegm. Incorporate the Spleen Qi diet, avoiding refined carbohydrates, sweeteners, and dairy products. Eat lots of seaweed. Use herbs like Atractylodes (Bai Zhu), magnolia bark (Hou Po), coix (Yi Yi Ren), fluorite (Zi Shi Ying), Epimedium (Yin Yang Huo), and Poria (Fu Ling). Strengthen the Spleen energies with Sp 6, St 36, and Ren 6, and resolve dampness with Sp 9 and St 40.

BLOOD OBSTRUCTION AND STAGNATION

Main symptoms: Infertility after several years of trying to become pregnant. There is usually abdominal pain associated with the menstrual flow, which is often accompanied by blood clots. The tongue may or may not be dark, with small, flat blemishes or discolorations on the edges of the tongue or darkened papillae (bumps). The pulse will usually be taut or wiry, like a guitar string, and "choppy" — coming and going roughly.

Pattern diagnosis: Blood stasis (**Bl X**), Liver Qi stagnation (**Lv Qi X**)

Treatment methods: Move the Qi, invigorate the Blood, and transform stasis. Herbal treatments include Salvia root (Dan Shen), red peony (Chi Shao), peach kernel (Tao Ren), Corydalis (Yan Hu Suo), cattail pollen (Pu Huang), rhubarb (Da Huang), and Aucklandia (Mu Xiang). The herbal formulas Frigid Extremities Powder (Si Ni San) and Four Substances Decoction with Safflower and Peach Pit (Tao Hong Si Wu Tang) together resolve this type of scenario. Use points to invigorate the Blood like UB 17 and Sp 10, and resolve the Liver Qi stagnation with Lv 3 and Lv 14. Supplement the diet with fish oil or evening primrose oil, and take pycnogenol.

This treatment method would be appropriate for women diagnosed with endometriosis who have the characteristic pelvic pain; clotty, dark menstrual blood; and infertility. They also may have higher levels of circulating immunoglobulins found in their blood.

YIN DEFICIENCY WITH HEAT

Main symptoms: Lack of conception after one year of unprotected intercourse. Symptoms include short cycles, profuse menstruation, afternoon tidal fever, dry mouth, sore throat, constipation, red eyes, dizziness, tinnitus, low back pain, lower leg weakness, heart irritation, easy anger, a thin, red, dry tongue, and a fine, rapid pulse.

Pattern diagnosis: Kidney Yin deficiency (**Ki Yi–**), excess heat (**^H**)

Treatment methods: Enrich Yin and clear heat to bring the fire down. Take the herbal formula Anemarrhena, Phellodendron, and Rehmannia Pill (Zhi Bai Di Huang Wan) with the following modifications: Anemarrhena (Zhi Mu), Phellodendron (Huang Bai), fresh Rehmannia (Sheng Di Huang), Alisma (Ze Xie), moutan (Mu Dan Pi), Poria (Fu Ling), Cornus (Shan Zhu Yu), Angelica (Dang Gui), Scrophularia (Xuan Shen), Lycium (Gou Qi Zi), Ligustrum (Nu Zhen Zi), and Eucommia bark (Du Zhong). Supplement the Kidney Yin and clear heat with Ki 3, Ren 3, Sp 10, and LI 11. Do not eat hot, spicy foods; avoid caffeine; and exercise only in moderation.

DAMP HEAT

Main symptoms: Lack of conception after one year of unprotected intercourse. Profuse, yellow vaginal discharge, possibly with a foul odor. Sometimes there is a lack of menstruation, or there may be early menstruation. The blood flow can be profuse or diminished, sometimes with slimy clots. Other symptoms include vaginal or rectal itching (especially premenstrually); chronic pain in the lower abdomen increasing with the menstrual period; lower back pain; a red tongue with a moist yellow coating; and a fine, slippery, rapid pulse.

Pattern diagnosis: damp heat (**DH**)

Treatment methods: Clear heat, drain dampness, and supplement and move the Qi. Herbs that resolve damp heat include Scutellaria (Huang Qin), Coptis (Huang Lian), and Phellodendron (Huang Bai). Ginseng (Ren Shen) and Atractylodes (Bai Zhu) supplement the Qi, and herbs like black cohosh (Sheng Ma) and Bupleurum (Chai Hu) move it. Acupoints Lv 2, Sp 6, Sp 9, and Sp 10 would be beneficial.

OTHER DIETARY AND
LIFESTYLE
RECOMMENDATIONS

Beyond the use of herbal formulas to treat immunologic reactions, some health care professionals recommend the use of PABA (para-aminobenzoic acid) to treat immunologic factors affecting fertility. PABA affects the formation of red blood cells and protein metabolism, and stimulates the production of folic acid in the intestines. It is therefore recommended in disorders of folic acid production. Supplementation with 300 to 400 milligrams of PABA daily has been found to prevent or correct aspects of certain autoimmune conditions like Crohn's disease, ulcerative colitis, scleroderma, and infertility. PABA is found naturally in organ meats like liver, as well as in eggs, rice, wheat germ, bran, molasses, and dark-green vegetables.

When treating immunologic concerns, include antioxidants (vitamins C, E, beta-carotene, selenium, and zinc) and super-antioxidants OPC/pycnogenol (found in grape seed extract, pine bark extract, red wine extract, and bilberry extract). Fish-oil supplements keep the blood clear and moderate NK cell activity. The bulk of your diet should consist of whole, organic foods, supplemented with green foods, wheatgrass, spirulina, flower (bee) pollen, and royal jelly. Blue-green algae has been found to trigger the movement of NK cells from the blood into the tissues. I usually recommend taking blue-green algae with OPC and fish oil. You can also include reishi and shiitake mushrooms, and Kombucha tea.

THE EFFECT OF MEDICATIONS

Drugs like cortisone, prednisone, prednisolone, dexamethasone, and methylprednisolone are glucocorticoid medications used by Western physicians to inhibit immunologic reactions within the body. All of these medicines would be categorized in Chinese medicine as exterior-resolving medicinals, which can deplete the Essence if used in abundance. Their known side effects include insomnia and anxiety (because of the depletion of Essence in the body). The increased appetite and water retention associated with glucocorticoid use are caused by disturbances in the Yang Qi. If Spleen Qi and Kidney Yin are problematic to begin with, glucocorticoids will exacerbate this deficiency. Those with Qi deficiency and Kidney Yin deficiency, therefore, should be wary of long-term glucocorticoid administration as it may damage the ability to conceive.

One natural alternative to glucocorticoids like prednisone may be the Chinese herb taibo. A 1997 study from the Xiyuan Hospital in Beijing compared results of using taibo and prednisone to inhibit the cytotoxic effects of antisperm antibodies in mice. Mice that were infertile because of immunologic factors (antisperm antibodies) were divided into four groups. One group received saline injections; one was injected with prednisone; a third was administered high levels of taibo; and a fourth was given low levels of taibo. The mice were then artificially inseminated. The pregnancy rates for the four groups were as follows.

- ◆ Saline group   38.89 percent
- ◆ Prednisone group   47.06 percent
- ◆ High-dose taibo   70.00 percent
- ◆ Low-dose taibo   75.00 percent

Low doses of taibo actually produced a higher rate of pregnancy than high doses. It's also important to note that the levels of cytotoxic antibodies to sperm were much lower in the prednisone and taibo groups than in the saline group. If you are diagnosed with antisperm antibodies, taibo may be a viable, natural alternative treatment.

YEAST

The negative consequences of overuse of antibiotics, glucocorticoids, and birth control pills brings us to the topic of excess yeast. While we have come to rely on antibiotics as a treatment for many conditions, these drugs are often prescribed for circumstances that may not warrant their use, including respiratory and intestinal viruses on which they have no effect. Antibiotics do not kill viruses; antibiotics kill bacteria — nothing more. The problem is that they also kill intestinal bacterial flora, which keep organisms like yeast in check.

Most women can relate to the experience of developing a vaginal yeast infection after a bout of antibiotics. Candida albicans is a yeast that occupies the large intestine; its function is to clean up cellular debris. Candidiasis is an overgrowth of this intestinal yeast. When the yeast proliferates beyond its role of cleaning up dead cells, it can wreak internal havoc. And if, because of the yeast's unchecked multiplication, the intestinal wall becomes permeable to its infiltration, then yeast can enter the bloodstream and cause all kinds of endocrine and immunologic problems.

Gastrointestinal signs of overproliferating candida albicans include indigestion, gas, and bowel irregularities like constipation and diarrhea. Evidence of candida albicans outside the intestine includes vaginitis, sinusitis, certain skin manifestations, and oral thrush. Fatigue and depression also are commonly involved. Disruptions in the menstrual cycle often occur with yeast proliferation and provide evidence of the hormonal effects of this problem.

Traditional Chinese medicine states that whenever there is excess yeast in the system, the Spleen is always involved. Luckily, an anticandidal diet can help individuals with yeast overgrowth return to a normal state of health. If you believe you have too much yeast in your system, follow these dietary recommendations.

◆ Consume plenty of organic vegetables.
◆ Eat brown rice as your staple grain.
◆ Tofu and tempeh are good sources of protein.
◆ Consume only organic, hormone-free meats.
◆ Do not eat dairy products.
◆ Avoid yeast breads and all forms of alcohol, vinegar, and fermented beverages.
◆ Yeast thrives on sugar, so avoid sweets. Also avoid refined carbohydrates, which almost immediately turn into glucose within the body.
◆ Do not consume sugary fruits that mold easily, like grapes, oranges, and strawberries. Don't eat bananas. Apples and pears are permissible. Do not drink fruit juices.

◆ Acidophilus supplementation helps to repopulate the bacterial flora and control the yeast. Active-culture yogurt contains acidophilus as well, but the dairy in yogurt usually promotes a condition of dampness, which can damage the Spleen.

Herbs that have an antimycotic (anti-fungal) nature include Coptis (Huang Lian), Scutellaria (Huang Qin), Phellodendron (Huang Bai), Sophora root (Ku Shen), Dictamnus root bark (Bai Xian Pi), Houttuynia (Yu Xing Cao), Cnidium seeds (She Chuang Zi), Areca seed (Bing Lang), and Melia (Chuan Lian Zi). Herbs that help cleanse the blood of toxins include Angelica (Dang Gui), white peony (Bai Shao), Astragalus (Huang Qi), Polygonatum (He Shou Wu), and Acanthopanex root bark (Wu Jia Pi).

🐾 NOTE: Strict adherence to this diet and herbal regimen may cause a phenomenon known as a Herxheimer reaction: as the yeast population dies, it produces large amounts of histamine, which can cause symptoms like feverish, flulike feelings, headaches, nausea, vomiting, and diarrhea. These symptoms should not last more than one to two days and can be alleviated by taking antihistaminic herbs like dried ginger (Gan Jiang), Amomum (Sha Ren), Galanga root (Gao Liang Jiang), Galanga seeds (Cao Dou Kou), white Atractylodes (Bai Zhu), and black Atractylodes (Ang Zhu). You can also take rhubarb (Da Huang) to help purge the bowels and rid the body of the toxic buildup. When the histamine-induced symptoms subside, the symptoms caused by yeast overgrowth also should be ameliorated. When yeast overgrowth is experienced in women with endometriosis, the patent herbal formula Mume Pill (Wu Mei Wan) has been found effective.

It's important to note once more that infertility caused by immunologic factors may have a wide variety of TCM patterns at its root. A few minutes spent reviewing your symptoms, diagnosing your pattern based on the principles in chapter 4, and then choosing the appropriate treatment for your particular pattern will save you a lot of time, energy, and emotional investment. In addition, as your condition resolves you may find you have to adjust your treatments accordingly.

TCM IN ACTION: CLAUDIA'S ORDEAL

Claudia and her husband, Jerome, were both thirty-seven and had been married for four years. Claudia was petite and sophisticated, and Jerome was handsome and humorous. They were devout Catholics who desperately wanted a family. Unfortunately, Jerome's sperm analysis revealed an overall low sperm count, marginal motility, and very poor morphology (abnormally shaped sperm). He was diagnosed with a slight varicocele (dilation in the spermatic cord that creates swelling and can impair male fertility). Claudia had been diagnosed with endometriosis but was told she was fine otherwise. She had previously undergone a full

fertility workup, a laparoscopy, six unsuccessful Clomid cycles, three hormonally stimulated IUIs, and one failed IVF treatment. She and her husband experienced difficulty with their decision to try ART because of religious considerations but were told it was their only hope because of Jerome's sperm quality. They were tired, frustrated, and frantic for answers.

Claudia and Jerome scheduled separate appointments, and I treated each of them weekly. Jerome was a corporate lawyer and suffered from intense stress and tension headaches. He had difficulty sleeping and had been prescribed Ambien (a sleeping aid). He lived on ibuprofen to control his headaches. I gave him a list of supplements to purchase (vitamins A, C, E, selenium, zinc, L-arginine, and L-carnitine) and treated him with acupuncture for his headaches, which were caused by stress manifesting as Liver Qi stagnation, which created heat. Within two weeks, his headaches were gone, and he could function without sleep disturbances. He dealt with his stress and quit taking ibuprofen and Ambien. I told him he could stop seeing me. Six weeks later, his next sperm analysis was normal. His sperm quantity and quality improved on its own when his body was in balance. Both Jerome and Claudia were hopeful that they might have finally found the answer to their fertility problems.

Claudia, a flight attendant, suffered from severe PMS: about a week before her period, she became extremely depressed and irritable. She experienced lower back pain and abdominal cramping up until her menses arrived, then spent a full day in bed with a heating pad and her own ibuprofen-and-Coke cocktail. Her menses were regular, coming every thirty to thirty-two days. She bled rather heavily, and the menstrual blood was dark red and clotty. She was always cold, especially her feet. She had occasional itchy vaginal discharge that worsened after intercourse. She had already eliminated coffee and alcohol and ate a fairly healthy diet, except for her monthly menstrual Coke. Her pulse was full and taut, like a vibrating metal guitar string.

I prescribed two herbal formulas, one during the follicular phase to tonify the Yang aspect of her Kidney and clear damp heat, and a luteal phase formula to clear the Liver, move the Qi, and invigorate the Blood. We reinforced her herbal therapy with weekly acupuncture treatments. Although Claudia didn't modify her diet, she did supplement it with acidophilus capsules to control the yeast infections she thought she was experiencing. Within three months the menstrual pain and premenstrual irritability were greatly improved. But she still had not conceived.

In their desperation, the couple sought out another reproductive endocrinologist for further treatment. Claudia was told to quit taking herbs. One more laparoscopy was performed, and very little new endometrial tissue was found in the abdominal cavity. Both Claudia and Jerome were found to carry and exchange a bacterial infection called Ureaplasma, which was blamed as the culprit for implantation failure. They were jointly prescribed antibiotics for one month, after which another hormonally stimulated insemination was performed, to no avail.

Claudia returned to me for treatments. Her symptoms had not worsened in the interim, but the vaginal itching never had ceased. We discussed the potential immunologic nature of her implantation failure, and I prescribed a formula to clear damp heat. I modified the formula slightly by adding Liver-rectifying herbs like Bupleurum. During one visit, Claudia offhandedly told me she was experiencing vision changes premenstrually. She had told her gynecologist and reproductive endocrinologist that her vision would dim and that she saw "floaters" just before her period arrived, but they both told her it was insignificant. According to Chinese medicine, however, the Liver governs the eyes and vision, and also supplies Blood to the Uterus. This clue allowed me to home in on another aspect of Claudia's menstrual disharmony: although the Liver Qi had been rectified, the Blood exchange from the Liver remained relatively weak. Her vision changed because there wasn't enough Liver Blood to supply both the eyes and the Uterus. So I further modified the herbal formula she was taking to include Lycium (Gou Qi Zi) and white peony (Bai Shao) to tonify the Liver Blood after ovulation. The floaters went away.

Meanwhile, the clock was still ticking. Jerome and Claudia, who both had turned thirty-eight, decided to go out of state for reproductive immunologic treatments. Claudia received a more complete laboratory analysis of immunologic factors and started preparing for another IVF. (She again was advised to stop the herbs.) This time, in addition to her hormonal stimulation, she was prescribed a blood thinner (Lovenox), intravenous immunoglobulin injections, and the steroid dexamethasone. Her blood analysis revealed that she had conceived during this cycle, but twelve days after the embryo transfer, her beta-hCG was negative and she got her period. Hopeful because Claudia's uterus at least had allowed implantation, they geared up for another cycle. Same treatment, same result: the first blood test was positive for pregnancy, the second negative. The road toward parenthood for Claudia and Jerome was looping back around itself, with more forks and dead ends. More complex lab work revealed that the couple's DNA was so similar that Claudia's immune system was unable to mask the presence of the implanting embryos. (The immune system needs to be "tricked" by pregnancy hormones to allow the invading embryo entrance.) Her body, thinking the embryos were harmful, was rejecting them.

Claudia's PMS and depression had returned, now in the form of despair. She resumed acupuncture treatments because she wanted to feel hopeful again. One last modification to the herbal formula, incorporating treatments for Liver Blood deficiency, Liver Qi stagnation, and damp heat, brought Claudia's body into balance within weeks.

She never had another period. To their utter disbelief, the couple discovered Claudia had become pregnant naturally. They never had to hear another nurse's voice over the phone tell them they were unsuccessful yet again. They experienced the joy of discovering the appearance of the double line on a home pregnancy test. All laboratory tests during Claudia's pregnancy were normal. In due course, Claudia gave birth to a healthy baby girl. They since have had another child — naturally.

RECURRENT MISCARRIAGE

There are few more devastating events than the loss of a pregnancy at any stage, especially after a woman has suffered from fertility impairment. Women who experience this loss go through the stages of grief just as if they have lost a loved one — and they have. It is a continuum: the most overwhelming loss a woman can experience is the loss of a child she has given birth to, but next is the loss of a child she has carried within her womb.

While miscarriages resulting from genetic defects and fetal developmental failures cannot and should not be thwarted, those caused by maternal reactions are preventable. Numerous pregnancy losses are the result of the same immunologic factors and hormonal imbalances preventing pregnancy from occurring in the first place. Unfortunately, women with these problems all too often receive dismal results from their Western medical caregivers.

One of the most common reasons for early pregnancy loss is inadequate progesterone production, the same factor that causes luteal phase defect. Incorporating the treatments for the specific pattern that underlies the progesterone deficiency — be it Kidney Yang (**Ki Yan–**) or Spleen Qi deficiency (**Sp–**) — will also enhance a woman's ability to carry the pregnancy until the placenta takes over its own progesterone production. Herbs to improve progesterone production and prevent miscarriage differ according to the pattern underlying the deficiency. If your progesterone deficiency is caused by Spleen Qi deficiency, taking a Blood deficiency formula won't resolve the condition.

Here are the herbal formulas prescribed for the different patterns. (Consult chapter 8 for more specific information.)

- *For Spleen Qi deficiency* (**Sp–**): Take Atractylodes (Bai Zhu), Astragalus (Huang Qi), Codonopsis (Dang Shen), and Dioscorea (Shan Yao).
- *For Kidney Yin* (**Ki Yi–**) *and/or Yang* (**Ki Yan–**) *deficiency:* Take Eucommia bark (Du Zhong), Dipsacus (Xu Duan), Loranthus (Sang Ji Sheng), and Cuscuta (Tu Si Zi).
- *For Blood deficiency* (**Bl–**) *symptoms:* Take fleeceflower root (He Shou Wu) and gelatin (E Jiao).
- *To clear excess heat* (**^H**) *from the upper part of the body and prevent miscarriage:* Take Scutellaria (Huang Qin).

Some premade TCM herbal formulas for miscarriage prevention can be obtained through an herbal pharmacy or an acupuncture/herbal clinic. These prescriptions have helped many maintain their pregnancy. Remember, however, they are designed for specific patterns and should not be taken indiscriminately. These preparations are not commonly purchased over the counter; they usually must be specially made through an herbal pharmacy or by an acupuncture/ herbal clinic.

- *For Spleen Qi deficiency (**Sp−**) with Liver Qi Stagnation (**Lv Qi X**):* Take Protect the Fetus and Aid Life Formula.
- *For cold Uterus (**CW**):* Take Warm the Menses Decoction (Wen Jing Tang).
- *To supplement Spleen Qi (**Sp−**) and Blood (**Bl−**), and to calm the Fetus:* Take Powder that Gives the Stability of Mount Tai (Tai Shan Pan Shi Shan).
- *To dispel Blood stasis (**Bl X**) in the womb during pregnancy:* Take Cinnamon Twig and Poria Pill (Gui Zhi Fu Ling Wan).

The key to treating recurrent miscarriage is twofold: first, prepare the body before conception; second, provide whatever assistance is necessary to encourage the body to retain the child until it is ready to be born. Sometimes this assistance can be minimal; at other times consistent care is required. In the following story, we meet Laura, a woman who was able to carry her child to term with TCM treatments.

TCM in Action: Laura's Failing Ovaries

Laura was thirty-eight years old when she first consulted me. She had been pregnant twice before, both through hormonally stimulated inseminations. She miscarried the first time at nine weeks, the second time at seven weeks. On each occasion the pregnancy seemed to be going fine, but during her ultrasound scan, she found the embryo had stopped growing. She received the dreaded pronouncement that her FSH levels were high and was given a diagnosis of premature ovarian failure. She was told that her ovaries had quit responding to hormonal stimulation, and therefore, the quality of her eggs was poor, resulting in inferior-quality embryos.

After her last miscarriage, Laura's FSH was measured at 18 milligrams on cycle day 3. (Normal FSH should be below 10 milligrams on cycle day 3.) Her periods ceased, and her body was immediately thrown into what seemed like menopause. She sweated all the time. She was always tired because she was so hot and miserable at night that she couldn't sleep. She was experiencing heart palpitations, general irritability, and lethargy. She reported vaginal dryness but wasn't overly concerned because her libido was nonexistent. Just before she came to see me, her FSH was 29 milligrams, and she had been given a prescription for hormone replacement therapy.

When Laura came to my clinic, I noticed her hands were ice cold and her skin was clammy. Her pulse was very frail, almost undetectable, and her tongue was bright red and quivered. She had a classic presentation of Spleen Qi and Kidney Yin deficiency with deficient heat in the Heart. She was sweating out all the fluids in her body, making her hot, dry, and miserable. I knew her condition would respond best to herbal therapy, so I saw her in the clinic every two weeks for herbal modification. I prescribed raw herbs, which are stronger than the powdered concentrates. I gave her a formula consisting of oystershell (Mu Li), Astragalus (Huang Qi), Ephedra root (Ma Huang Gen), unripened wheat (Fu Xiao Mai), and cooked Rehmannia (Shu Di Huang). She boiled up the ingredients daily and drank the resulting tea. She reported that although it tasted and smelled "less than appealing," her body began to crave it.

Within a month, her sweating stopped, and she was sleeping and feeling better. Her vaginal discharge returned, and two weeks later she had a period. Within three more weeks, the vaginal discharge appeared to be the clear, fertile type she remembered, and she used an ovulation kit, which indicated she was indeed ovulating again.

Laura became pregnant, but soon after, she started to experience feverlike sensations, which caused profuse sweating from her chest. She recalled that she had felt this way when she had miscarried previously. She was still drinking her herbal tea, but had cut down on it dramatically. I urged her to continue drinking the tea, that it was more important now than ever. However, I modified the prescription to clear heat from the Heart by adding Scutellaria (Huang Qin), an herb that clears heat from the upper body and also has an empirical effect of "calming the fetus" to prevent miscarriage.

Laura's body calmed down, and her pregnancy continued. She came to the clinic for acupuncture treatments every week throughout the first trimester, and then returned only for assistance in preparing for labor. She soon became the proud mother of a healthy baby girl.

With autoimmune disorders and recurrent miscarriage, our own bodies are fighting against our intense desire for motherhood. But if we wish our wombs to nurture the children we want so much, we need to provide the same kind of gentle care to every aspect of our bodies. Once we have restored balance and health, our immune systems can do only what they are meant to do — keep us healthy — even as they welcome the new energy of a child to take up residence within us.

13

Endometriosis and Fibroids: Cleansing Your Uterus So a Child Can Grow

The lotus springs from the mud.

— CHINESE PROVERB

What do endometriosis and fibroids have in common? Both conditions are characterized by inappropriate tissue growth within the reproductive system, causing damage to the reproductive organs and preventing conception. There is no Western cure for either. In Eastern medicine, however, they are both considered processes of inhibited, stagnated uterine Blood. The menstruate has become blocked, and the normal reproductive cycle is therefore obstructed. Women with either of these conditions often experience a sedimentlike menstrual flow with dark, brown, clotted blood that has been allowed to oxidize. The immune system reacts to this silty, old blood, recognizing its toxic state and mounting chemicals to clean up the debris. (Remember, our body's immunologic priority is to keep us safe from external or internal insults.)

Luckily, both conditions respond very well to Chinese medicine. Given time and the proper treatment, the blood flow will improve, the sediment will clear, and the body will overcome its immunologic protective mechanisms. Our psychoneuroendocrine system will settle down, and our body can relax so conception can take place.

❧ ENDOMETRIOSIS: THE RIGHT TISSUE IN THE WRONG PLACE

Endometriosis affects millions of women, and while it is most commonly diagnosed in women between thirty and forty years of age, it can begin as early as the teenage years. The condition is classified according to its severity — mild (small, flat patches of endometrial tissue growing outside the uterine lining), moderate (larger, often somewhat raised implants), or severe (inflammation and scarring caused by the unabsorbed blood creates bands of fibrous scar tissue — adhesions — that bind pelvic organs together). Symptoms of endometriosis include painful periods (women with endometriosis have higher prostaglandin levels, one of the causes of menstrual pain), pathological uterine bleeding, and bleeding at sites other than the endometrium (sometimes as distant as the nasal cavity) during menstruation. Other symptoms include back pain or severe abdominal cramping during menstruation, painful intercourse, painful intestinal upset or urination during menstruation, and, of course, infertility. In some cases, the high levels of pain caused by endometriosis can deplete a woman's energy and cause depression and anxiety. However, there may be no symptoms at all associated with the condition. Around 40 percent of women diagnosed with endometriosis report no symptoms other than infertility.

In endometriosis, the endometrial cells somehow migrate and implant in areas outside the uterus. Common sites of implantation include the cervix, the vaginal-rectal space, the ovaries, the fallopian tubes, the colon, and the bladder wall. Endometrial cells also have been found in the abdominal wall muscles, the lungs, the nose, even the brain. These misplaced endometrial cells respond to the hormonal stimuli of estrogen and progesterone just like the endometrium is supposed to: they bleed during menstruation. But there is no way for this blood to leave the body, so it stagnates at the site of the endometrial implantation, causing inflammation and possibly scarring in the surrounding tissue.

Retrograde menstruation is one theory that explains endometrial tissue migration. When a woman is supposed to menstruate, the blood should be discharged through the cervix. But sometimes it can seep back up the fallopian tubes and flow into the abdominal cavity. Endometrial cells in the menstrual blood then can attach to sites in the abdominal cavity, outside the uterus. Western medicine theorizes that anatomic abnormalities such as a retroverted uterus or a smaller than usual cervical opening (which does not allow the blood to pass through freely) cause menstrual blood to back up into other areas of the pelvis. However, many women have some degree of retrograde menstruation or anatomic abnormality and yet do not have the endometriosis reaction.

Some researchers believe that endometrial cells are transported through the blood and lymph systems to different sites in the body. Others theorize that embryonic cells outside of the uterus are transformed by some unknown stimulus into endometrial cells. It is clear there is a lack of consensus on the cause of this disease.

Western science is also somewhat at a loss when it comes to understanding why women with endometriosis have fertility problems. Certainly, the scarring and adhesions associated with severe endometriosis can obstruct the path of the egg to the uterus, but women with milder cases can suffer impaired fertility as well. It is possible that dysfunction in the ovaries or the hormonal issues producing luteal phase defect causes problems leading to endometriosis. (Approximately 27 percent of women with mild endometriosis also have ovulatory dysfunction or luteal phase defect.) Another theory holds that endometrial implants secrete prostaglandins, which can cause muscle spasms in the reproductive organs and hinder their proper functioning.

It's probable that endometriosis is yet another autoimmune disease. Some women who are diagnosed with endometriosis have high levels of autoantibodies, which are associated with recurrent miscarriage (see chapter 12). Endometriosis creates an inflammatory reaction in the body, in response to the endometrial tissue growing outside its intended site. In an attempt to "clean up" this tissue, the immune system is reprogrammed to react to *all* endometrial cells as if they were not part of the body. This reaction can cause the endometrial cells in the uterus to cease production of the protein marker (beta-integrin-3) needed to encourage a fertilized egg to implant. It can also cause the endometrial glands to fail to respond to the progesterone produced during the luteal phase of the reproductive cycle.

Regardless of the cause of endometriosis, current Western medical treatment for the condition can be risky when it comes to fertility. Usually, pain-relieving medication is prescribed to mitigate discomfort, and then the patient either undergoes surgery or is prescribed hormone-controlling drugs to remove the excess endometrial tissue. Sometimes the endometrial growths are surgically excised or burned off with a laser. In severe cases (many growths or extensive adhesions), major surgery may be required, after which fertility may or may not be restored.

Hormonal treatments like birth control pills and testosterone-enhancing or menopause-inducing drugs are sometimes prescribed to halt menstruation altogether, the theory being that when menstruation ceases the misplaced endometrial tissue will "starve" to death. Of course, ovulation is also halted in the process. In addition, the masculinizing side effects of increased testosterone are difficult for women to endure. Even if the displaced endometrial tissue is surgically removed, the toxic effects may remain. The lingering presence of endometrial cells can continue to contaminate the fallopian tubes, affecting the egg's ability to become fertilized as it travels toward the uterus.

If tests reveal inflammation as a result of endometriosis, the only Western treatment is to use GnRH agonists like Lupron. These drugs are designed to inhibit the release of pituitary hormones, which then don't stimulate the ovaries to produce their hormones, thus depriving the endometrium of hormonal stimulus. A course of Lupron is often followed quickly with an IVF procedure in the hope that the endometrium cooperates and an embryo can implant. However, GnRH agonists can cause unpleasant menopausal symptoms like hot flashes, night sweats, and general irritability. And, of course, the underlying inflammation caused by the endometrial disorder has not really been addressed.

THE TCM VIEW AND TREATMENT OF ENDOMETRIOSIS

While endometriosis is not a disease category in TCM, Eastern healers have recognized this disease for far longer than Western medicine. In TCM, endometriosis is known by its symptoms and is referred to as "menstrual movement pain." In the *Jin Gui Yao Lue* (*Essentials from the Golden Cabinet*), the chapter on "Women's Miscellaneous Diseases' Pulse, Pattern and Treatment" describes this condition as follows: "The menstrual blood is inhibited and there is (resulting) lower abdominal fullness and pain." Just as Western medicine believes retrograde menstruation is created by pelvic and uterine anomalies including cervical stenosis (when the cervical canal doesn't open), congenital pelvic defects would be characterized as a general Kidney deficiency in TCM. Kidney deficiency is commonly diagnosed in conjunction with Blood stasis (**Bl X**) in women with endometriosis. Therefore, we must treat both patterns for complete resolution.

Chinese medicine categorizes endometrial lesions as static Blood, or Blood that is not flowing as it should. (This is not so different from our Western understanding of endometriosis.) However, since the compromised Blood is located in an area where normal blood flow is often absent or minimal, the body has a tougher time resolving it. The Chinese say the static Blood has entered the network vessels (offshoots of the major meridians, like energetic capillaries), which are more difficult to reach. When an enduring disease enters the network vessels, it is wise to employ the use of resins like frankincense and myrrh with treatment. The Chinese say these resinous herbs infiltrate into the deeper meridians, just as sap penetrates a tree.

As we discussed earlier, static Blood may also trigger an inappropriate immune system response to the endometrial cells growing outside the uterus. If the immune system detects endometrial cells in the wrong place, an inflammatory reaction is mounted to protect the rest of the body from this perceived "invader." When the immune system is unable to eradicate the misplaced tissue, it reacts to *all* endometrial tissue, creating a toxic environment for an implanting embryo. In TCM, this process is almost always categorized as Blood stasis with excess heat (^H) or Blood stasis with damp heat (**DH**), and is treated accordingly.

When I treat a woman with these patterns, I put her on a pure macrobiotic-type diet, free of dairy, wheat, and most animal products, to calm the immune system. I also have her supplement with flaxseed, evening primrose or fish oil, and bioflavonoids like pycnogenol, a superantioxidant helpful in muting immune responses. I then prescribe an herbal formula to clear internal Blood heat (which is a Chinese approach to resolving immunologic processes), and I calm the Uterus with acupuncture. Within a few months, pregnancy usually will occur naturally. Sometimes the body responds immediately; other times it takes up to eight months for some of my patients to conceive after beginning treatments.

HERBAL TREATMENTS FOR ENDOMETRIOSIS

Chinese herbal formulas have been tested against common Western medical treatments for endometriosis, with some surprising results. One such study, conducted at Osaka City University Medical School in Japan, measured immune factors in the blood of a group of women diagnosed with endometriosis. The women were found to have elevated serum levels of anti-endometrial immunoglobulin M (IgM) antibody titers, indicating an immune response to the endometrial tissue. One group of women received treatment with leuprolide acetate (Lupron) to suppress hormonal production. A second group received the herbal formula Cinnamon Twig and Poria Pill (Gui Zhi Fu Ling Wan), which historically has been used in China to treat bleeding during pregnancy caused by Blood stasis (**Bl X**) in the womb, or to prevent miscarriage.

At the conclusion of the study, the Lupron-treated group had lower levels of estradiol but no change in the IgM antibody titer. The group treated with herbs had no changes in estradiol levels, but the levels of IgM antibody titer were decreased and the patients remained symptom-free for months. It would appear the herbal formula was able to reduce the body's immune response to the endometriosis — a hopeful sign when it comes to restoring a woman's fertility.

Another study, done in China, treated women with severe menstrual pain. (The authors stated that the primary disease mechanism related to dysmenorrhea is Blood stasis [**Bl X**] — the same pattern that often creates endometriosis.) A group of 125 women were diagnosed using the principles of TCM and were categorized into four groups depending on the patterns they were exhibiting.

- **Group 1:** Qi stagnation with Blood stasis
- **Group 2:** Qi stagnation, Blood stasis, and cold
- **Group 3:** Qi stagnation, Blood stasis, and heat
- **Group 4:** Qi stagnation, Blood stasis, and deficiency

The study began by comparing serum levels of various prostaglandins (a contributing factor in menstrual cramps) in the bloodstreams of all three groups. Then the women were given either Eastern or Western medical treatment. The women treated with Eastern methods received an herbal formula whose intended purpose is to invigorate the Blood, transform stasis, and move the Qi. (From a Western medical point of view, the formula achieves its effect by regulating serum prostaglandins.) The herbs were taken as a decoction and administered twice a day beginning two weeks before the anticipated start of the period. The other women were given the Western medicine indomethacin, a nonsteroidal anti-inflammatory analgesic. In both groups, treatment was administered for three months.

In the group treated with herbs, 80.4 percent of women experienced relief from their menstrual pain, compared to 73.3 percent for the indomethacin group. Further, the herbs seemed to help balance the reproductive cycle, as indicated by markedly lower levels of a negative type of estrogen. The herbal decoction also increased the content of late-phase progesterone secreted by the corpus luteum (essential to creating a proper climate for implantation). Indomethacin, on the other hand, had no marked effect on either estrogen or progesterone.

It is clear that Chinese herbal medicines can play an important part in balancing the complex interrelated factors contributing to both the treatment of endometriosis and the promotion of a normal reproductive cycle. But what is most important, of course, is to discover the pattern of imbalance that has caused the individual patient's problem. If you have endometriosis, please refer to the pattern diagnosis section of chapter 4 to evaluate your underlying imbalance, and then use the herbs recommended in chapter 8 to restore your system to health.

OTHER PATTERNS THAT MAY CONTRIBUTE TO ENDOMETRIOSIS

Like many conditions related to the reproductive cycle, endometriosis involves imbalances in several of the body's energetic systems and Organs. According to TCM, contributing patterns include:

- Liver Qi stagnation (**Lv Qi X**)
- Heat (**^H**)
- Damp heat (**DH**)
- Blood stasis (**Bl X**)
- Cold conditions (like Kidney Yang deficiency [**Ki Yan–**]) causing stagnation and severe menstrual pain
- Spleen Qi deficiency (**Sp–**)

◆ Kidney Yang deficiency (**Ki Yan–**)

◆ Blood deficiency (**Bl–**)

◆ Mixed heat and cold, deficiency and repletion — includes Spleen Qi (**Sp–**) and/or Kidney Yang (**Ki Yan–**) deficiency, Blood stasis (**Bl X**), and Liver Qi stagnation (**Lv Qi X**) (If symptoms include digestive complaints, and the tongue has a patchy coating, the herbal formula Mume Pill [Wu Mei Wan] has been found to be very effective.)

In each case, the pattern must be addressed using dietary principles, herbal categories, and acupressure treatments based upon the diagnostic presentation.

Endometriosis also is related to hormonal imbalances such as estrogen dominance. Estrogen feeds endometriosis; it is therefore important to help the body rid itself of excess estrogen. Since the liver metabolizes estrogen, using methods that resolve Liver Qi stagnation (**Lv Qi X**) will assist the body in clearing surplus amounts of the hormone. To resolve Liver Qi stagnation, you can stimulate the acupuncture points Lv 2, Lv 3, and Lv 14 (see chapter 7). You can also use the dietary recommendations and herbal preparations in chapters 6 and 8 to move Liver Qi and resolve Blood stasis (**Bl X**).

In both Eastern and Western medicine, endometriosis is seen as an effect of retrograde menstruation, so we need to view the therapy of endometriosis as supporting the downward, outward flow of the menstrual blood. Avoid breathing exercises emphasizing concentration on the upward energetics, like certain forms of yoga and Qi Gong, during menstruation. Also, use pads instead of tampons. Tampons block the flow of the menstrual blood, especially if the blood flow is clotted and not smooth already.

TCM IN ACTION: ANTHONY AND MARGARET FIND A WAY

Anthony and Margaret came to my clinic together, hopeful that I would offer them a chance to become parents. A few months earlier, they had been looking forward to their next IVF attempt when they attended a lecture I had given on TCM and infertility. Just prior, they had consulted a new doctor, who diagnosed Margaret with endometriosis after a laparoscopy. Although there were no obstructive problems or sperm issues, Margaret and Anthony had gone through many months of IUIs and one IVF prior to the discovery of her endometriosis.

They found the information in my lecture interesting but thought it didn't pertain to their situation; they held much hope for their IVF. Margaret said she liked the "immediacy" of the IVF procedure and that they were aggressively attacking the infertility problem. However, as with so many of my patients who take the assisted reproductive route, this attempt did not bear fruit. While the couple was trying to remain positive, they were becoming disillusioned with what Western reproductive endocrinology had to offer.

Margaret could tell that time was closing

in on her, not only from the desperation she was experiencing but also because her cycles were becoming shorter. She was ovulating earlier than she used to (about day 9 or 10 of her cycle), she was having night sweats, and, most ominous, her physician reported her day 3 FSH level was above the acceptable limit for future IVFs.

When Margaret came to my clinic, her pertinent symptoms were early ovulation, night sweats, short cycles of about twenty-three days, constipation, extreme breast discomfort, bad premenstrual tension, premenstrual headaches, excruciating back pain that worsened with the onset of menstruation, and severe, stabbing uterine cramps. She slept poorly and urinated frequently before and during her period. Her menstruation was bright red with black clots and normal in amount and duration. Her pulse was thready, rapid, and taut, and her tongue was red and peeled.

My diagnosis was Yin deficiency with deficiency heat, Liver Qi stagnation, and Blood stasis. The treatment plan was to nourish Kidney Yin, invigorate and cool the Blood, resolve Liver Qi stagnation, and clear heat. I began with acupuncture treatments, stimulating Sp 6, Ki 3, Sp 10, LI 11, Lv 2, Lv 3, LI 4, Yintang, auricular spirit point (ear triangular fossa), and ear intertragic notch, at various times in her menstrual cycle. Within a month, she had no PMS, breast tenderness, or headaches. I also gave her two herbal formulas — Six Flavor Pill with Rehmannia (Liu Wei Di Huang Wan) with red peony (Chi Shao) and moutan (Mu Dan Pi) to be taken before ovulation, and Rambling Powder (Xiao Yao San), Epimedium (Yin Yang Huo), and red peony (Chi Shao) to be taken premenstrually.

Each month, Margaret noticed new improvements in her cycle. The night sweats went away completely, her BBT graph became more consistently biphasic with less sawtooth temperature variations, and, even more important, her ovulation became delayed and her entire cycle lengthened to twenty-seven and twenty-eight days. I knew her FSH level would be in the normal range now.

Margaret became pregnant for the first time when she was thirty-nine years old. Her pregnancy was uneventful, and she gave birth to a healthy little boy.

UTERINE FIBROIDS

Uterine fibroids, or myomas, are the most common neoplasm (abnormal growth) of the female reproductive organs. They are benign tumors found in approximately 20 percent of women over thirty-five years of age. They can occur on the inner and outer wall of the uterus, or anywhere else in the pelvic cavity. They range in size from small (the size of a pea) to large (the size of a cantaloupe). Some women have only one small fibroid, whereas others have several.

Many women with fibroids report menstrual pain, heavy menstrual bleeding, and fertility problems. Fibroids on the back wall of the uterus can contribute to constipation, urinary tract difficulties, and heavy menstrual periods. Larger fibroids can cause pain with intercourse and pelvic pressure. Fibroids may impair conception if they obstruct the uterine cavity or the entrance into the uterus from the fallopian tubes. They also can block an embryo from implanting in the uterine wall. Fibroids can increase in size during pregnancy because of the increased hormone levels, causing pressure in the uterus and, in some cases, premature labor. Many fibroids have enough mass to be detected by a routine pelvic exam. To determine their extent and exact location, ultrasound, sonohysterography (a vaginal ultrasound using sterile salt water inside the uterus), hysteroscopy, and MRI are sometimes used.

Just as pregnancy hormones can cause a fibroid to grow, a lack of reproductive hormones can cause it to shrink. Western medical treatment occasionally uses drugs like Lupron to create the condition of pseudo-menopause. In many cases, drug therapy is accompanied by surgical removal of the fibroid. If the fibroids are small and accessible from inside the uterus, a laparoscopic procedure can be done, in which the surgeon uses a probe threaded through the cervix to destroy the fibroid using either heat or cold. Another technique is arterial embolization, when the blood vessels feeding the fibroid are cauterized. However, as this cuts off blood flow to the uterine lining as well, it is not recommended for women who wish to have children. In more complicated cases, when the tumors are larger or located on the outside of the uterus or in the pelvic cavity, a laparotomy may be necessary. This procedure, which involves an incision either through the abdominal wall or uterus, requires a three- to six-month healing process before pregnancy should be attempted. If the fibroids are too large or in a location that compromises a woman's health, hysterectomy — removal of the uterus — is the last line of treatment. With her uterus gone, a woman's only remaining means for parenthood are gestational surrogate or adoption.

❧ SHRINKING FIBROIDS THE EASTERN WAY

TCM provides far gentler and more effective remedies for fibroids. Like the tissues formed by endometriosis, fibroids are considered lumpy nodulations within the body caused by hardening static Blood (**Bl X**). This condition can be treated with means similar to those used for endometriosis, with equally dramatic results. One Chinese study used traditional Chinese medicinals to treat 223 cases of uterine fibroids. All patients had measurable symptoms, such as heavy menstrual bleeding, and were diagnosed clinically by pelvic examination confirmed by ultrasonography. Treatment involved invigorating the Blood and eliminating Blood stasis (**Bl X**), clearing heat, and softening the indurations (hardening of surrounding tissue caused by new growth, such as fibroids).

The basic herbal formula used in the study contained herbs to resolve Blood stasis and move Liver Qi stagnation (**Lv Qi X**). Additional specific herbs were added based on the different patterns (Yin deficiency, Qi stagnation, or heat) diagnosed as contributing to the formation of the fibroids. The appropriate herbal combinations were administered after menstruation. Following treatment, most of the patients' symptoms, like heavy blood flow, abnormal vaginal discharge, and backache, improved or were eliminated. The fibroids themselves were either diminished or disappeared in 72 percent of patients.

Acupuncture and acupressure are also recommended in the treatment of fibroids, using the points recommended in chapter 7 for Blood stasis (**Bl X**) in the Uterus. The stimulation provided by acupuncture has been found to reduce pathologically proliferating cells through local stimulation near the site of the growth. Stimulating points like Sp 10 and UB 17, which invigorate the Blood throughout the body, will help shrink fibroids.

TCM in Action: Maggie's Story

Maggie came to my clinic after being diagnosed with a grapefruit-size fibroid. She had been experiencing lower abdominal discomfort, bloating, and frequent urination, which prompted her to consult with her gynecologist. His solution was a hysterectomy, to which she was adamantly opposed.

I was newly in practice when Maggie came to see me, and not having much diagnostic experience, I relied on the knowledge that uterine fibroids usually mean Blood stasis. I provided acupuncture and herbal treatments to invigorate the Blood, but six weeks later had achieved no effect. So I went back over Maggie's symptoms to see what I had missed. I found she had signs of damp accumulation like phlegm production and postnasal drip, breast nodules, and vaginal discharge, which I previously hadn't considered significant. However, when I switched the focus of my treatment to supplementing the Spleen Qi to help resolve dampness and included some drying herbs with the Blood-moving formula, Maggie responded dramatically. Within a month, her discomfort had resolved, and when she went back for a follow-up appointment with a (new) gynecologist, the fibroid was completely gone.

OTHER NATURAL TREATMENTS FOR ENDOMETRIOSIS AND UTERINE FIBROIDS

Here's a list of recommendations for using TCM to treat your endometriosis or uterine fibroids. You'll find more specific information in chapters 6, 7, and 8.

- Rest and wear loose, comfortable clothing.
- Perform deep-breathing exercises and meditative practices.
- Take warm baths (with aromatherapy if you wish).
- Use essential oils like frankincense, myrrh, clary sage, peppermint, lavender, rosemary, juniper, and thyme.
- Use a heating pad or hot water bottle on your abdomen during and after menstruation.
- Apply warm castor-oil packs on your abdomen to invigorate the Blood, assist the lymphatic system, and balance hormone levels. Apply warm castor oil to the lower abdomen and cover with plastic wrap two to three times per day during the premenstrual and menstrual period. (If you are actively trying to conceive, use only during the menstrual period.)
- Follow dietary recommendations according to the immune-calming, Spleen-supplementing diet in chapter 6.
- Massage the acupressure points for resolving Blood stasis (Sp 6, Sp 8, Sp 10, UB 17) and for whichever other diagnostic categories apply. Ki 3 and Ki 7 increase circulation of the reproductive organs, and Lv 2 and Lv 3 help detoxify excess hormones and resolve stagnated Qi.
- Regular, moderate daily exercise helps improve circulation and ease symptoms. Meditation, Qi Gong, and yoga are also helpful. (However, you should not perform inversion techniques during menstruation, especially if you have endometriosis. The energetic flow must always be descending.)
- Take herbal supplements to invigorate the Blood, as well as those for resolving your particular pattern presentation (see chapter 8). Bupleurum (Chai Hu) and Angelica (Dang Gui) have been used together for millennia to regulate hormones and relax the nervous system. Safflower (Hong Hua) and peach kernel (Tao Ren) decrease inflammation in the lower abdomen. Nettle is also good after menstruation.
- Avoid all foods that have been treated hormonally.
- Consume soy and soy products like tofu.
- Eat only organic fruits and vegetables.
- Avoid refined and hydrogenated oils.
- Use only unprocessed plant sources of essential fatty acids.

◆ Use oils rich in both linoleic and alpha-linolenic fatty acids such as flaxseed, pumpkin-seed, and chia-seed oils, but *only* if they are recently cold-pressed and refined.

◆ Include dietary spirulina, evening primrose oil, and oil from black currant and borage seeds.

◆ Avoid sources of arachidonic acid, which comes from animal meats, dairy products, eggs, and peanuts.

◆ Avoid all animal products, except fish. If you do consume meat, make sure it is organic and not hormonally treated.

◆ Eat walnuts, dark greens, saffron, and cold-climate root vegetables like squash.

◆ Foods that are especially good for resolving Blood stasis (**Bl X**) include kelp, lemons, limes, onions, Irish moss, and bladder wrack.

◆ Supplement your diet with B vitamins and antioxidants like vitamins C, E, beta-carotene, selenium, and zinc. Include OPC superantioxidants (grape seed extract, pine bark extract, red wine extract, bilberry extract), which contain procyanidins and caffeic and ferulic acid. These substances have demonstrated anti-inflammatory and antispastic effects.

◆ Both fibroids and endometriosis benefit from the use of omega-3 fatty acids in the diet. Fish oil and linseed oil are good sources of these omega-3 fatty acids. Fish oil prevents abnormal blood clotting. If your menstrual blood contains clotty tissue, supplement with fish oil, linseed oil, and evening primrose oil (which also contains gamma-linolenic acid, known as omega-6).

For conception to occur, all the energies of the body must be free-flowing and moving, like water in the river bringing life to the land through which it passes. Fibroids and endometrial growths are like rocks in that river, preventing the embryo from mooring safely within the walls of your womb. By eliminating Blood stasis, balancing the body's other energies, and softening the concretions within your reproductive organs, you can restore the flow of the "river of life" through you and provide a clean, clear harbor for your unborn child.

14

PCOS and POF:
You *Can* Heal Your Ovaries

The little seed cracks, and the spirit of heaven emerges.

— SCANDINAVIAN PROVERB

The ripening of eggs within the follicles of our ovaries is a miracle. From birth, women are filled with all the eggs they will ever have — one to two million of them. For most of us, the eggs we possess at birth, and the 400,000 or so we still have when we begin menstruating, are more than enough to ensure the possibility of pregnancy before we enter menopause. However, even though our ovaries are the "nests" holding our eggs and allowing them to ripen and release every month, the "weather" permitting ovulation — the cascade of hormones that must happen in the right amounts at the right time — can very easily fail to do its job. Then our ovaries are left without the support they need to nurture our potential children. If our hormones are out of whack long enough, the ovaries themselves can become afflicted with disease or fail altogether. There can be many causes for the hormonal interference that saps vitality from our ovaries. In this chapter, we'll look at two specific conditions, polycystic ovarian syndrome (PCOS) and premature ovarian failure (POF), both of which are manifestations of hormonal imbalance.

❧ POLYCYSTIC OVARIAN SYNDROME

Polycystic ovarian syndrome, or PCOS (also known as Stein-Leventhal syndrome), is defined as a disorder of ovulation, but it also can affect the skin, hair, body weight, reproductive system, and endocrine system, including the pancreas, hypothalamus, pituitary gland, and adrenal glands. Polycystic ovarian syndrome was first recognized as a medical disease, or syndrome, in 1845 in France. It is said to affect up to 10 percent of women of reproductive age and up to 90 percent of women with irregular menstrual cycles.

The primary outward indication of possible PCOS is irregular or absent periods, often dating back to menarche. Yet PCOS has a multitude of other symptoms, including obesity (about 50 percent of women with PCOS are overweight), acne, excess facial hair and/or increased body hair, and thinning of the hair on the head. There also may be high lipid levels in the blood (an indication of possible cardiovascular disease in the future) and disturbance of sugar metabolism. Women with PCOS are also at risk for other health hazards like vascular disease and cancer. Of course, infertility is one symptom experienced by many women with PCOS. (It's important to note, however, that some women with PCOS have none of these symptoms.)

In 1990, a National Institutes of Health conference stated that the two most consistent elements of PCOS include elevated androgenic hormones and chronic lack of ovulation. In PCOS, multiple small cysts, which are actually tiny follicles, develop inside the ovaries. The cysts are not the same as active follicles but instead have been arrested in their development, never growing to full size or releasing healthy eggs. The cysts and the connective tissue surrounding them produce male hormones called androgens. Androgens block follicular development and cause the follicles to degenerate, preventing the release of mature eggs.

In addition, androgen produced by the cysts enters the bloodstream and alters the feedback mechanism within the HPO axis. The amount of estrogen circulating in the bloodstream increases in relation to other hormones like progesterone, causing increased production of LH and testosterone. Because of this hormonal cascade, ovulation is prevented. Yet many women with PCOS think they're ovulating because each time they use an ovulation predictor test it turns positive. That's because the urine test detects LH, which in some women with PCOS remains elevated. Diagnostically, the most distinctive signs of PCOS are changes in the ovaries, which are larger than average and appear to have a thick, shiny, white coating over the many rows of cysts on their surface.

If your Western medical doctor suspects PCOS, he or she will undoubtedly order a series of tests. You may have your ovaries examined by ultrasound or undergo blood tests to evaluate a number of hormonal factors.

In some cases, women with PCOS can have very long cycles and very heavy bleeding; in other cases, they don't ovulate and have little to no bleeding. With PCOS, if an egg is released it is often later in a woman's cycle, and it is of poorer quality because of the unhealthy surroundings in which it has been developing.

Western medical doctors and scientists have been unable to pinpoint the actual cause of PCOS and thus have been unable to treat it effectively. One contributing factor appears to be abnormal insulin and glucose (sugar) interaction. Excess insulin circulating in the bloodstream stimulates enzymes that help manufacture androgens in the ovaries. High insulin levels may also over-stimulate androgen receptors, leading to follicular atresia (basically "starving" the follicles of the correct hormonal food for the developing eggs). Improper insulin production or insulin resistance can contribute to obesity, which is one of the reasons many women with PCOS are overweight. Glucose intolerance and diabetes also are associated with insulin resistance.

Women diagnosed with PCOS often are prescribed a series of drugs such as clomiphene, hCG, and gonadotropin. If these drugs fail, IVF and other ART are recommended. However, most women with PCOS don't respond well to any hormonal manipulation that does not address both the health of the egg and the state of the ovary's endocrine balance over the previous three or more months of development.

Remember, follicular development within the ovary is a process that takes many months. Eggs are meant to develop in an estrogen- and progesterone-rich environment, not in an androgenic setting. Therefore, even if a woman's body is forced to ovulate with ovulation-stimulating drugs, the quality of her eggs may be poor. If women with PCOS do become pregnant, they have a higher risk of miscarriage, presumably because of the health of the egg and its effect on the developing embryo. In addition, women with PCOS run the risk of possible ovarian hyperstimulation syndrome (OHSS) triggered by the medication. Ovarian hyperstimulation syndrome can be life threatening, resulting in painful enlargement of ovaries, fluid retention in the abdominal cavity, nausea, and fever.

Other treatments for PCOS focus on surgically eliminating follicular cysts, or balancing hormone levels using drugs and / or supplements, such as dexamethasone, an oral steroid. However, long-term use of such drugs can cause bone changes in the hip joints. Drugs like Glucophage or Actos are often prescribed to control insulin and blood sugar levels. Still, the current knowledge of Western reproductive medicine offers few options and little hope for women with PCOS.

✿ POLYCYSTIC OVARIAN SYNDROME: THE EASTERN VIEW

Chinese medicine seeks to redress the entire hormonal milieu that produces the changes in a woman's ovaries seen in PCOS. The most common manifestation of PCOS is dampness or phlegm. Going back to our checklist from chapter 4, the symptoms for phlegm (considered dampness) include:

◆ feeling tired and sluggish after a meal
◆ fibrocystic breasts
◆ cystic or pustular acne
◆ urgent, bright, or foul-smelling stools
◆ menstrual blood containing stringy tissue or mucus
◆ being prone to yeast infections and vaginal itching
◆ aches in the joints, especially with movement
◆ being overweight
◆ a wet, slimy tongue

However, with some conditions like PCOS, even if you do not fit the diagnostic criteria perfectly, we assume there is some element of phlegm that is very deep and does not necessarily produce external symptoms. In TCM, this condition is seen as a disorder consisting of quite a few possible linked patterns of deficiency and excess. All the patterns have different manifestations in the way the body ovulates.

(Remember, most women with PCOS ovulate later in the cycle, if at all.) For example, phlegm obstruction can produce a BBT graph that does not exhibit the typical two-phase pattern but is more of an erratic, flat line across the graph (a typical PCOS presentation). It may also reveal a long follicular phase (indicated by low basal temperatures) with a shortened luteal phase (indicated by high basal temperatures). Yang Qi deficiency may produce phlegm because the fluids aren't moving but condensing.

Treatment must be based upon these different patterns as well as on the different ways these patterns show up as symptoms. You may categorize your symptoms in any combination of these diagnostic categories. While your treatment should be based first and foremost on your diagnostic pattern, here are some general recommendations for patterns related to PCOS.

DIETARY THERAPY

Most women with PCOS have endocrine abnormalities affected by diet. If you are overweight, you can help treat your PCOS by losing weight. Fat cells store estrogen, and usually there is relatively too much circulating estrogen and LH in women with

PCOS. The liver metabolizes these hormones, so a healthy functioning liver is also mandatory for proper insulin balance. To keep the liver healthy, include dietary sources of the B vitamins, like meats and organ meats, leafy green vegetables, and whole grains.

Because of the insulin resistance and impaired glucose metabolism often found with PCOS, it is very important to modify your diet if you have this condition. The best natural management for insulin resistance and impaired glucose metabolism is to lower the level of sugar intake and eliminate the ingestion of any food the body utilizes as simple sugar. The following list outlines an insulin-managing diet.

◆ Cut out all forms of refined sugar.

◆ Cut out all forms of refined carbohydrates, as the body immediately turns them into sugar. Refined carbohydrates include white bread, pasta, white rice, most breakfast cereals, rice cakes, or any starchy, low-fiber food.

◆ Do not follow fertility diets advocating massive yam consumption. The high starch and sugar content in yams exacerbates the impaired glucose metabolism and can actually delay or prevent ovulation if you have PCOS.

◆ Avoid soda, fruit juice, and any drink that rapidly raises the blood sugar level.

◆ Consume adequate amounts of protein, either in vegetarian form or in the form of lean meat that has not been treated hormonally.

◆ Eat as many fresh vegetables as you wish.

◆ Eat only complex, whole grains like oatmeal, brown rice, and whole wheat.

◆ Eat fruits like berries, which are not too sweet.

◆ Avoid milk and dairy products, which tend to exacerbate the condition of internal dampness.

◆ Eliminate alcohol and caffeine.

◆ Increase your dietary fiber intake.

◆ Get adequate amounts of exercise.

◆ Do the exercises listed in chapter 6 to increase blood flow to the ovaries.

❧ NOTE: Adhering to a low-carbohydrate diet and eliminating sugar and starches may make you prone to hypoglycemia (low blood sugar) until your body gets used to its new metabolic regime. The addition of chlorophyll helps reduce the symptoms of hypoglycemia without raising your blood glucose level. Chromium also increases the sensitivity of insulin receptors within the cell to fluctuations in blood sugar levels. Recommended chromium dosage is approximately 300 micrograms per day. Other supplements that improve insulin resistance include the B vitamins, magnesium, alpha-lipoic acid, and conjugated linoleic acid.

One novel treatment for insulin imbalance is the antioxidant N-acetylcysteine (NAC). In a study done at the Università Cattolica del Sacro Cuore in Rome, Italy, women with impaired glucose tolerance and hyperinsulinism were given between 1.8 and 3 grams of NAC per day. As a result of treatment, they exhibited statistically significant decreases in total circulating testosterone levels and free androgen index, as well as total cholesterol, plasma triglycerides, low-density lipoproteins, insulin, pancreatic C-peptide, and insulin sensitivity. (In TCM, NAC would be categorized as a Liver-clearing substance.)

USING HERBS TO TREAT PCOS

If you choose to supplement with herbs, include Gleditsia (Zao Jiao Ci) during the first half of your menstrual cycle, before ovulation. Gleditsia is categorized as a phlegm-resolving medicinal in TCM and is known to dissolve the waxy capsule that forms around the ovaries in PCOS. Gleditsia also promotes ovulation.

Most women with ovulatory pain have Blood stasis (**Bl X**) on ovulation, and Leonurus seed (Chong Wei Zi) is a Blood-quickening medicinal that encourages ovulation in those who have any element of Blood stasis. Other herbs are given to address the concurrent patterns of imbalance that were introduced in earlier chapters. Using the combination of diet, acupuncture, and herbs, anovulatory women should begin to notice signs of ovulation, like increased fertile vaginal discharge followed by an elevation in their BBT, after a couple of months of treatment. Women with belated ovulation will often notice that their ovulation comes earlier and earlier in the cycle, indicating healthier egg production.

TREATING PCOS WITH ACUPUNCTURE

Studies done in Europe in the 1990s on anovulatory women with PCOS showed that electroacupuncture restored ovulation in one-third of the test subjects. Acupuncture also reduced endocrine indicators of PCOS, including LH/FSH ratios, mean testosterone concentrations, and beta-endorphin concentrations. Researchers theorized that this improvement was caused by an inhibition of hyperactivity in the sympathetic nervous system (see chapter 11). A more recent Swedish/Italian study described in *Biology of Reproduction* (2000) validated this theory. This study involved using injections of estradiol valerate (a kind of estrogen) to induce a state of polycystic ovaries in rats. Increased activity of the sympathetic nervous system resulted, followed by increased concentrations of nerve growth factor in the rats' ovaries and adrenal glands. Within sixty days, the rats developed polycystic ovaries.

The rodent subjects were separated into two groups. The control group received no therapy and maintained features of PCOS. The other group was treated with acupuncture and showed a decrease in the hyperactivity of the ovarian sympathetic nerve fibers, reduction of the increased nerve growth factor concentrations within the ovaries to normal, and shrinkage of the weight of the polycystic ovaries. All these are indicators of a diminished "stress" reaction within the nerve and blood supply of polycystic ovaries. Acupuncture treatments were effective in resolving this condition because they reduced the level of hypersympathetic nervous system response, relaxing the whole neuroendocrine system.

In other words, acupuncture works to restore the entire sympathetic nervous system to health and balance. The result is a normalization of the hormonal system directly tied to ovulation and reproduction; then the entire hormonal cascade allowing an egg to develop and be released can occur on schedule. With PCOS, I often include acupuncture treatments that normalize the hormonal environment, stimulating Yintang, ear intertragic notch, Sp 6, Zigong, Ren 3, Ren 4, Ren 6, and St 40 to resolve phlegm. Then I use electroacupuncture treatment to the lower back (UB 23, UB 32, UB 52) along with Sp 6 and ear triangular fossa to reduce the sympathetic activity to the ovaries. And, as always, I address the underlying pattern.

With all treatments, however, it's important to remember the hundred-day time line for the production of a healthy egg. To ensure follicles are healthy and capable of nurturing healthy eggs, I recommend that my patients wait three cycles before they start trying to get pregnant. Give your body (and your future child) the chance for the healthiest conception and pregnancy possible.

TCM IN ACTION: MARTY'S "CURE" IS MORE THAN A HEALTHY BABY

Marty, thirty-eight, and her husband had been trying to conceive for three years. Her gynecologist had given her the diagnosis of anovulation caused by PCOS. This diagnosis was based upon ultrasound examination that showed thickened ovaries containing multiple cysts, and a laboratory blood analysis that revealed elevated levels of testosterone, LH, and prolactin, as well as insulin resistance.

Marty was short in stature with more than adequate body fat, yet she had minimal secondary sexual characteristics — small breasts and narrow hips. She began to menstruate just before she was eleven years old (early menarche indicates strong Kidney function) and had become sexually active at age thirteen. She had been on oral contraceptives from age eighteen through thirty-five. Her cycles used to be around 29 days, but now they were typically 40 to 50 days apart. Her periods were extremely painful. The pain was preceded by intestinal discomfort, especially above and behind the rectum; she experienced relief with a bowel movement. Afterward, the pain moved to the front. This sensation lasted two to three days, was heavy and stabbing, and was not relieved by heat, cold, or pressure. (This told me her condition was excessive rather than deficient in nature.) She suffered from premenstrual migraine headaches (severe, stabbing, behind one eye) and had premenstrual tension and irritability. She bled for five days, and the blood was heavy and dark red with clotting. During the first day of her period, she experienced dizziness with blurred vision. There was no spotting between periods.

Marty had excessive facial hair and very

oily skin, and also had experienced discharge from her nipples. She had a stressful occupation, did not exercise regularly, and described her sexual energy as low. She suffered from allergies, fatigue, irritability, nervousness, sinus headaches, and cold hands and feet. She reported eating a lot of sweets. She had a history of high blood pressure and elevated cholesterol levels. Her tongue was wet and pale pink, with an underlying purple hue and a slightly red tip. Her pulse was thready but taut.

My diagnostic impression of Marty was that she suffered from anovulation, delayed menstrual cycles, and menstrual pain caused by Spleen Qi deficiency with excess damp accumulation, Blood stasis, and Liver Qi stagnation, along with depressive heat (caused by Liver Qi stagnation). I asked her to start monitoring her BBT. I treated her weekly with acupuncture and prescribed several different herbal formulas to be taken at the different phases of her cycle. I used the energetic principles of each phase of the cycle but also addressed the components of her specific diagnostic pattern throughout.

Over the following weeks, Marty's pulse became stronger and no longer had the thready quality. (It did, however, remain tight in quality, an indication of internal stress.) Her tongue also developed more color. She still experienced symptoms of cold feet, premenstrual lower back pain, and low libido. Her next period contained no clots, and the blood was a brighter red. She continued to have slight premenstrual tension and breast tenderness, but the migraine

headaches went away. Her menstrual flow was still heavy, and she was cramping just as much. Her BBT graph was sawtoothed throughout the 35-day cycle (fig. 14.1).

We continued the same regimen, using acupuncture to balance weekly symptoms as they arose and to clear internal heat, a common recurring manifestation. After six months, Marty's symptoms seemed to stabilize. She suffered less irritability, and the menstrual blood seemed "healthier." But the cramps had not lessened, the periods were still 35 days apart, and, most important to her, she was still not ovulating.

Marty had all the signs of endometriosis (see chapter 13), which would have been a further impediment to conception if we had not addressed this aspect of her imbalance. I treated the Blood stasis further with herbs during the menses and acupuncture treatments (Sp 6, Sp 8, and ear triangular fossa) before and during menses to alleviate the menstrual discomfort. She supplemented her diet with pycnogenol and fish-oil capsules. After two more months, Marty's cycle shortened to 32 days, and her cramps were greatly lessened. She also said she felt better overall. Notably, her BBT graph started to reveal an ovulatory pattern. However, it was not yet totally biphasic.

The following month, I asked Marty if she would be willing to go on a carbohydrate-restrictive diet to control the insulin resistance. She cut out all refined sugars, sweeteners, starches, sodas, and fruit juices while she continued on the same herbal regimen. She also added the supplement NAC to her

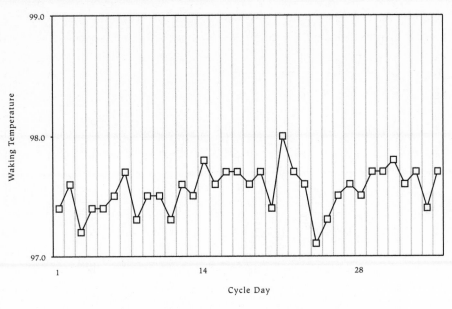

Figure 14.1: Marty's BBT Graph — Polycystic Ovarian Syndrome

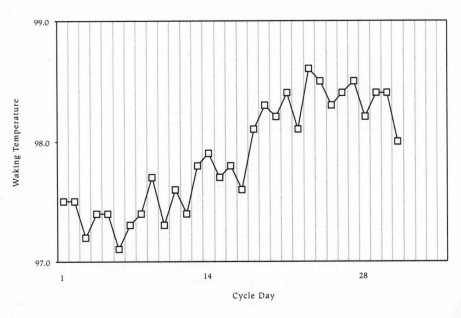

Figure 14.2: Marty's BBT Graph — Ovulation on Day 17

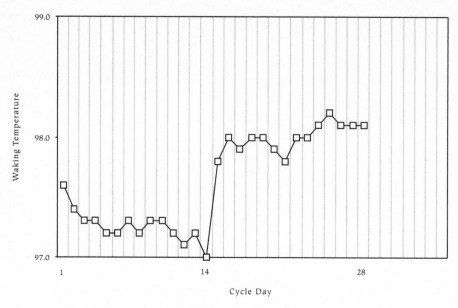

Figure 14.3: Marty's BBT Graph — Ovulation on Day 14

diet. The following month, she ovulated on day 17 (fig. 14.2). She continued on this regimen until ovulation occurred on day 14 (fig. 14.3).

Marty became pregnant in two more months. In addition to being a contented mother today, she is very happy about the alleviation of her menstrual symptoms. Most important, however, is that her overall endocrine imbalance has been addressed and resolved. She is ovulating on her own, her blood pressure and cholesterol levels are lower, and she feels healthier than ever before in her adult life.

🌺 PREMATURE OVARIAN FAILURE

Premature ovarian failure (POF) is essentially very early menopause, occurring before a woman reaches the age of forty. Remember I said that most women have hundreds of thousands of eggs at the time of menarche? By the time we hit full-blown menopause, that supply of eggs has dwindled.

This gradual loss of eggs during our fertile years is normal, but in POF, for some reason, either the loss of eggs is accelerated or the follicles themselves become less responsive to hormonal stimulation (of course, these conditions contribute to each other). Unfortunately, POF is one of the more common conditions affecting a woman's fertility — one in every thousand women between the ages of fifteen and twenty-nine, and one in every hundred women between the ages of thirty and thirty-nine is diagnosed with POF. Women with POF will have stopped menstruating altogether, or will have short cycles characterized by early (or no) ovulation. Sometimes periods do not occur at all, and menopausal symptoms — hot flashes, amenorrhea, and vaginal dryness — may appear suddenly over one to two months, or gradually over several years.

As ovulation occurs increasingly early in women with POF, the cycle is often accompanied by elevations in FSH, indicating that the ovaries are not responding to clues from the brain. This lack of communication causes hormonal "confusion." The hypo-thalamus gives the pituitary gland messages to try harder to stimulate the ovaries. More FSH is produced to invigorate the ovaries, but the ovaries, whose receptors are down, have become less responsive to this message. A BBT graph will typically show the pattern seen in fig. 14.4.

In such a case, estrogen production is reduced, the uterine lining is often too thin for implantation, and the follicles have not had time for their residing egg to fully mature, leaving no chance for conception.

Premature ovarian failure is an extremely frustrating diagnosis, as Western medicine cannot pinpoint its cause with any degree of accuracy. Some theories include chromosomal defects; damage from pelvic surgery, chemotherapy, or radiation therapy; or pelvic inflammatory disease (PID). One promising

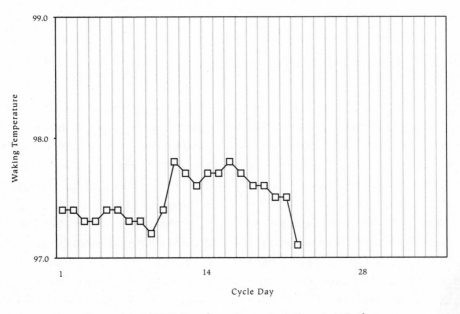

Figure 14.4: BBT Graph — Premature Ovarian Failure

avenue of investigation has to do with auto-immune disorders, in which a person's immune system attacks the body's own tissues, including (in theory) the ovaries. Often, a woman diagnosed with POF will have a concurrent diagnosis of conditions like autoimmune thyroiditis, Graves' disease, or Addison's disease (involving the adrenal glands).

Unfortunately, no matter what the cause of POF, Western medicine can do little to help it. Sometimes treating the associated autoimmune disorder (hypothyroidism, for example) will restore function to the ovaries, but this doesn't always work. If there is evidence of ovarian antibodies indicating an autoimmune disorder, high doses of steroids may be given in an attempt to restore ovarian function. However, the side effects of this treatment are severe. The treatment of choice for POF is usually estrogen replace-

ment therapy (a version of hormone replacement therapy, or HRT). However, this is not an option for women who are attempting to conceive because the estrogen tells the hypothalamus that it doesn't need to prompt the pituitary to stimulate the ovaries to produce estrogen. The whole hormonal system then goes to sleep.

Women with POF who consult reproductive endocrinologists are usually given one option: IVF with donor eggs. While this might give a woman a baby, it does nothing to address the underlying failure of the ovaries and all of the menopausal symptoms occurring as a result. And since the average age of POF onset is twenty-seven, most women with POF prefer a treatment that will restore their ovaries and hormonal system to full, functional health.

❧ THE CHINESE MEDICAL VIEW

Although treatment of POF may be challenging for the TCM practitioner, it is also rewarding because Chinese medicine offers one of the most effective ways to address POF. Traditional Chinese medicine views most cases of POF as a combination of excess and deficiency patterns causing the Penetrating and Conception meridians to become "empty." The lack of menstrual bleeding tells us there is also a deficiency in Blood (**Bl–**). Blood deficiency may be caused by an obstruction, but in most POF cases it is because of defi-

cient Blood *production*, usually from faltering Spleen energies (**Sp–**) or insufficient Kidney Yin (**Ki Yi–**). If a woman is experiencing short cycles, early ovulation, and heat signs like night sweats and hot flashes, there is also concurrent heat.

I view the condition of POF as a failure of communication: messages from the brain just aren't getting to the ovaries, which stop performing. As a result, the whole system increases its (Yang) energy to try to evoke a response from the ovaries, producing a frenetic cycle of stimulation with no effect. The result is depletion of Yin and deficiency heat. Most POF cases I have treated have presented with a severe Kidney Yin deficiency (**Ki Yi–**), usually accompanied by (Liver or Heart) Blood deficiency (**Bl–**), and Spleen Qi deficiency (**Sp–**) with deficient heat. It also is not unusual to see concurrent Kidney Yang deficiency (**Ki Yan–**).

A typical treatment will consist of the following recommendations:

♦ Follow dietary modifications from the Spleen-fortifying diet, avoiding wheat, refined carbohydrates, sugars, dairy, and most animal products (see chapter 6). It's also wise to avoid hot, spicy foods if signs of internal heat are present. We want to calm the body down to make it less reactive. Dietary insults can set off aggravations in autoimmune conditions.

♦ Take herbs like Astragalus (Huang Qi) to fortify the Spleen; herbs to nourish Yin and Blood like the formulas Six Flavor Pill with Rehmannia (Liu Wei Di Huang Wan) or Four Substances Decoction (Si Wu Tang) or the individual herbs cooked Rehmannia (Shu Di Huang), Angelica (Dang Gui), white peony (Bai Shao), Ophiopogon (Mai Men Dong), and herbs to resolve Blood stasis and obstruction, such as peach kernel (Tao Ren), moutan (Mu Dan Pi), and red peony (Chi Shao).

♦ Stimulate the acupressure points to regulate the Penetrating and Conception meridians, and to supplement Yin and Blood, including ear intertragic notch and triangular fossa, Sp 4, Pc 6, Ren 3, Ren 4, Zigong, Yintang, Sp 6, and St 36. Points to invigorate the Blood include Sp 8 and Sp 10 (see chapter 7).

TCM IN ACTION: DANNETTE OVULATES AGAIN

Dannette, thirty-three, a school librarian, had been pregnant once before when she was twenty-seven but had miscarried at six weeks. She bled profusely for two weeks afterward, had to go in to the hospital for a D & C, and continued to bleed for another three weeks before she finally stopped. Afterward, her cycles never returned to normal. She developed a red facial rash known as rosacea and always felt like her face was hot. Night sweats became commonplace as well, although her hands and feet were always cold and her BBT remained about 96 degrees. Every three weeks or so, she experienced light-brown vaginal discharge, which could barely be called "blood," for a day and a half at most. She had no vaginal discharge anymore, and had been told she was no longer ovulating because her FSH levels were elevated and her ovaries were not responding.

Perhaps you can begin to recognize Dannette's pattern of imbalance. Her miscarriage and incessant bleeding had robbed her reproductive system of its precious Blood, which is Yin. Because her fluids had exhausted (dried up) the Penetrating and Conception meridians, the production of heat (Yang) was the result. All body processes are Yang in nature, requiring and producing energetic heat. But when the basic substance Yin (in this case, estrogen) is deficient, Yang (in the form of FSH) will be unchecked, producing pathologic heat.

Dannette wanted children more than anything else, so she obtained a referral to a reproductive endocrinologist. He informed her that her uterine lining was extremely thin; nevertheless, he put her on Clomid to test her response. (You may recall that Clomid invigorates Yang at the expense of Yin, further thinning the endometrium and drying up cervical mucus.) Dannette produced one visible follicle, but her FSH rose even higher and made her feel horrible. The treatment left her with more night sweats, and now she also experienced cramping, bloating, and PMS, which she had never had before. Her doctor proclaimed her "irreversibly" infertile but said he could help her undergo IVF using a donor egg. However, Dannette could not afford this treatment, nor was she amenable to the idea of using someone else's egg if there were any way she could produce her own.

Dannette consulted me about four years after her miscarriage. She told me that she still wanted a child, but also that she had put that dream to rest. Now she just wanted her periods back. She didn't sleep well and woke up with a sore jaw because she was grinding her teeth. She suffered from occasional heart palpitations and had become irritable and anxious. The most frustrating element, however, was that she still was experiencing hormonal fluctuations. Every three weeks, her abdomen would become gassy and distended, and she would feel a burning, ripping pain in her lower abdomen, which sometimes was followed by brownish discharge. But there was no blood, no ovulation, and no relief, just a constant reminder of what she had lost. Her tongue was red and dry, and her pulse was weak and wiry.

Dannette's recent symptoms had become excess in nature, indicating too much Liver Qi and too much heat, both of which were affecting her Heart and spirit. Because of her history, I knew the nature of the imbalance stemmed from deficient Yin and Blood, so I began by supplementing them as I cleared the internal heat. I prescribed the herbal formula Anemarrhena, Phellodendron, and Rehmannia Pill (Zhi Bai Di Huang Wan), which supplements Yin and clears heat, for two weeks, followed by a modification of Rambling Powder (Xiao Yao San), which regulates Liver Qi and supplements the Spleen, to which I added red peony (Chi Shao) to cool and invigorate the Blood. I used acupuncture points Sp 4, Pc 6, Lu 7, and Ki 6 to redirect her body's attention to the Penetrating and Conception meridians. I gave her other treatments to supplement the Yin and Blood, stimulating points like Ki 3, Sp 6, and St 36. I also worked to calm the Heart using points Ht 7 and Yintang, and to clear heat with Sp 10 and LI 11, while rectifying the Liver with Lv 2, Lv 3, Lv 8, and Lv 14.

When Dannette's Liver Qi and heat

were resolved, her irritability and sleepless, hot nights vanished. Afterward, I strongly supplemented the Blood with the herbal formula Four Substances Decoction (Si Wu Tang). Her periods came back, and her cycles lengthened. When the school year started again, we had to eliminate Dannette's acupuncture treatments, but she continued with the herbs. Gradually, her body started to take over, and the next three months were characterized by incremental improvements. She began producing normal amounts of fertile cervical fluid. She ovulated the next month on day 12 and held a 14-day luteal phase. Her follicular phase lengthened next, and then she conceived.

Dannette is now back for occasional acupuncture treatments to keep her system in balance during this pregnancy. Her last ultrasound showed a strong little heartbeat in a fetus developing in a plush endometrial home.

Mechanical Infertility: Clearing the Path to Conception

I thank God for my brokenness;
only then may I heal.

— Anonymous

In the preceding chapters, we addressed the hormonal causes of infertility. Sometimes, however, a woman can't get pregnant because the path from the ovary to the uterus is compromised. For instance, the ovary could be covered with adhesions blocking the mature egg from entering the pelvic cavity; the fallopian tube could be narrowed or even completely obstructed; or perhaps the uterus is bound up with scar tissue, keeping it from holding the fertilized egg successfully. Such blockages may be caused by congenital defects, scarring from past infections, and even surgical procedures like tubal ligation and D & C.

Some cases of blockage can be resolved through surgery. In other cases, however, surgery results in a relatively small improvement in fertility, if any. In that case, IVF may be a woman's only choice. In this chapter, we'll discuss some causes and symptoms of mechanical infertility and review how TCM can provide support in healing your reproductive system.

PELVIC INFLAMMATORY DISEASE (PID)

Pelvic inflammatory disease, or PID, is one of the most heartbreaking causes of mechanical infertility, simply because it can destroy a woman's fertility without warning, long before she even considers getting pregnant. Pelvic inflammatory disease is usually the result of a bacterial infection that can involve the ovaries, fallopian tubes, uterus, and cervix. The bacteria commonly enter the body through the vagina and cervix, and from there spread throughout the pelvic cavity. More than one million women in the United States — most of them in their teens and twenties — are diagnosed with acute PID every year.

The best-known causes of PID are sexually transmitted diseases (STDs), especially chlamydia and gonorrhea. Pelvic inflammatory disease also can result from intrauterine device (IUD) use, complication from earlier pregnancy, or infection following any surgery of the reproductive tract. Depending on the infectious organism and the severity of infection, the acute phase of the disease may be characterized by lower abdominal pain, fever, painful sexual intercourse, irregular bleeding, and profuse vaginal discharge. As with any bacterial infection, signs such as these should be treated as quickly as possible with antibiotics. On the other hand, some PID infections, like chlamydia, may be silent (without symptoms of any kind) yet can cause extensive damage to the reproductive organs, especially the fallopian tubes. Untreated, chronic PID creates a condition of long-standing inflammation within the pelvic cavity, and this sets up a reactionary environment within the reproductive organs, especially the fallopian tubes. If antibiotics are not prescribed or have not been effective, PID may produce chronic scarring. Indeed, most fertility problems associated with PID are caused not by active infection but by scarring from past infections. If a woman suspects she has (or has had) PID, it's important to consult a Western medical doctor for a diagnosis and possible treatment with antibiotics.

TREATING PID WITH CHINESE MEDICINE

Since my specialty is infertility, it is rare for me to see a patient with active PID — I usually see them only long after the damage has been done. However, there are ways to use TCM to treat both the symptoms and infection of active PID. Once again, in addition to treating the manifestation of the problem, we must address the underlying imbalance.

When PID is in its acute form, it often produces a condition of damp heat (**DH**) in the body, accompanied by Blood stasis (**Bl X**) and Liver Qi stagnation (**Lv Qi X**). (This is also a common pattern seen with fallopian tube obstruction, as we will discuss later.) To diagnose PID according to TCM, we begin by looking at the symptoms that this particular kind of inflammation produces. Since most cases of PID involve abnormal vaginal discharge, TCM practitioners start by examining its quality and quantity. If the discharge is profuse and watery and without any smell or irritating sensation, it would be categorized as being damp and cool in nature. This does not mean the organism itself is "cold" per se, but the body's response to it creates a pattern of cold. Any treatment, therefore, would need to resolve dampness (by drying) and cold (by warming).

On the other hand, if the discharge appears puslike, discolored, and foul-smelling and causes irritation, itching, or burning, it would be characterized as damp heat. (Again, it is our physiologic response to the inflammation that is "hot" in nature, not the pathogen itself.) Traditional Chinese medicine treatment would be based on balancing the damp cold or damp heat conditions created by the body's response to infection. It is important to note, however, that our inflammatory response to the infection may remain for some length of time after symptoms have been resolved. In the same way a course of Western antibiotics usually must be continued for several days after symptoms of the underlying infection disappear, it is equally essential that TCM treatment continue until the inflammatory

response has quieted and the body's balance has been fully restored.

A primary means of treating excess discharge is through one of the Extraordinary meridians known as the Girdle meridian (Dai Mai). The *Nei Jing* describes the Extraordinary meridians as a system of "drainage ditches" that tap in to the main meridians and allow their excesses to run off and discharge. We drain excesses like profuse vaginal discharge through the Girdle meridian. (The Girdle meridian is described as a belt that cannot be too tight or too loose.) Although the Girdle meridian does not have any points of its own, it does tap in to points on other meridians, like the Gallbladder and Triple Warmer, so treating points like GB 26, GB 41, and SJ 5 (see chapter 7) will help clear the Girdle meridian.

Other TCM treatments for excess vaginal discharge include the following:

◆ *Herbs to resolve (cold) dampness:* Chinese herbal formula Cinnamon Twig and Poria Pill (Gui Zhi Fu Ling Wan), with the addition of herbs like mugwort (Ai Ye) to warm the channels, fennel fruit (Xiao Hui Xiang) to expel cold, and Hypoglauca (Bei Xie) to clear dampness.

◆ *Herbs that warm:* dried ginger (Gan Jiang), cinnamon bark (Rou Gui), Evodia (Wu Zhu Yu), clover (Ding Xiang), and fennel fruit (Xiao Hui Xiang).

◆ *Herbs to resolve dampness:* Poria cocos (Fu Ling), Polyporus (Zhu Ling), coix (Yi Yi Ren), and Kochia fruit (Di Fu Zi).

◆ *Acupoints to resolve dampness:* Sp 9, St 30, St 40, and Lv 8.

◆ *Herbs to resolve damp heat:* Scutellaria (Huang Qin), Coptis (Huang Lian), Phellodendron (Huang Bai), and Gentiana (Long Dan Cao).

◆ *Acupoints to clear heat:* UB 40, Sp 10, and LI 11.

If pelvic pain is the predominant problem, TCM diagnoses its underlying pattern by assessing the nature of the pain. If it is sharp or stabbing, it involves Blood stasis (**Bl X**), and we apply the principles of invigorating the Blood. If the pain is more strangulating and distending, then it involves obstruction of the Qi mechanism, and we treat to resolve Qi stagnation. Some treatment options include the following:

◆ *Herbs to invigorate the Blood:* Ligusticum (Chuan Xiong), Salvia (Dan Shen), Corydalis (Yan Hu Suo), Leonurus (Yi Mu Cao), Lycopus (Ze Lan), red peony (Chi Shao), peach kernel (Tao Ren), safflower (Hong Hua), Curcuma (E Zhu), Scirpus (San Leng), frankincense (Ru Xiang), and myrrh (Mo Yao).

◆ *Acupoints to invigorate the Blood:* UB 17, Sp 10 with Sp 6 and St 29.

◆ *Herbs to rectify (move) the Qi:* citrus peel (Chen Pi), green tangerine peel (Qing Pi), immature fruit of bitter orange (Zhi Shi), Cyperus (Xiang Fu), Aucklandia (Mu Xiang), Lindera (Wu Yao), and Melia (Chuan Lian Zi).

◆ *Acupoints to rectify the Qi:* Lv 3, Lv 2 (if heat is present), and Lv 14.

FALLOPIAN TUBE OBSTRUCTION

One of the more common results of PID is fallopian tube obstruction. The fallopian tube is the "golden path" the egg must travel to get from the ovary to the uterus. It is also the most common location for egg and sperm to meet and for fertilization to occur. The tubes contain two specialized kinds of cells: those producing mucus, glucose, and other substances needed to nourish the egg before and after fertilization, and tiny, hairlike structures called cilia that move the egg through the tube and into the uterus.

Unfortunately, the fallopian tubes are often the first location attacked by opportunistic bacteria coming from the uterus in cases of PID or other infection. And because the tubes are such narrow structures, it doesn't take much to block them. They can become inflamed within, a condition called salpingitis. They may become filled with fluid (hydrosalpinx) or pus (pyrosalpinx), creating a bulge and/or possibly destroying the lining and musculature needed to nurture the egg and move it along. (Some researchers suspect the fluid from a hydrosalpinx can seep into the uterus and have an adverse effect on implantation.) The tubes may develop adhesions and thickened walls, and close off completely. In that case, a woman's hormones can be fine, her eggs can mature, and she can even release healthy eggs every month, but the sperm may not be able to reach them. Further, if the tubes are open just enough to allow the sperm through, fertilization may occur in the fallopian tubes. Then the fertilized egg (which is much larger than a sperm) may get stuck on its journey through the obstructed tube and actually implant in the fallopian tube itself, resulting in an ectopic pregnancy, causing loss of the embryo and, possibly, further tubal damage.

Since most fallopian tube obstructions produce no overt symptoms other than infertility, most women discover the state of their fallopian tubes as a result of a laparoscopy, laparotomy, or a hysterosalpingogram (when dye is injected into the uterus, and the uterus is examined via X-ray to see if any dye spills into the pelvic cavity). Treatment for tubal blockage is always some kind of surgery, either to remove or reduce the blockage or, in the most drastic cases, to excise the occluded part of the tube itself, followed by sewing the two healthy ends of the tube together. Advances in micro- and laser surgery are making success rates higher for tubal blockage treatment. If a woman still cannot get pregnant, however, the final treatment recommendation is IVF, in which a fertilized egg is implanted directly into the uterus, bypassing the blocked tube and allowing pregnancy to occur.

❧ TREATING FALLOPIAN TUBE OBSTRUCTION WITH TCM

When the fallopian tubes are closed off, it takes powerful measures to open them. Chinese medicine employs a number of techniques to help remedy fallopian tube inflammation and obstruction. Herbs to invigorate the Blood are typically given orally to help diminish active inflammation. To eliminate tubal blockages in China, herbal concoctions are sometimes injected directly into the uterus, as in a hysterosalpingogram procedure. The herbs then flow to and through the fallopian tubes, bringing the healing effect of the herbs directly to the site of obstruction. However, in the United States, our medical/legal system will not allow any procedure involving this kind of internal delivery of herbs. Therefore, we must utilize alternatives that treat the pattern imbalance using less direct but still effective means.

Most fallopian tube obstructions have Blood stasis (**Bl X**) as an underlying pattern.

When we use Chinese herbal therapy to treat enduring diseases like fallopian tube obstruction, the stasis-resolving medicinals prescribed must be both powerful and capable of reaching the closed-off environment of the fallopian tubes. Chinese medicine calls this "resolving stasis in the network vessels" (which lie between the major vessels and are thus harder to reach). To treat Blood stasis in network vessels, we use resins like myrrh and frankincense, which are known for reaching the deepest meridians and their offshoots.

In the case of conditions residing in the uterus or fallopian tubes, women can ingest herbs that then find their way through the digestive system to the fallopian tubes. Or they can use herbal enemas (decoctions taken rectally) or suppositories (herbal concentrates in a glycerin or cocoa-butter base), both of which bypass the need for harmonizing the herbal formula for digestion. Specific acupoints can help resolve Blood stasis in the fallopian tubes: Sp 10, St 30, Zigong, St 29, Ren 3, Ren 4, and the ear triangular fossa (see chapter 7).

In terms of diet and lifestyle, cigarette smoking paralyzes the cilia, the small hairs in the fallopian tubes that help propel the eggs to the uterus. Therefore, if you smoke, stop now. I also recommend a tubal obstruction massage using a deep, kneading technique on the lower abdomen. In some cases, this deep massage can apply enough friction to the fallopian tubes to resolve the adhesions manually.

FALLOPIAN TUBE MASSAGE

The fallopian tubes extend outward from both sides of the uterus. The points most closely correlated with the fallopian tubes are located just above the pubic bone, approximately five inches down from the navel and about two inches out from the midline (see acupoint St 30 in chapter 7). Massage this area in circular, clockwise motions with your fingertips, going outward from the midline at the uterus area toward the ovary, then return to St 30. Note any areas of tension and congestion and apply deeper pressure, holding at the tighter regions. (This may be somewhat painful.) Continue the massage outward toward the ovary and back again. End with a pumping motion with the heel of the hand.

⚘ NOTE: These massage techniques should be practiced only between menstruation and ovulation, not during menses or during the luteal phase.

PELVIC ADHESIONS

Most mechanical infertility is caused by adhesions and / or scar tissue found inside or outside the organs of the reproductive tract. Adhesions form naturally within the body as a healing response to tissue trauma. They may form after injury (such as a fall or physical or sexual abuse), inflammation or infection (such as endometriosis, yeast or bladder infection, or PID), or surgery (such as D & C, abortion, cesarean section, or appendectomy). The damaged connective tissue creates a series of vascular and cellular changes that cause cross-linkage of the collagen fibers, contracting the tissue and resulting in adhesions. Wherever adhesions form, they act like a glue on neighboring structures. Unfortunately, the female reproductive structure is so delicate that it doesn't take much "glue" to severely restrict its movement and function.

Adhesions may impair the mechanical functioning of the ovaries, the fallopian tubes, and the passage between the two, blocking the egg from entering the uterus. When adhesions form within the uterus, they tend to make an inhospitable surface for implantation, often resulting in miscarriage or infertility. Adhesions on the outer surfaces of the organs in the pelvic cavity can attach these organs to each other or to neighboring structures, restricting their movement and their proper function.

Where adhesions are present, you can feel the restriction in the deeper tissues through manual palpation. Adhesions are usually detected during pelvic exams and then confirmed by laparoscopy or laparotomy. Western medical treatment is inevitably surgical and may or may not restore fertility. In some cases, however, the adhesions are so extensive that they make pregnancy impossible.

USING TCM TO TREAT MECHANICAL OBSTRUCTION

To decrease adhesions of the female reproductive tract, Chinese medicine prescribes manual massage of the pelvic organs. Applying a deep pressure to knead and stretch the abdominal area can help break up scar tissue and slowly and gently pull adhesions apart. As the adhesions decrease, function improves. These massages often are given on points related to acupuncture and acupressure meridians (see chapter 7).

In addition to the fallopian tube massage described earlier, here are some specific massage techniques to release adhesions in the uterus and ovaries.

🌿 NOTE: Please do not perform after ovulation or during menstruation.

UTERINE MASSAGE

Your uterus is located just above the pubic bone, the bony part beneath the upper part of the pubic hair. You can locate it by making an upside-down triangle with your two thumbs and index fingers. Place your thumbs at your navel and extend your fingers downward. Beneath this, at the midline, is the uterus. Place your fingers on either side of the uterus and apply a deep, kneading type of massage, pressing and lifting while massaging any tight spots. (You'll be massaging acupoints Ren 3, St 29, and St 30.) Finish with a pumping motion with the heel of the hand.

OVARIAN MASSAGE

The ovarian massage location is approximately three inches from the midline, about four inches down from the navel (the Zigong point — see chapter 7). Massage in a circular (clockwise) motion. If you note any areas of tension or congestion, knead deeply, apply increased pressure, and lift with the fingertips. Finish with a pumping motion with the heel of the hand to resolve conges-

tion and improve circulation. (If you have ovarian cysts, this massage may be very uncomfortable. Do not apply excessive force to the point of pain.)

I also like to employ the use of light or laser therapy to help resolve adhesions through electromagnetic radiation. Laser acupressure is a beautiful blending of modern technology with ancient tradition. Low-energy photonic therapy applies light to stimulate acupoints without penetrating the skin. The resulting effect of red spectrum light absorption is photochemical and aids in the production of adenosine triphosphate (ATP), the fuel of the cell. The light therapy realigns the electrical potential of collagen, which is responsible for adhesions and scar tissue. Ovarian cysts, fibroids, blocked fallopian tubes, and adhesions all have collagen constituents and can benefit from electromagnetic stimulation. (Laser pens or photonic-stimulating devices can be obtained through alternative health supply providers on the Web — see chapter 7.)

TCM IN ACTION: PAIGE'S PELVIC DAMAGE

Paige and her husband, J.D., came to see me when Paige was thirty-two. She had a history of PID when she was in college. She and J.D. had married eight years ago, and they had been trying to have a baby ever since. After two years, Paige had consulted her gynecologist for a preliminary fertility workup. When the doctor injected dye into her uterus and then viewed it on an X-ray, they knew immediately that Paige had partial fallopian tube obstruction because the dye barely seeped into the pelvic cavity on one side. Paige was referred to a reproductive endocrinologist, who performed laparoscopic surgery and removed some of the adhesions covering the pelvic cavity, fallopian tubes, and ovaries. The doctor told Paige she had endometriosis in addition to the adhesions.

After the surgery, her reproductive endocrinologist told Paige and J.D. that the most conservative course of action would be to start with injectable hormonal stimulation and IUIs. The fifth IUI worked, and she became pregnant. However, the embryo had embedded itself in the fallopian tube (an ectopic pregnancy). Paige had to take a drug that caused her to abort the embryo. Afterward, the doctor would not perform any more inseminations; it was simply too risky. Their only remaining option was IVF. Paige and J.D. decided to go for it, but the IVF was not successful. The doctor said Paige's harvested eggs were not fully mature and therefore couldn't be fertilized.

Paige's close friend was a reproductive clinic nurse who had become pregnant with my treatments. Both Paige and J.D. came to the first visit, which was ideal, as I could show J.D. how to perform some of the pelvic massage that improves pelvic circulation. From my evaluation, I was concerned about Paige's short monthly cycles (shorter than ever since the hormonal stimulation of IVF), painful ovulation, and crampy periods, with dark, clotty menstrual blood. Every month, Paige experienced a couple of days of brown spotting before her periods arrived. She also had a history of bleeding hemorrhoids, increased nighttime urination, low libido, and constant fatigue. My diagnosis was Spleen Qi deficiency contributing to a Kidney Yang deficiency with Blood stasis. I saw her once per week for acupuncture, and I stimulated pelvic points like St 30, Zigong, Ren 3, Ren 4, Ren 6, ear triangular fossa, St 36, Sp 6, Ki 7, and Sp 10. I prescribed the herbal formula Tonify the Middle and Augment Qi Decoction (Bu Zhong Yi Qi Tang) to supplement the Spleen Qi, added red peony (Chi Shao) to invigorate the Blood, and suggested she take Epimedium (Yin Yang Huo) to tonify the Yang. I also advised her to supplement her diet with fish oil and pycnogenol every day. Within a couple of months, her cycle had lengthened, and she had no pain at ovulation or menstruation. Four months after Paige began treatment, she and J.D. conceived, this time with a thriving intrauterine pregnancy.

16

Male-Factor Infertility: It Still Takes Two to Make a Baby

Unless a man asks, "Will this help? Will that help?"
I know not how to help him.

— CONFUCIUS

The number of men who come to my clinic is a fraction of my patient load, but I feel as much compassion for them as I do for my female patients. If women can feel a loss of identity and a sense of being less feminine when they can't get pregnant, men can feel less virile and even ashamed if they can't father a child. Most men are better at hiding their feelings, but based on the joy I see in their eyes when their fertility factors resolve and their partners become pregnant, I know how important fertility can be to a man's self-worth.

In the United States, approximately 15 percent of the population fall into the category of being unable to conceive. In these couples, male and female factors are equally accountable for the problem, and one in four couples has multiple factors contributing to their failure to conceive.

In men, infertility is defined as the inability to fertilize the ovum, whereas sterility is defined as the lack of sperm production. Male fertility depends upon three things: (1) adequate production of spermatozoa by the testes, (2) unobstructed transit of sperm through the seminal tract, and (3) satisfactory delivery to the ovum. Diagnosing male infertility issues usually begins with a doctor taking a thorough medical history to see if factors in the patient's past, such as mumps, failure of the testes to descend, or any sexually transmitted infections, could contribute to the problem.

The medical history is followed by a physical exam, during which the doctor looks for possible structural and / or congenital abnormalities that may cause obstruction of the seminal tract. The size and shape of the testicles are evaluated to see if they are within the normal range. Of particular interest is the presence of a varicocele — essentially, a varicose vein in the blood vessels serving the testicles, sometimes causing scrotal swelling. Occasionally the swelling caused by a varicocele obstructs the vas deferens (the passage from the scrotum to the ejaculatory duct); more often, the abnormal backflow of blood into the scrotum causes the temperature in the testes to rise, which may interfere with testosterone levels and sperm production. Around 40 to 50 percent of men who report infertility are found to have a varicocele, although it's possible this condition can be found in upwards of 10 to 15 percent of all men.

After examining the genital area, the doctor usually conducts a general evaluation of secondary sex characteristics such as breast size, amount and location of body hair, etc., as these may provide clues to an underlying endocrine disorder. Any results of the doctor's exam are usually confirmed with further tests, including a semen analy-

sis, blood hormone levels, or radiographic exams to determine if there are any conditions that could prevent the sperm from being ejaculated. One such condition, retrograde ejaculation, is caused by a weakening of the muscles surrounding the bladder and the urethra. When these muscles are too weak to close the bladder's sphincter, the ejaculate can flow backward into the bladder instead of through the ejaculate tube.

Analysis of the semen requires a sample of the ejaculate to be sent to a laboratory and analyzed for the following factors:

◆ deficient sperm count (less than 20 million per milliliter; volume should be 1 to 5 milliliters of ejaculate)
◆ insufficient sperm motility (over 50 percent should be motile and demonstrate purposeful forward movement)
◆ poor sperm morphology (less than 30 percent normal forms)

In 40 percent of cases of male infertility, sperm abnormalities are either *a* factor or *the* factor in the condition. The average ejaculate sample contains almost 200 million sperm, but amazingly enough, only a few dozen sperm actually reach the egg for a chance at penetration. This makes for some pretty ominous statistics for sperm overall. Sperm numbers must be high just to have a modicum of hope of reaching the vicinity of the egg traveling down the fallopian tube. However, sperm counts have dropped 50 percent in the last thirty-five years. (Sperm are at least as susceptible as eggs to environmental influences.) Sperm production may be affected by factors such as radiation and other environmental toxins, an undescended testis, trauma-induced or infectious testicular atrophy, drug effects, prolonged fever, and endocrine disorders affecting the hypothalamic–pituitary–gonadal axis. Low sperm counts can be aggravated, if not caused, by factors such as tight-fitting underwear or hot baths (which raise the scrotal temperature), urogenital infections, poor diet, and prescription drugs (antihypertensives and anti-inflammatories can drastically reduce sperm count). Even antihistamines can affect sperm count negatively by diminishing the quantity of seminal fluid. Stress, lack of sleep, and overuse of alcohol, nicotine, and marijuana decrease sperm production as well. If semen analysis shows results within normal parameters, and if physical examination has indicated no possible obstructions, hormone levels will be measured.

In certain couples, antisperm antibodies also may be a factor in reduced fertility. We discussed antisperm antibodies in women in chapter 12, but these cells may be produced by either partner. In both cases, the antibodies will attack the sperm as if they were dangerous invaders, killing them off before they can reach the egg. Other tests of the sperm include measuring its ability to penetrate both the cervical mucus and the outer layer of the egg.

Male infertility factors are easier to diagnose with Western methods than female infertility, but often harder to treat. In cases of mechanical obstruction, the only potential remedy is surgery. New microsurgical techniques have made it possible to repair obstructions and other problems within the narrow spaces of the vas deferens and the epididymis (the duct leading from the testes and the place where sperm mature). In cases of varicocele, the affected vein or veins are tied off surgically, or a balloon or other support is implanted in the vein to allow blood to flow freely through it again. Unfortunately, surgeries can worsen sperm counts because with every surgery there is a risk of scarring and adhesion formation.

In cases of poor sperm production or quality, some dietary and lifestyle changes can help. However, when it comes to hormonal abnormalities, Western medicine has little to offer, as supplementation with testosterone, FSH, LH, or other hormones rarely improves sperm production significantly. If a man has some healthy sperm present, the doctor may recommend that he and his partner try either an IUI or IVF procedure. In both cases, a man's sperm is retrieved either from ejaculate or by extracting the sperm surgically from the epididymis. Then the healthy sperm are separated out, and the sperm sample is placed in the woman's uterus through IUI or mixed with or injected into her retrieved eggs in an IVF procedure.

❧ THE TCM VIEW OF MALE INFERTILITY

Some men may be skeptical about treating their fertility with Chinese medicine. A few years ago, one man came to see me because his wife made him. He had low sperm count with lower back pain, as well as several other symptoms that told me his Kidney Yang was deficient. However, he told me right up front, "I don't believe this will do me any good. I told my wife I'm giving it two months, no more, and then I'm out of here." While I could understand his attitude, I also didn't want to treat someone who didn't want to be at my clinic — my waiting list is too long and there are far too many couples who *do* want to consult me. Nevertheless, I agreed to work with him, and he agreed to follow my instructions for two months. The very day the two months had passed, he declared he wouldn't be seeing me anymore because he knew the treatments were useless. Then his wife made him get another sperm analysis. Afterward, he called me and said, "I don't know what you did, but it worked!" His sperm counts were normal for the first time. He was so pleased that he referred one of his friends to me.

From a Chinese perspective, the main causes of male infertility fall under two broad categories: (1) deficiency of the Kidneys (**Ki Yi−** or **Ki Yan−**) or the Spleen (**Sp Qi−**), or (2) excess of stasis, stagnation, or damp heat (**DH**) in the pelvic organs. Even when symptoms indicate patterns of damp heat, Qi stag-

nation, and Blood stasis, they are usually superimposed upon or even caused by Kidney deficiency. Therefore, tonifying the Kidneys almost always produces an improvement in sperm production and quality. Yet building the Blood, clearing heat, or moving the Qi if the pattern fits is essential for optimum improvement. In Chinese medical diagnosis, the presence of a varicocele translates to Blood stasis (**Bl X**); it is therefore necessary to invigorate and move the Blood so the sperm can develop normally.

Almost all aspects of male infertility can benefit from TCM treatment. Certainly, sperm production and quality can be increased, some mechanical blockages can be dissolved or reduced, and even hormonal factors can be resolved by restoring balance to the entire body. While specific elements of diet and lifestyle, acupuncture, and herbs will be addressed later, here are some general recommendations.

◆ *To improve overall health:* Take the antioxidant formulas described below in "Diet and Lifestyle Changes" and add L-arginine (an amino acid involved in cellular replication) and L-carnitine (found in very high levels in sperm, this amino acid transports fatty acids into the mitochondria and assists sperm motility).

◆ *To improve poor morphology and decrease high levels of oxidants in the seminal fluid:* Take antioxidants and superantioxidants like pycnogenol. Invigorate the Blood with Blood movers.

◆ *To increase sperm counts:* Take Blood and Qi tonics and seeds like Lycium (Gou Qi Zi) and Cuscuta (Tu Si Zi).

◆ *To improve testosterone levels:* Take Qi tonics like ginseng (Ren Shen).

◆ *To improve sperm motility:* Tonify Qi and Yang. Take Cornus (Shan Zhu Yu).

◆ *To improve liquefaction:* Supplement Kidney Yin with asparagus root (Tian Men Dong), Ophiopogon (Mai Men Dong), or the formula Six Flavor Pill with Rehmannia (Liu Wei Di Huang Wan).

◆ *To resolve varicoceles:* Apply a cold pack to the scrotum twice per day and take a Blood-moving herbal formula like Cinnamon Twig and Poria Pill (Gui Zhi Fu Ling Wan).

DIET AND LIFESTYLE CHANGES

To nourish the sperm, the seminal vesicles secrete substances including fructose (which feeds the sperm), fibrinogen (which holds or coagulates the fluid together), and prostaglandins (which help the sperm penetrate the cervix). The prostate adds an alkaline fluid to the ejaculate. Seminal fluid in normal, fertile men contains antioxidant factors. However, in many subfertile men, the seminal fluid may not contain these protective elements, or the circulating free radicals may be so abundant that the seminal fluid is not capable of eliminating the damaged cells. Therefore, men with suboptimum sperm counts should include dietary sources of antioxidants like wheat and barley grass, sprouts, and dark-green vegetables.

The plasma membrane of human sperm contains high levels of polyunsaturated fatty acids, making it extremely susceptible to damage by free radicals, which can lead to lower motility and poor morphology. Adding unsaturated fatty acids like those found in sesame, almonds, flaxseed, hazelnuts, pecans, pumpkin seeds, sunflower seeds, pine nuts, walnuts, olives, avocados, soybeans, and quinoa as well as omega-3 fatty acids found in fish oil to the diet can improve sperm integrity.

Many environmental and dietary factors are hostile to the production of healthy sperm. For example, estrogen is important in sperm formation, but consuming too much synthetic estrogen in the diet can be harmful. Unfortunately, most red meat, dairy products, and even poultry and eggs contain substantial quantities of synthetic estrogens. Some reports have shown the presence of synthetic estrogen in sources of drinking water as well. Therefore, eating only hormone-free meat, poultry, eggs, and dairy products and drinking only purified water is suggested.

Many environmental toxins such as pesticides and other chemicals found in nonorganically grown produce also can impair spermatogenesis, so men should consume organic fruits and vegetables whenever possible. To support cardiovascular and reproductive health, avoid saturated fats, hydrogenated oils, coconut, palm, and especially cottonseed oil (it contains gossypol, a chemical inhibiting sperm formation). Include polyunsaturated vegetable oils and essential fatty acids like fish oil, flaxseed oil, and pumpkin-seed oil, as these contribute to the health of the sperm and seminal fluid.

A variety of natural supplements can be used to promote fertility in men. For instance, soy products contain isoflavones, or phytoestrogens with a weak estrogenic effect that actually inhibits the production of excess estrogen in the body. I do not recommend high-dose soy concentrates, however, as too much estrogen from any source can be counterproductive. Soy, other legumes, nuts, and seeds also contain phytosterols that promote testosterone production.

Almost half of the diagnosed cases of insufficient sperm count also reveal oxidative damage. The seminal fluid contains high levels of antioxidants, but when the development of healthy sperm becomes impaired because of environmental toxins, stress, or pharmaceutical agents, the seminal fluid will be found to have elevated levels of oxidants. To halt this process and prevent further free-radical damage to developing sperm, the following nutritional supplementation should be used by most, if not all, men.

◆ Vitamin C: 2,000 milligrams per day (in divided doses)
◆ Vitamin E: 800 international units per day
◆ Beta-carotene: 100,000 international units per day
◆ Selenium: 200 micrograms per day

Other important nutritional supplements include:

◆ Zinc: 60 milligrams per day (necessary for sperm production and testosterone metabolism)
◆ Vitamin B12: 1,000 milligrams per day (involved in the replication of cells)
◆ L-arginine: 2 to 4 grams per day (helps promote cellular replication)
◆ L-carnitine: 1,000 to 1,200 milligrams per day (assists sperm motility)

One of the most potent bioactive antioxidant sources, pycnogenol, is made from pine bark extract, red wine extract, grape seed extract, and bilberry extract. Pycnogenol also enhances the effects of other antioxidants. I recommend 125 milligrams per day from various sources.

If the seminal fluid is too viscous, the sperm cannot travel freely through the cervix. Men with overly viscous seminal fluid should consider taking herbs that supplement the Yin, like Ophiopogon (Mai Men Dong), or the herbal formula Six Flavor Pill with Rehmannia (Liu Wei Di Huang Wan). Guaifenesin, an expectorant found in some cough syrups, reduces the surface tension and, therefore, the viscosity of mucous secretions. I recommend men take pure guaifenesin (without other ingredients) a day or two before their partners ovulate.

Finally, since elevated temperatures in the testes can lower testosterone and compromise sperm production, I suggest men keep their scrotal temperatures between 94 and 96 degrees Fahrenheit by wearing loose underwear, avoiding hot baths, and applying daily cool packs (ice water in a plastic bag, wrapped in a thin towel, applied for ten to twenty minutes).

ACUPUNCTURE AND ACUPRESSURE TREATMENTS

Acupuncture has been shown to help balance the hormonal system and restore higher levels of virility in men. A study conducted by the College of Acupuncture and Moxibustion at the Shanghai University of Traditional Chinese Medicine in China reported on thirty-five cases of infertility caused by sperm abnormalities and treated only with low-frequency electroacupuncture. Points Sp 6, Ren 12, and Ren 4 were stimulated and moxibustion (heating the acupoints in conjunction with needle insertion) was applied. The men showed improvement in their symptoms of lumbosacral aching, frequent urination, and emission. Activity and quantity of sperm and semen quality also improved, as did spermatogenic environment (indicated by significant decreases of mucosity and liquefaction time). Equally

important, sex hormones were normalized as follows:

33.5 percent improvement in FSH levels
35.3 percent in LH levels
57.1 percent in estrogen levels
65.1 percent in testosterone levels

TREATMENT WITH CHINESE HERBS

As stated earlier, most cases of male infertility involve some element of Kidney deficiency (**Ki Yi–**, **Ki Yan–**), which can be treated effectively with Kidney-tonifying herbs. A study at the Institute of Acupuncture and Meridians, Anhui College of TCM, Hefei, China, reported that eighty-seven cases of male infertility with semen abnormalities were treated with the herbal formula Kidney Qi Pill from Formulas to Aid the Living (Ji Sheng Shen Qi Wan). Semen analysis after treatment showed sperm parameters improved in eighty-three of the eighty-seven cases, or over 95 percent of the time. By the end of the study, forty-nine of the men's wives (56.32 percent) were pregnant.

Different studies have shown that another herb, Cornus fruit (Shan Zhu Yu, used to stabilize the Kidney Essence and tonify the Liver and Kidneys), has been found to improve sperm motility. Kidney Yang tonics like Eucommia (Du Zhong), Epimedium (Yin Yang Huo), Morinda root (Ba Ji Tian), and deer antler (Lu Rong) have been found to decrease impotence, fatigue, low back pain, urinary frequency, and spermatorrhea.

Other energetic patterns and conditions that improve with TCM herbal treatment include:

◆ *Source Qi* — This is an important component in a man's reproductive health, as source Qi (our genetic constitution, which is affected by diet and lifestyle) is considered the basis of all life and cellular function. Ginseng (Chinese, Korean, or Siberian) supplements the source Qi and has been shown to promote testicular growth, testosterone levels, and sperm formation.

◆ *Sperm antibodies* — The presence of antisperm antibodies in men is treated according to the pattern creating the antibodies, whether Spleen Qi deficiency (**Sp–**), damp heat (**DH**), or Blood stasis (**Bl X**). See chapter 12 for a discussion of treating female antisperm antibodies. The same recommended dosages apply to men.

◆ *Varicocele* — Most men I treat for varicoceles respond to the use of cool packs applied twice a day to the scrotum. Men also derive great improvement from Cinnamon Twig and Poria Decoction (Gui Zhi Fu Ling Wan), which consists of cinnamon twig (Gui Zhi), Poria (Fu Ling), moutan (Mu Dan Pi), peach kernel (Tao Ren), and red peony (Chi Shao). This formula, which is traditionally used for gynecologic disorders of Blood stasis

(**Bl X**) in the Uterus, has proven very promising in treating sperm abnormalities resulting from varicocele. A study from the *American Journal of Chinese Medicine* reported thirty-seven infertile patients with varicocele were treated with 7.5 grams per day of Gui Zhi Fu Ling Wan for three months, after which semen qualities such as sperm concentration and motility were graded. A varicocele disappearance rate of 80 percent was obtained with forty out of fifty varicoceles. In addition, sperm count improved in 71.4 percent of patients, while sperm motility increased in 62.1 percent. This formula invigorates the Blood and inhibits the pooling mechanism that causes poor sperm quality.

Below you will find descriptions and symptoms of the different patterns that may contribute to male infertility, along with suggested herbal medicines and acupuncture treatments.

KI YAN– KIDNEY YANG DEFICIENCY

Signs/symptoms: aversion to cold, low back pain, coldness in the scrotum, deep and thready pulse, thin and white tongue coating, low libido, and poor erectile function.

TCM herbal prescription: Restore the Right Pill (You Gui Wan), which includes cooked Rehmannia (Shu Di Huang), Dioscorea (Shan Yao), Cornus (Shan Zhu Yu), Cuscuta (Tu Si Zi), Lycium (Gou Qi Zi), deer antler glue (Lu Jiao Jiao), Eucommia (Du Zhong), Angelica (Dang Gui), cinnamon bark (Rou Gui), and aconite (Fu Zi). For patients with aspermia: remove Eucommia (Du Zhong), cinnamon bark (Rou Gui), and aconite (Fu Zi); add Ligusticum (Chuan Xiong) and red ginseng (Hong Shen). For patients with absence of sperm liquefaction: add Hypoglauca (Bei Xie). For patients with dead sperm: add Dipsacus (Xu Duan).

Another Kidney Yang supplement is the prescription Five Seeds Developing the Ancestors Pill (Wu Zi Wan Zong Wan). This includes Lycium (Gou Qi Zi), Cuscuta (Tu Si Zi), Schisandra (Wu Wei Zi), Plantago (Che Qian Zi), and Rubus (Fu Pen Zi).

Acupuncture: Stimulate acupoints Ki 7, Sp 6, St 36, UB 23, UB 52, Du 4, Ren 4, and Ren 6.

✿ NOTE: Lack of ejaculation and/or erectile function is usually seen as Kidney Yang deficiency (**Ki Yan–**). However, we can't make this assumption automatically. Sometimes we need to calm the spirit or resolve Liver Qi stagnation (**Lv Qi X**) if present. Erection is a function of the parasympathetic nervous system, and high internal stress may block blood flow to the pelvis. We need to diminish sympathetic (fight or flight) overdrive and allow the blood vessels to relax. This may be accomplished with spirit-calming acupoints and herbs (see chapters 7 and 8), as well as by applying deep massage to the upper thighs and lower abdomen.

KI YI– KIDNEY YIN DEFICIENCY

Signs/symptoms: emaciation, lower back pain, poor sperm liquefaction, irritability, weak, frail pulse, and red tongue body.

TCM herbal prescription: Preserve the Left Pill (Zuo Gui Wan) variation, which includes cooked Rehmannia (Shu Di Huang), Dioscorea (Shan Yao), Cornus (Shan Zhu Yu), Cuscuta (Tu Si Zi), turtle shell glue (Gui Ban Jiao), deer antler glue (Lu Jiao Jiao), and Cyathula (Chuan Niu Xi). For patients with aspermia: add Angelica (Dang Gui), Ligusticum (Chuan Xiong), Ligustrum (Nu Zhen Zi), and Eclipta (Han Lian Cao). For patients with absence of sperm liquefaction: add Salvia (Dan Shen), Hypoglauca (Bei Xie), and Phellodendron (Huang Bai).

Acupuncture: Stimulate acupoints UB 23, UB 52, Sp 6, Ren 3, Ren 4, Ki 3, and Ki 7.

BL X STASIS OF QI AND BLOOD

Signs/symptoms: distended scrotum, morphology problems, diagnosis of varicocele, high levels of stress, falling and painful testicles, wiry pulse, and dark tongue.

TCM herbal prescription: Frigid Extremities Powder (Si Ni San) variation, which includes Bupleurum (Chai Hu), immature bitter orange (Zhi Shi), red peony (Chi Shao), licorice (Gan Cao), Salvia (Dan Shen), and citron fruit (Fo Shou). For men with falling and painful testes: add Vaccaria seeds (Wang Bu Liu Xing), Gleditsia (Zao Jiao Ci), tangerine seed (Ju He), and sweet gum fruit (Lu Lu Tong). For men with impotence: add Six Flavor Pill with Rehmannia (Liu Wei Di Huang Wan).

Acupuncture: Stimulate Sp 6, Lv 3, Lv 14, Sp 8, Sp 10, and UB 17.

DH DAMP HEAT

Signs/symptoms: frequent urination, pain in lower abdomen and loins, slippery pulse, signs of phlegm in throat, and yellow tongue coating.

TCM herbal prescription: Gentiana Drain Fire Decoction (Long Dan Xie Gan Tang) and Four Marvel Pill (Si Miao San) for damp heat. It contains Gentiana (Long Dan Cao), Scutellaria (Huang Qin), gardenia fruit (Shan Zhi Zi), Alisma (Ze Xie), Clematis (Mu Tong), Plantago seed (Che Qian Zi), fresh Rehmannia (Sheng Di Huang), Angelica (Dang Gui), Bupleurum (Chai Hu), licorice (Gan Cao), Atractylodes stem (Cang Zhu), Phellodendron (Huang Bai), Cyathula (Chuan Niu Xi), and coix (Yi Yi Ren).

Acupuncture: Stimulate Sp 6, Sp 9, Sp 10, LI 11, St 36, Ren 12, and UB 40.

WHEN TCM IS NOT THE CURE

Congenital absence of sperm, a condition known as azoospermia, has no known cure, and TCM treatments are not effective in resolving this condition. However, lack of sperm production caused by extreme stress does respond to the TCM principles of pattern identification and treatment with lifestyle changes, acupuncture, and herbs.

TCM IN ACTION: SCOTT AND TRINA'S IVF

Scott and Trina, both in their late thirties, were scheduled to undergo an IVF after four failed stimulated inseminations. They came to see me two months prior to their IVF to help them prepare physically for the procedure. Trina had a healthy hormonal and reproductive system, but Scott's sperm had been found to have very poor morphology (they were abnormal in shape and function). Both sperm count and motility were also well below normal levels. Scott and Trina had been told by their Western medical doctor that their only chance for a pregnancy was washing Scott's sperm to ensure only healthy ones were left and then injecting those sperm into Trina's retrieved eggs.

Scott was a chemical engineer who worked at an oil refinery, and he thought it likely that environmental toxins had played a role in his sperm parameters. However, it was not feasible for him to leave his work-place, so he went on the antioxidant regimen described above, taking daily doses of vitamins B12, E, and C, beta-carotene, zinc, selenium, L-arginine, and L-carnitine. He also supplemented twice daily with 125 milligrams of pycnogenol. I saw him once a week for acupuncture — "just for stress reduction," I told him. In addition to calming the spirit with the Yintang, the ear spirit point in the ear triangular fossa, and the ear intertragic notch (endocrine point), I harmonized the Qi with Lv 3 and LI 4, and stimulated Sp 6. Trina also received acupuncture to help her tolerate the stressful effects of hormonal stimulation and to improve blood flow to her uterus in preparation for the IVF. They left Houston a few days before egg retrieval to go to their IVF clinic, which was in another state.

They called me the following week, elated. Scott had donated his sample, and it was completely normal — count, motility, and morphology. They still proceeded with the IVF, but they did not need to do intracytoplasmic sperm injection (ICSI), which forces fertilization by injecting the sperm directly into the egg. In fact, if Trina and Scott hadn't already been committed to the IVF cycle, they would have been able to conceive naturally — and they have done so since then. Trina had an uneventful pregnancy, and I did not see her again until she brought her first son by the clinic to meet me. They now have two young boys.

17

Using Chinese Medicine to Complement Assisted Reproductive Technology

There are many paths to the top of the mountain, but the view remains the same.

— CHINESE PROVERB

Western medicine's ART applies some of the world's most advanced medical technology to help women with fertility problems become pregnant. I respect not only the expertise of practitioners of ART but also the courage, faith, and commitment of the men and women who use ART in their quest for children.

Obviously, my focus is, first and foremost, to help women restore balance to their bodies so they can become pregnant without such techniques. However, complete resolution of severe, long-term tubal obstruction (for example) using only massage, acupuncture, and herbal therapy is often unrealistic. Yes, improvements can be made, but *resolution* may not be possible. In such cases, ART is the only option for women who wish to give birth to their own genetic offspring. Applying TCM principles can help you prepare your body for an ART, support you physically and mentally during and after the procedure, and mitigate some of the difficult side effects caused by some of the medications.

The Centers for Disease Control (CDC) in Atlanta, Georgia, is the agency supervising and regulating ART use in the United States. (They also report reproductive clinics' success rates at www.cdc.gov.) The CDC defines ART as "all treatments or procedures that involve handling of human eggs and sperm for the purpose of helping a woman become pregnant." The very first successful ART pregnancy occurred in 1978. Since then, thousands of children have been born as a result of ART.

While the first ART pregnancy involved no hormonal stimulation of the mother, today most ART uses a combination of hormonal therapy and egg retrieval, followed by a meeting of egg and sperm outside a woman's body. However, the hormonal therapy tends to have side effects and undesirable symptoms, the surgical procedures can be uncomfortable, and the level of success a woman can expect may not inspire optimism. For instance, 10 to 20 percent of ART cycles have to be canceled either because a woman has not produced enough eggs or because her ovaries have become overstimulated, affecting the quality of eggs available for retrieval. Even when eggs are produced, retrieved, and fertilized, overall success rates for IVF procedures are around 28 percent in women under thirty, about 8 percent for women age thirty-nine, and 3 percent for women age forty-four. On average, women go through seven cycles of ART before they either conceive or quit. Therefore, anything you can do to increase your chances of success will definitely be worthwhile.

You need to prepare yourself in the best way possible for a successful ART procedure. Most women know they have only a certain window of time in which they can become pregnant, and each failed cycle is a lost opportunity. In addition, with IVF procedures costing upwards of ten thousand dollars per cycle, financial resources can quickly become a consideration. Therefore, you need to do everything possible to ensure you are hormonally healthy *before* you begin pursuing pregnancy through ART. The hormonal medications given during ART are designed to increase your production of eggs but are not going to help those eggs be healthy. Remember, giving birth is the goal, not pregnancy. Miscarriage rates are significantly higher for pregnancies in which hormonal stimulation has been used. (Women with mechanical fertility issues like fallopian tube obstruction who use IVF are much more likely to give birth than those with unexplained infertility or ovulatory disorders. These women account for 25 to 40 percent of those who seek reproductive assistance. I believe this is because most women with mechanical fertility issues don't have hormonal imbalances that affect the quality of their embryos.)

The need for hormonal health prior to ART applies to men as well. Conceptions resulting from fathers with sperm issues — low count, poor morphology, or impaired motility — also have higher rates of miscarriage, as well as increased instance of genetic defects. A study in the *New England Journal of Medicine* in spring 2002 reported the risk of birth defects doubles when IVF procedures include ICSI (intracytoplasmic sperm injection, which is used when sperm are not healthy enough to penetrate the egg on their own).

A woman's best response to any ART will depend upon her overall endocrine status in the few months preceding the procedure, when the follicles are developing within the ovary. Before you begin an ART, you should use any means possible to improve the quality of your eggs, rather than the number of eggs produced per cycle. *You must do everything you can to ensure you are as hormonally healthy as possible before you attempt medical reproductive assistance.*

TCM TECHNIQUES TO IMPROVE ART PROCEDURES

Time and again, TCM has helped women embarking on ART procedures improve their chances for conceiving and carrying healthy children to term. At one clinic where I often refer patients, the statistical success rate is typically around 60 percent. However, for the patients I send there, the success rate reaches 90 percent. Traditional Chinese medicine can improve the outcome of ART even in women with mechanical and anatomical obstructive factors. Indeed, as you've seen from the stories in this book, many of my patients get pregnant during the TCM treatment they are undergoing in *preparation* for a reproductive procedure. Once the underlying pattern that had been preventing pregnancy was addressed, conception occurred naturally.

NOTE: If you are currently preparing for an ART procedure or are already under treatment by a reproductive endocrinologist, you must consult your doctor before adding anything to your health-care regimen. Your reproductive endocrinologist is "driving the ship," so to speak: the doctor has to know what is going on so he or she can steer it correctly. Any TCM treatment you choose will have an effect on your hormones and your reproductive system, ideally while increasing your fertility. However, such treatments may necessitate changes in your reproductive endocrinologist's prescription. For your well-being and your relationship with your doctor, let your medical team know what else you are doing.

I prefer that my patients start their TCM treatment three months before their ART cycle, especially if there are hormonal, age, or implantation factors. That usually gives us enough time to restore adequate balance to the body's energies and organs so the ART will produce the best possible response. However, in most cases, I will tell patients to stop their herbs and acupuncture treatments when they start their ART cycle. After all, if the soil is well prepared, you don't have to keep giving it fertilizer every single day. If a woman is in good balanced health before the ART, perhaps she won't even need the procedure. But if she does, it's important for her to go through it with a good conscience and good medical guidelines.

DIET AND LIFESTYLE

Everybody who has been through a cycle of hormonal stimulation knows how difficult this process can be. Numerous visits to the clinic, daily injections, suffering through the side effects, hoping for a good response to the medication, anticipating a smooth insemination, praying implantation is successful, and the dreaded waiting for a positive or negative blood test . . . almost every aspect of the process is out of your control, and the stress is enormous.

Putting an embryo, which has been developing in an artificial laboratory setting, into the uterus changes its environment, and a change in the environment adds more stress. Therefore, you want the surroundings in which your embryo will hopefully find its home for the next nine months to be free of the toxic results of stress and tension. Even though ART procedures create tremendous hormonal and emotional demands, for the sake of your embryo you need to lower your tension level as much as possible.

You can use the principles of TCM to lower stress levels through diet and lifestyle. Begin with the following suggestions:

- Perform the femoral massage techniques in chapter 6 to improve blood flow to the pelvic organs before and during the ART, but *not* after embryo transfer.

- Do not smoke, use nicotine patches, or chew nicotine gum.

- Do not drink any alcohol.

- Do not drink any coffee.

- Eat well, using the pattern discrimination dietary guidelines listed in chapter 6.

- Take wheatgrass supplements, blue-green algae; co Q-10, pycnogenol, fish oil, and royal jelly. (You may take these all the way through your hormonal stimulation if your physician allows.) These nutritional supplements will help keep you from depleting your Essence (and taxing your Kidneys) any further.

- Exercise daily before an IVF transfer, but do not *begin* any exercise program just before or during a cycle. If you do exercise, avoid sit-ups or any jarring, high-impact, or heavy weight-lifting exercises that make you grunt and raise intra-abdominal pressure. I recommend walking, except on the days immediately following embryo transfer.

- After the egg retrieval, you may feel very uncomfortable and bloated. This is because follicular fluid may spill into the abdominal cavity during the procedure. The best remedy for this is to drink lots of water and avoid sodium after retrieval.

- After transfer, remain as calm and stationary as possible. Meditate. Breathe deeply. Listen to soothing music. Order takeout.

- Avoid straining with a bowel movement in the days following transfer. If you are prone to constipation, increase dietary fiber or take a mild stool softener (but not a cathartic/laxative).
- Listen to yourself. How will you feel best about this time? Will taking time off from work help? Do your best to keep stress hormones out of the equation. Give the embryo within you as much help as you can to settle in to its new home.

In some cases, specific supplements can help you respond better to the hormonal medications of ART procedures. For instance, patients who are diagnosed as "poor responders" (meaning they fail to produce enough hormones or mature eggs in response to the hormonal medications used during their ART protocol) are usually told their only hope is to use donor eggs. One method to improve ovarian response in poor responders is to increase blood flow to the uterus and ovaries. A study in the *Journal of Human Reproduction* reported that supplementing with 16 grams daily of oral L-arginine (taken from day 1 of the menstrual cycle until the dominant follicle reached over 17 millimeters in diameter) improved hormonal response. Another European study endorsed giving "poor responder" patients 80 milligrams per day of oral DHEA for two months to improve their response to ovarian stimulation.

Another way to improve uterine blood flow is through massage and exercise. Before and during hormonal stimulation, I recommend you perform exercises that directly increase blood flow to the pelvic organs. I especially like the femoral massage technique described in chapter 6. You also may find that the Qi Gong breathing helps you relax while directing energy to your pelvic area. (However, do not perform this exercise once embryo transfer has occurred.)

One final reminder: you are creating a healthy environment to welcome and nourish a new life within you. This new life needs every ounce of your support — physical, mental, and emotional. But one of the best ways you can support yourself and your child is to *relax*. Do what you need to do in terms of exercise, massage, supplements, diet, and herbs — but also think of the kind of mother you want to be. Remember your goal. Think of holding your sleeping child in your arms. Relax into the love you will share. Then hold that image and love in your heart as you undergo your ART procedure. That is the most welcoming environment you can create in your body and womb.

ACUPUNCTURE

Acupuncture can help improve dramatically the outcome of ART in four ways. First, it can alleviate the side effects of medical treatments and improve response to hormonal stimulation. Second, acupuncture can improve the blood flow to the uterus and ovaries. Third, it can alleviate some of the tension inherent in these extremely stressful procedures. Fourth, it can calm the uterus to prepare it for implantation.

You can use the general stress points listed in chapter 7 to lower your stress levels. You can gauge the acupuncture's effectiveness by measuring changes in hand skin temperature. Biodots (heat-sensitive adhesive strips that change color as hand skin temperature increases) are a very inexpensive form of biofeedback monitoring. As you stimulate your acupoints or do any of the breathing and meditative techniques described earlier, put a biodot on your hand to see if you can increase the heat there. An increase in hand skin temperature tells you your sympathetic nervous system response is being calmed, and so is the rest of your body.

To improve blood flow to the uterus and ovaries before retrieval, Swedish researchers used electroacupuncture on points UB 23, UB 32, Sp 6, and UB 57. You could get a similar effect by vigorously massaging UB 23, UB 52, UB 31, UB 32, UB 33, UB 34, and Sp 6 daily, prior to retrieval.

I suggest a specific pretransfer protocol on the day of embryo retrieval to regulate the Liver and Blood flow, and calm the spirit and Uterus (making the uterus nonreactive to the catheter, and therefore more receptive). I stimulate Lv 3, LI 4, Pc 6, ear triangular fossa, ear intertragic notch, Du 20, Sp 6, Sp 8, Sp 10, St 36, and St 29. Using magnets, light, or massage to activate these points will work, but I recommend acupuncture as a proven treatment. These points are stimulated only the day before and day of transfer.

HERBAL TREATMENTS BEFORE OR DURING ART

Depending upon your reasons for undergoing an ART, there are different herbal preparations you may use — always, of course, basing treatment on the underlying pattern of imbalance. For example, if you fall under the category of anovulation caused by Liver Qi stagnation (**Lv Qi X**), then you should adhere to the dietary guidelines and take the herbal preparations to help resolve stagnated Liver Qi. You also should perform the exercises described in chapter 6 to alleviate stress.

Many women who are undergoing an ART, however, are already somewhat deficient in nature, especially if they are older. Hormonal stimulation will deplete the Kidneys, and the Kidneys govern reproduction. Kidney Essence is responsible for underlying egg quality, as well as for uterine lining and other measurable responses to hormonal stimulation. Therefore, if there is one supplement I believe would best prepare the average woman for ART, it would be Six Flavors Decoction (Liu Wei Di Huang Wan), perhaps with the addition of the five seeds Cuscuta (Tu Si Zi), Rubus (Fu Pen Zi), Lycium (Gou Qi Zi), Plantago seed (Che Qian Zi), and Schisandra (Wu Wei Zi), or Eight Treasure Decoction (Ba Zhen Tang) if the deficiency involves Qi and Blood.

If your reproductive endocrinologist will allow the use of herbs during your hormonal cycle, it is important to support the Yin during the follicular phase, when the follicles are developing. The uterine lining also may be helped with Blood-tonifying herbs like white peony (Bai Shao) or Four Substances Decoction (Si Wu Tang). Certain herbs that harmonize the Qi, like Cyperus (Xiang Fu), can be used during the follicular phase, as well for those who have severe Liver Qi stagnation, and will help the body handle the stress of the procedure successfully. Cyperus (Xiang Fu) also helps to support the production of estrogen.

HORMONAL MEDICATION SEEN THROUGH THE EYES OF TCM

All hormonal medications can be categorized by their inherent energetic effects. This section will cover some of the most commonly used drugs in reproductive medicine and describe their energetic functions according to the principles of TCM. We can then apply the techniques of TCM to enhance the drugs' intended effects while reducing their unwanted side effects. When we treat side effects, the patient often responds more effectively to the medication, thus greatly improving the statistical outcome.

One important note: Weight gain can be a distressing side effect of the hormonal medications women receive. This is caused by the imbalance of excess estrogen (Yin) with too much FSH. But this is not something you want to fix, because you don't want your hormone levels balanced at this point in time — you want them high. Realize that not all side effects should be mitigated by TCM — the condition underlying the side effect (in this case, excess Yin) may be necessary for conception and implantation.

CLOMIPHENE CITRATE (CLOMID, SEROPHENE, FEMARA)

Clomiphene citrate is an orally administered nonsteroidal ovulatory stimulant, one of a group of drugs categorized as selective estrogen receptor modulators (SERMs). It is prescribed to help correct irregular ovulation (or induce ovulation in anovluatory patients), increase egg production, and correct luteal phase defect. Clomid is one of the drugs given most frequently for infertility. Originally, Clomid was intended as a form of birth control because it prevents the pituitary from perceiving circulating estrogen levels. According to Hoechst Marion Roussel (the manufacturer of the drug), Clomid is indicated for the treatment of ovulatory dysfunction in patients with PCOS and various forms of amenorrhea. Femara, a newer estrogen inhibitor, acts like Clomid but is used to treat hormonally responsive breast cancer. Recently, Femara has been used to replace Clomid in ovulation induction.

In TCM, the ovulatory stimulation provided by Clomid is viewed as having Yang-invigorating effects. It raises the Yang, lifts the Qi, and up-bears and out-thrusts the Qi (rectifying the Qi and Blood). However, by overinvigorating the Yang, Clomid disturbs the Qi and depletes the Yin. Accompanying disturbances and deficiencies in other organ systems include night sweats and hot flashes; nausea and vomiting; breast distension; ovarian enlargement; pelvic pain and discomfort; visual changes like blurred vision, lights, floaters, and photophobia; headache; and abnormal uterine bleeding. Clomid can also cause cyst formation, thin the endometrium, and thicken cervical fluid — all barriers to conception.

If a person already has damaged Yin, she is more at risk for experiencing the side effects associated with Kidney and Liver Yin deficiency. Those with Liver Qi stagnation (**Lv Qi X**) or heat symptoms will be more susceptible to experiencing the side effects (headaches, stomach upset, abnormal bleeding) but not the therapeutic benefits of this drug. Further, if the person with damaged Yin (already hot and dry) with a constitutional Blood or Yin deficiency takes a Yang-invigo-

rating drug, there is a much greater chance of failure during the Clomid-stimulated cycle. If a woman on Clomid experiences symptoms of severe hot flashes, night sweats, headaches, and irritability (all symptoms of Yang excess/Yin deficiency), this indicates that her body cannot properly adapt to the Yang-invigorating effects of the drug. Indeed, in such cases, Clomid actually can deplete a woman's fertility, and she will most likely be in the great majority of patients who do not become pregnant on Clomid.

Who, then, should receive Clomid? According to Chinese medicine, the only patients who would respond favorably to Clomid are women who have a Kidney Yang deficiency (**Ki Yan–**), Spleen Qi deficiency (**Sp–**), or cold and dampness in the Uterus (**CW**). In these patterns, the Yang-stimulating effects of Clomid can help restore a woman's ovulatory response.

There have been some studies of the effects of Chinese herbal medicines given in conjunction with Clomid. For instance, a 1989 Japanese study reported on a group of anovulatory women who previously had not responded favorably to Clomid and were given the uterine warming formula Warm the Menses Decoction (Wen Jing Tang). The dosage was 5 grams per day starting on cycle day 2 along with Clomid administration. Ovulation occurred in 49 percent of the cycles with concurrent administration of Clomid with Wen Jing Tang. However, no pregnancies resulted. This study illustrates how Chinese medicine can enhance the effects of Western fertility drugs, yet it provides further evidence that if medicine is not given according to the specific diagnostic pattern, the real aim of treatment — pregnancy — is not achieved.

If you have experienced some of the above side effects with Clomid, what should you do? If a woman with a Kidney Yin deficiency (**Ki Yi–**) scenario (especially if she has scant cervical mucus and shorter cycles) is prescribed Clomid, I recommend she supplement her Kidney Yin with formulas like Six Flavors Pill with Rehmannia (Liu Wei Di Huang Wan) or herbs like Ophiopogon (Mai Men Dong). I would stimulate the Yin-tonifying acupoints like Ki 3, Sp 6, Sp 4, Pc 6, Ren 3, Ren 4, Lu 7, and Ki 6. If she further experiences deficiency heat, I would prescribe Anemarrhena, Phellodendron, Rehmannia Pill (Zhi Bai Di Huang Wan) to tonify Yin and clear heat. In addition to the above points, I would also stimulate Sp 10 and LI 11 or UB 40 to clear heat. If you experience more of the Liver Qi stagnation (**Lv Qi X**) side effects — irritability, headaches, and visual disturbances — I would clear Liver heat with points including Lv 2 and Lv 3, LI 11 and LI 4, and take herbs such as Cyperus (Xiang Fu) and black cohosh (Sheng Ma) or the herbal formula Rambling Powder (Xiao Yao San) with added ingredients to clear heat: Anemarrhena (Shan Zhi Mu), Phellodendron (Huang Bai), gardenia fruit (Shan Zhi Zi), red peony (Chi Shao), or moutan (Mu Dan Pi).

One final word: A Clomid challenge test is often used by reproductive endocrinologists to test a woman's ovarian reserve (whether she has enough eggs left to make her a candidate for IVF). In the test, a woman's FSH levels are measured on day 3 of her cycle, she is given Clomid for approximately five days, and then her FSH is measured again on cycle day 10. If it is still high, this means there are not enough responsive eggs left in her ovaries — she has "failed" the test. Usually she will be told IVF with donor eggs is her only option. However, if a woman has recently undergone any kind of hormonal regimen preparing for an IUI or other ART procedure, for example, her ovaries are exhausted and will need time to recover. With such a patient, I will say, "Maybe you want to hold off a month before you take the test. Until then, we can work on getting more blood flow to the ovaries so they'll respond better." I've had many women who fail Clomid challenge tests come to me for treatment and then find they start to ovulate naturally. And they pass their next Clomid challenge with flying colors.

HUMAN MENOPAUSAL GONADOTROPIN (HMG) (PERGONAL, REPRONEX, HUMEGON)

Pergonal, Repronex, and Humegon are purified preparations of human menopausal gonadotropin (hMG) extracted from the urine of postmenopausal women. The drug is given by injection, and each ampule contains both FSH and LH, plus lactose.

Human chorionic gonadotropin (hCG), a naturally occurring hormone in pregnant and postmenopausal urine, is also present in Pergonal. Administration of hMG followed by hCG is used for the induction of ovulation and pregnancy in anovulatory women, but only when the cause of anovulation is functional and not the result of primary ovarian failure. Human menopausal gonadotropin is also used to stimulate increased production of follicles and eggs in women undergoing IUI or other ART.

Human menopausal gonadotropin acts directly on the ovaries to stimulate follicle development. It is administered for seven to twelve days (different clinics have differing protocols) starting at the beginning of the cycle and should result in follicular growth and maturation. To cause the mature eggs to be released, however, hCG must be given when clinical evidence of sufficient follicular maturation has occurred.

There is a 25 percent risk of ovarian hyperstimulation syndrome (OHSS) during hMG therapy, resulting in ovarian enlargement, abdominal distension, and/or abdominal pain. Adverse reactions to hMG are numerous, including pulmonary and vascular complications, adnexal torsion (twisting of the fallopian tubes), and ovarian cysts, as well as a host of other "lesser" symptoms.

Pergonal is a Yang-invigorating, warming medicinal, and its effects are similar to those of Clomid. It will offer greater therapeutic benefit to women who are not deficient in Yin, Qi, or Blood, and those whose Qi is not obstructed. If you fall under any of these categories, follow the dietary, acupressure, and exercise guidelines for your specific pattern treatment.

FOLLITROPINS/FOLLICLE-STIMULATING HORMONE (FSH) (FOLLISTIM, FERTINEX, BRAVELLE, GONAL-F)

Follicle-stimulating hormone (FSH) is required for normal follicular growth, maturation, and ovarian steroid production. Increases in the level of FSH are critical for follicular development and, consequently, for the timing and number of follicles reaching maturity. Follistim, Fertinex, Bravelle, and Gonal-F are used to stimulate ovarian follicular growth in women who do not have primary ovarian failure. These pure FSH drugs are used for women with PCOS (who have too much LH in proportion to FSH) and to increase follicle and egg production in preparation for ART procedures. The FSH present in both Follistim and Gonal-F has been manufactured by recombinant DNA technology, which ensures the purity of the genetic material and prevents possible allergic reactions. These drugs are given by injection.

Overstimulation of the ovary may occur with the use of FSH drugs as well. Adverse reactions include miscarriage, OHSS, ectopic pregnancy, abdominal pain, injection-site pain, and vaginal hemorrhage. These side effects are caused by the Qi- and Yang-invigorating nature of the drugs.

Follistim, Fertinex, Bravelle, and Gonal-F will provide greater therapeutic benefit to those who are not deficient in Yin, Qi, and Blood, and whose Qi is not obstructed. If these are your patterns, follow the dietary, acupressure, and exercise guidelines to balance your system.

HUMAN CHORIONIC GONADOTROPIN (HCG) (PREGNYL, PROFASI, NOVAREL)

Pregnyl, Profasi, or Novarel is used in conjunction with hMG or FSH treatment to induce ovulation and pregnancy in anovulatory women when the cause of anovulation is not the result of primary ovarian failure. When patient monitoring indicates appropriate follicular development has occurred after a course of hMG/FSH, one shot of hCG is given to simulate a pre-ovulatory surge in LH, which then triggers release and final maturation of eggs. Human chorionic gonadotropin also stimulates the corpus luteum of the ovary to produce progesterone, which acts on the endometrium and provides a receptive environment for embryo implantation.

Human chorionic gonadotropin should be used in conjunction with hMG/FSH only by physicians experienced with infertility problems and familiar with the criteria for patient selection, contraindications, warnings, and precautions. Adverse reactions include OHSS, rupture of ovarian cysts, multiple births, and arterial thromboembolism.

The indications, uses, and energetic category of hCG are the same as other Yang-invigorating medicinals. Those with deficient Yin or Blood, or Qi stagnation should develop a supplementing or Qi-rectifying program to improve this drug's therapeutic effect.

Human chorionic gonadotropin can also exacerbate OHSS. One study published in 1997 in the *Journal of Traditional Chinese Medicine* reported that a group of women who were prone to developing OHSS in hormonally stimulated cycles were given acupuncture instead of hCG to induce ovulation. The acupuncture caused ovulation and reduced the symptoms of OHSS.

GONADOTROPIN-RELEASING HORMONE (GNRH) AGONISTS (LUPRON)

When treating infertility, gonadotropin-releasing hormone (GnRH) agonists are often used to suppress the normal production of FSH, LH, and estrogens so that the patient's own hormones will not interfere with the medically controlled hormonal stimulation. The pseudomenopause caused by GnRH agonists produces a "clean slate" for the next drug-stimulated cycle.

Lupron, a synthetic version of GnRH, causes the pituitary to release FSH and LH initially; however, continued usage suppresses these hormones altogether. A lack of FSH and LH then shuts down ovarian estrogen production, effectively throwing a woman's body into menopause within two to four weeks of beginning treatment.

Lupron produces numerous side effects, including many associated with menopause. It can cause cardiovascular symptoms, intestinal tract problems, anemia, various pains, and other problems.

Since Lupron inhibits estrogen, or Yin, it often induces signs and symptoms of Yin deficiency and deficiency heat, like hot flashes, night sweats, and headaches. Headaches are typically located behind the eye or eyes and in the back of the head and neck, corresponding to heat rising along the Urinary Bladder or Gallbladder meridians. Chinese medicine can be used to alleviate the side effects of Lupron administration by clearing deficient heat in the channels in which it arises. Use the heat-clearing acupressure points described in chapter 7, and take herbs that nourish Yin (but not those with any estrogenic effects like Angelica [Dang Gui] and Cyperus [Xiang Fu]), in combination with those that clear deficiency heat.

Because it completely shuts down the body's estrogen production, Lupron is also used to "starve" the endometrium of estrogen in women who have been diagnosed with endometriosis. The theory is that if the endometriosis is not stimulated by estrogen, the growths will become malnourished and waste away, and so will the auto-endometrial antibodies that can prevent implantation. Unfortunately, while this approach is effective in decreasing estrogen production, it doesn't always control the auto-antibodies. The anti-endometriotic herbal formula

Cinnamon Twig and Poria Decoction (Gui Zhi Fu Ling Wan), which consists of cinnamon twig (Gui Zhi), Poria (Fu Ling), red peony (Chi Shao), Moutan (Mu Dan Pi), and peach kernel (Tao Ren), has been found to lower serum levels of immunoglobulins (thus controlling the auto-antibodies) without lowering the body's estrogen production.

When Lupron fails to down-regulate patients undergoing ART cycles, the estrogen level may remain elevated and the endometrium too thick. Since these women are not responding to the hormonal suppression of Lupron, they typically are not allowed to proceed with their ART cycle. Luckily, TCM may be able to help. Women who fail to respond to Lupron therapy are not metabolizing estrogen effectively, and any excess hormone can be cleared by invigorating the Liver channel with acupuncture and herbs. Vigorous stimulation to certain acupuncture points every other day, employing such points as Lv 2, Lv 3, Lv 14, and LI 4, can bring a woman's estrogen levels down to the desired range within just a few treatments. Herbal treatment aimed at draining the Liver channel can also help.

Before starting the down-regulation month before an ART cycle, sometimes it is necessary to bring on a woman's period. To do so, the same points listed in the above paragraph can be used, along with points such as Sp 6, GB 21, and Sp 10. Blood-invigorating medicinals added to this regimen help get the Blood moving and induce menstruation. (If your periods are scanty and short, take the Blood supplements listed in chapter 6.)

If ultrasound has shown the uterine lining or fallopian tubes are retaining fluid (which will delay or prevent your cycle because implantation cannot occur), use acupoints to drain dampness such as Sp 6, Sp 9, Ren 3, UB 66, ear triangular fossa, intertragic notch, and scalp Epang II. Herbs that help resolve fluid accumulation include algae, seaweed, coix (Yi Yi Ren), Poria (Fu Ling), Polyporus (Zhu Ling), Alisma (Ze Xie), and Hypoglauca (Bei Xie). This approach can also be helpful in resolving ovarian cysts. In such cases, direct the treatment to the ovaries with acupoint Zigong.

TCM IN ACTION: RHONDA'S ROAD

Rhonda didn't marry until she was forty-one but knew she wanted to have a family, so she and Robert began trying immediately. They were not successful, and after six months they went on to more aggressive treatments. Her doctor began by performing a Clomid challenge test. Her FSH levels, drawn on day 3 of her cycle, were higher than normal (indicating that her ovaries were not responding properly to the FSH produced by her body). She took Clomid for five days, and then her FSH levels were taken again to see how her ovaries responded. (The FSH levels should drop.) However, Rhonda's FSH levels had increased; she "failed" the test. Her doctor offered her little hope of ever being able to produce her own eggs.

When Rhonda consulted me, I diagnosed diminished ovarian reserve as a result of Kidney deficiency (a typical scenario for a woman trying to conceive in her forties). Rhonda also was developing signs of Kidney Yin and Liver Blood deficiency — sore low back, night sweats, vaginal dryness, visual changes, and hair loss. I prescribed acupuncture and herbs to nourish the Kidney Yin and Blood. As soon as we started to make a difference in these symptoms, however, Rhonda was eager to see if she could proceed with hormonal stimulation. She took another Clomid challenge test, and this time she "passed."

Rhonda was determined. She declared she was going to go through one last IVF cycle and give it her all. She went on a diet consisting of only pure, macrobiotic, organic foods and nutritionally pure substances. She took Kidney Yin- and Yang-tonifying herbs and Blood supplements every day for three months. She took a leave of absence from her job; her new job became maximizing her fertility. She diminished the stress in her life; she meditated, got massages, and took yoga classes. We worked on improving the Blood supply to her ovaries and Uterus with acupressure techniques. When Rhonda finally had her IVF, she had a fabulous response to the medication — according to her doctors, a response typical of a much-younger woman. She became pregnant during her forty-third year and gave birth to a baby girl when she was forty-four.

LIFE AFTER ART

It may be hard to imagine when you're preparing for or in the middle of your ART procedures, but there will be life after ART. Your path will take one of four directions. First, you may be pregnant (hooray!). Second, you may not be pregnant and may opt to try another ART procedure. Third, you may not be pregnant and may decide to seek other ways to have a child — through alternative medical means, donor egg or sperm, and so on. Fourth, you may decide not to try to conceive again. (If this is the case, please see chapter 18.)

If your ART procedure has resulted in successful conception, congratulations! But conception is not the end of the road. It takes quite a while to fully grasp the fact that there is a developing fetus inside you. Many of the women I treat prior to their ART procedure return to me afterward, and they are almost always in a state of disbelief. Now a whole new concern arises: the fear of miscarriage. True, the risk of miscarriage is greater with children conceived through ART. Even in a normal pregnancy, miscarriages resulting from improperly developing embryos are unavoidable. If either the egg or sperm is genetically abnormal, the pregnancy will result in a miscarriage. But there is no way to determine the health of your egg and sperm unless you have had pre-implantation genetic studies performed on the developing embryo.

If you are carrying a genetically abnormal embryo, no amount of bed rest, acupuncture, or herbs will curtail the inevitable. However, if you have cared for your hormonal status, if the blood flow to the ovaries and uterus has been good, and healthy eggs and sperm were the result of your adherence to this program, you should be able to ease your mind about the health of your embryo. Enjoy your expectant state and continue to take your vitamins (pycnogenol, and fish oil, too, if your obstetrician does not object). Use the acupressure and meditations described in chapters 6 and 7 for stress reduction.

If you are worried about miscarriage resulting from factors other than the genetic health of the embryo, there are things you can do. If ever you experience signs of cramping, bleeding, and low back pain during pregnancy, you should seek help *immediately*. We discussed miscarriages resulting from maternal factors (which are usually immunologically based) in chapter 12. If you choose to support your pregnancy with natural means, you may need to consult a licensed acupuncturist who is experienced in gynecology and obstetrics.

If you have not had success with ART, fortunately your body can recover from the extreme hormonal and physical shifts. I see many women in my clinic both before and after their ART procedures, and it takes comparatively little time and treatment before their bodies are back to normal — assuming they were healthy in the first place. However, if you have used ART for more than one cycle, it's vital that you understand the effects of hormonal manipulation on a woman's reproductive health. Drugs that compel the ovaries to produce more eggs have a long-term energetic effect of depleting the Essence of the Kidney. (This becomes more important in women age forty and older, because after forty our reproductive energies are beginning to decline anyway.) It is therefore wise to give your body a break between hormonal cycles to recover the Kidney Essence. Regardless of age, I recommend that women allow *two months or more* between rounds of ART.

Hormonal manipulation also includes birth control pills and other forms of hormonal supplements (like estrogen). Fertility is the natural expression of sufficient amounts and adequate flow (or coursing) of Qi and Blood; therefore, any environmental cause, psychological process, or drug that diminishes the amount or obstructs the free flow of Qi and Blood will inhibit the natural expression of fertility. Most forms of medical contraceptives operate either by inhibiting the production of Qi and Blood or obstructing its free flow. Some women who have been on oral contraceptives for many years or on any form of hormonal supplementation may experience permanent changes in their cycle. Treatment involves employing

methods to ensure the resumption of adequate production of Qi and Blood and its proper coursing.

No matter which procedure(s) you have been through, you should restore balance and healing to your body and soul. You have just been through a lot of physical, mental, and emotional stress. Whether you choose to start another ART cycle or take a break, or even stop trying altogether, it's absolutely vital to do everything you can to get your body as healthy as possible once more. But remember, the premises of TCM pattern diagnosis still apply. Most women who undergo ART procedures have depleted their physical resources, so begin by tonifying Qi, Yin, and Blood. Rectify the Qi, especially Liver Qi, which may have been depressed by the emotional strain of the procedure.

Finally, make sure to nourish your Heart, and not just with herbs or acupuncture. If you are still not pregnant, nurture the home of your spirit by allowing yourself to grieve. Although I truly believe there is a divine plan no matter what anguish or sorrow we bear, nothing I or anyone else can say will take away your loss. It must be felt, experienced, and mourned. The awareness of grief will eventually allow the light of acceptance to shine in so you may heal and, above all, so you may again become whole, with or without a child.

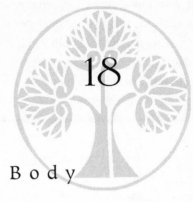

18

Healing the Soul and Body When All Else Fails

In the depth of winter, I finally learned that within me there lay an invincible summer.

— ALBERT CAMUS

We all strive for the miracle of letting life express itself through us. Some of us, however, have to take a different path to become mothers. And we may feel there is something missing: the experience of letting a life develop inside of us, of feeling the first kick, of holding our child the moment it comes into this world, of breast-feeding. For whatever reason, we have been programmed to believe motherhood is tied to these sensations. And choosing another route of becoming a mother often starts by grieving the loss of such experiences.

It is my blessing to be able to help most of the women who come to my clinic to conceive and bear healthy children — but not all of them. I believe all my patients will experience greater health by following the principles and treatments outlined in this book; yet nobody can predict if the spark of life will actually ignite. If there has been too much damage to a woman's reproductive organs, if she is approaching an age at which she no longer has healthy eggs, or if she or her husband has other medical conditions that preclude conceiving or giving birth to a child — not every couple is successful. In some cases, my role is more of a friend and guide, to support women in making difficult choices.

This chapter is about forgiveness, transition, letting go, and putting our maternal energies to use in new ways. It is about finding the invincible summer within your heart, even in the depths of winter. It is about discovering the truth of what love really means and how many ways there are to give and receive it. Most of all, this chapter is about healing your soul and body at the time they need it most.

❧ COMING THROUGH GRIEF

No grief so great as a dead heart.

— CHINESE PROVERB

When you're in the midst of trying to conceive, everything is overwhelming. All you know is you want to be a mother, and you can't. For women who have been on the infertility "treadmill" for years, making the choice to stop feels impossible. While the end of our fertility is something all women must face eventually, it is only natural to feel a sense of loss and sadness, mourning the children we will never have. But for those of us who have wanted children, making the decision to stop trying can feel like death. And the grief is real.

Grief and mourning are difficult emotions, especially in a culture like ours that prefers we do our mourning tidily and quickly. In addition, few people who have not experienced infertility can understand how much pain the unsuccessful pursuit of children engenders. They offer their seemingly simple solutions: "Maybe you're just not meant to have kids." "Have you thought of adopting?" "Isn't all this awfully expensive?" These and many other well-meaning comments can trigger new recriminations and fresh rounds of grief in those pursuing parenthood at any price. And, what's worse, showing our pain and anger to friends will usually result in blank stares or embarrassed looks.

However, for our own sanity we must be allowed to feel our grief and mourn our lost potential children. Our biggest mistake is not acknowledging our feelings as we experience them. In "Mourning the Losses of Infertility," Kim Kluger-Bell describes her own experience with infertility: "If you can't feel your grief, you can only move on by shutting a part of yourself down. . . . Although feeling your sadness won't kill you, not feeling it can harden your heart. . . . [W]hat will enable you to move on with an open heart is allowing your sadness to come and go as it pleases, rather than keeping the door locked tightly against it."

It is far better for us to experience the

small griefs along the way, to take the time to acknowledge our true feelings and their importance, and keep our hearts moist and fertile in the process. Let your monthly blood represent tears shed by the body to memorialize the passing of another opportunity. If you miscarry or fail to conceive after an ART procedure, start trying to conceive again immediately if you want, but create the space in your heart to mark what you have lost. And ask your partner to support you in the grieving process. No matter how much they may want children, men cannot feel the visceral level of loss women feel. But remember that your partner has lost something, too. In your loss, you may find consolation in each other. You may actually find each other in a new way.

Above all, remember to take care of yourself. Often, we're so busy taking care of the part of us that's going to make a baby that we forget we need to take care of the rest of us, too. Take time to pamper yourself. Get the emotional support you need, whether by talking to friends, not talking to the ones who don't understand, seeing a professional counselor, or even screaming into a pillow if that helps. Go for walks in nature. Ground yourself to the earth beneath your feet and breathe deeply. Nourish your heart and soul in as many ways as you can. Remember, if you are blessed with a child, he or she will require you to be the best mother you can be. If you are not

blessed with a child, *life* will still demand you to be the best *person* you can be.

If you choose to make children a part of your life through alternative forms of parenting like adoption, carrying a baby conceived from donor egg or sperm, or using a surrogate mother, then you must be comfortable with the fact that this child is not "related" to you biologically. However, I believe that whenever we choose to accept a child into our family, we are related to him or her on a far deeper level. First, we are related by choice. One of my patients once said to me, "Our children will always know they were wanted because we worked so hard to bring them into the world." This is equally true of the children we choose to make part of our family through adoption, surrogacy, donor egg or sperm, and so on. But in a spiritual sense, I believe these children are ours because they want us as their parents.

The way these children came to us — be it by our own eggs or ART or adoption — matters less than our tenacity, what we have gone through to make these children part of our lives. I believe the most important aspect of parenthood is letting our children know where they fit in the world, giving them a sense of belonging, no matter how they came to us. If they come *from* us, if they come *through* us, or if they come *to* us, being a parent means holding them and letting them know "This is where you belong."

🌿 CHOOSING TO LET GO AND MOVE ON

If you want to become whole,
let yourself be partial.
If you want to become straight,
let yourself be crooked.
If you want to become full,
let yourself be empty.
If you want to be reborn,
let yourself die.
If you want to be given everything,
give everything up.

— *TAO TE CHING*

Letting go is sometimes the easiest thing in the world: we know it's time to stop. "No more procedures," we say. "That's enough." But for most of us, the decision to let go is the most difficult one we have ever faced. How can we give up the dream that has consumed us day and night for years? We are not just giving up our own dream, we also are giving up the entire future that dream created. We are giving up a pursuit that has defined us for as long as we can remember. There is an identity in trying to conceive. We can even become attached to the label of "infertile." Our lives revolve around it, and it is difficult to release that obsession. As one of my patients said, "I know what it's like to be childless, but who am I if I let go of my pursuit of a child? Who will I be when I'm not pursuing this anymore? Who will I be if I am not a mother?"

Such questions can put us into a panic, or they can be the next step in a great adventure. Over and over I have seen the ending of the pursuit of fertility become an opening to a fuller idea of who we are. There will be grief and mourning, of course. We must move through the stages of grief — denial, anger, bargaining, depression, and acceptance — before we can take a look at what we would like the rest of our life to be. But in my experience, like the child who lets go of the table leg to take his or her first step, women who consciously choose to let go when they know the time is right find it much easier to step into life after infertility.

Sometimes the point where we find our souls is the point where we finally let go of our dreams. Shedding the identity of being a biological mother or of being an "infertile" woman can mean loss, or it can mean discovering the deepest truths about ourselves. Our ability to have children and our role as mother is only part of who we are. I believe one of the greatest things we can do to honor ourselves as we near the end of this path is to gently remind ourselves we are whole. Indeed, we are *more* whole because now we have more substance. As we release our fierce hold on external things and beliefs, we often come to a point of peace where we find we are not really lacking anything at all. In that place, our most fundamental needs are always met. At our core — without home, appearance, husband, profession, and, yes, even without children — *we already have all we will ever need*, and *that* is what life is trying to teach us.

The pursuit of a child is born of a deep longing of universal life to evolve — and isn't it rather grandiose of us to believe we have any control over the requirements of universal evolution? We can only manipulate our physiology; we can't control the expression of life itself. I believe that for God to breathe life into the developing cells that become fetuses and babies and human beings, harmony must be created in our physical environment; our physiologic condition; and our mental, emotional, and spiritual state. When these conditions have been met, then we must accept that if we are to become parents, we will.

I am reminded of the prayer "Grant me the serenity to accept the things I cannot change, the courage to change the things I can, and the wisdom to know the difference." We must accept our genetic constitu-

tion: there are certain aspects of our physical state that are not amenable to change. We cannot change the past, and we cannot change anybody else. We *can*, however, change our health and our experience of the present — what we put into our bodies, the environments in which we undergo stress, and our mental and emotional states.

This book has been an attempt to help you take control of everything possible that will help you have a child. But after we have done all we have control over, we must remember to breathe, and to recall we still have this present moment to allow Life to express itself through us, however it may.

Julie's "Success"

Throughout the chapters I have given examples of wondrous successes of children born under almost miraculous circumstances. Yet I consider one of my most rewarding clinical experiences what some couples might consider a "failure." Julie was lively, energetic, and fun. I immediately liked her, and we worked together for about two years. After a multitude of male and female reproductive difficulties, workups, probes, surgeries, and unsuccessful attempts to conceive, Julie decided the universe was not supporting her attempts to become a mother, the greatest dream of her life. She became depressed and angry, but out of her experiences with infertility, the most amazing spirit emerged. Julie and her husband, John, let go of their dream of becoming parents. After deciding to live her life without her own children, Julie found that her inner energetic potential became limitless. Julie is more happy and content than she has ever been in her life — not in spite of her struggle with infertility but, she says, *because* of it. Julie has since become one of my dearest friends. Like most people I admire, Julie has a depth that is borne of anguish and seemingly endless despair. But through it all she has become one of the world's wise women. And that's something you can't achieve by having your desires met.

From a "Mother of the Womb" to a Mother of the Heart

In Chinese medicine, menopause is described as the transition from our reproductive years into the "time of wisdom." At this point, the energy that has been pouring into our Uterus through the Penetrating meridian is redirected. And since the Penetrating meridian connects the Uterus to the Heart, the Heart is where our reproductive energy moves. We change from being reproductive mothers to being mothers of the Heart, where wisdom resides. Whether we are biological mothers or not, *all* women have the chance to be mothers of the Heart. We can choose to offer our love and maternal energies by creating a family with children, or we can choose to mother children, adults, groups, or organizations. Louisa May Alcott wrote, "Fatherly and motherly hearts often beat warm and wise in the breasts of bachelor uncles and maiden aunts; and it is my private opinion that these worthy creatures are a beautiful provision of nature for the cherishing of other people's children." You never know what place you will fill within

the universal plan, but I do believe with all my heart that the love that makes us want to be parents was not meant to go to waste. The *Tao Te Ching* says,

> *The Tao is called the Great Mother:*
> *empty yet inexhaustible,*
> *It gives birth to infinite worlds.*
> *It is always present within you.*
> *You can use it any way you want.*

When you become a mother of the heart, you tap in to the "Great Mother" that lies within you. That love is always there. And when you offer it to the world in any form, it will never go to waste.

If there is a divine plan and we are placed on this earth to learn and grow, then perhaps the lessons of our soul are taught through those who are put — and are not put — in our lives. Ultimately, however, we must recognize the children we wanted so much, and have done so much to bear, are not really ours to begin with. As Kahlil Gibran wrote:

Your children are not your children.
They are the sons and daughters of Life's
longing for itself.
They come through you but not from you,
And though they are with you, yet they
belong not to you.
You may give them your love but not your
thoughts,
For they have their own thoughts.
You may house their bodies but not their
souls,
For their souls dwell in the house of
tomorrow,
which you cannot visit, not even in your
dreams.
You may strive to be like them, but seek not
to make them like you.
For life goes not backward nor tarries with
yesterday.
You are the bows from which your children as
living arrows are sent forth.

The Archer sees the mark upon the path of
the infinite,
and He bends you with His might that His
arrows may go swift and far.
Let your bending in the Archer's hand be for
gladness;
For even as He loves the arrow that flies, so
He loves also the bow that is stable.

Perhaps the greatest lesson from our struggle to bear children is to find peace inside ourselves *no matter what.* I do know that finding a place of peace is the best gift we can receive. Those we love come, and yes, they go. Some don't come at all. But no matter what, we are whole and at peace. May you find that place of peace within yourself. May you find happiness. And may that happiness be unconditional.

Further Reading

Bensky, Dan, and Randall Barolet. *Chinese Herbal Medicine: Formulas & Strategies.* Vista, CA: Eastland Press, 1990.

Bensky, Dan, and Andrew Gamble. *Chinese Herbal Medicine: Materia Medica.* Vista, CA: Eastland Press, 1993.

Deadman, Peter, and Mazin Al-Khafaji, with Kevin Baker. *A Manual of Acupuncture.* Vista, CA: Eastland Press, 1998.

Flaws, Bob. *Fulfilling the Essence: A Handbook of Traditional & Contemporary Chinese Treatments for Female Infertility.* Boulder, CO: Blue Poppy Press, 1993.

Jin, Yu, M.D. *Handbook of Obstetrics & Gynecology in Chinese Medicine: An Integrated Approach.* Vista, CA: Eastland Press, 1998.

Kaptchuk, Ted J. *The Web that Has No Weaver: Understanding Chinese Medicine.* Lincolnwood, IL: McGraw Hill/Contemporary Books, 2000.

Maciocia, Giovanni. *Obstetrics & Gynecology in Chinese Medicine.* London: Churchill Livingstone, 1998.

Pitchford, Paul. *Healing with Whole Foods: Asian Traditions and Modern Nutrition.* Berkeley, CA: North Atlantic Books, 1993.

Pizzorno, Joseph E., and Michael T. Murray, eds. *Textbook of Natural Medicine.* London: Churchill Livingstone, 1993.

Te Velde, E.R., P.L. Pearson, and F.J. Broekmans, eds. *Female Reproductive Aging.* Studies in Profertility Series, Volume 9. London: CRC Press–Parthenon Publishers, 2000.

Glossary

acupoints Points on the skin where the body's energy network of meridians runs close to the surface.

acupressure Known as *Tui Na* in China, this form of stimulation energizes specific acupoints with vigorous manual massage.

acupuncture The means by which practitioners of TCM tap in to the energy system that enlivens and runs the body. Points along the meridians are stimulated using needles, normalizing the flow of Qi throughout the body.

adhesions Bands of tissue that form naturally within the body as a healing response to trauma such as injury, inflammation or infection, or surgery. Adhesions in the pelvic area can inhibit fertility.

amenorrhea Complete absence of menstruation.

androgen A male hormone, such as testosterone.

antiphospholipid and anticardiolipin antibodies These two kinds of antibodies moderate blood clotting at the placental attachment. They are thought to be associated with an immune reaction to an implanting embryo, preventing its implantation.

antral phase A stage of follicular growth when the follicle takes on a hollow, cavitylike appearance within the ovary, reaching a size of approximately 1 millimeter.

assisted reproductive technology (ART) Western medicine procedures designed to help women become pregnant. Assisted reproductive technology utilizes drugs and surgical procedures to overcome barriers to conception. Includes in vitro fertilization (IVF), gamete intrafallopian transfer (GIFT), intracytoplasmic sperm injection (ICSI), intrauterine insemination (IUI), and zygote intrafallopian transfer (ZIFT).

azoospermia A congenital absence of sperm.

basal body temperature (BBT) The temperature of a woman's body at rest.

beta-integrin 3 The protein marker that develops on the surface of the endometrium during the luteal phase and is needed to encourage a fertilized egg to implant.

biphasic A term used to describe a normal BBT chart.

blastocyst An embryo that has developed for approximately five days.

blastomere Formed when the single cell of a fertilized egg divides horizontally into two cells.

Blood A TCM term denoting one of the four vital substances of the body. It is similar to the Western medical definition of blood but has other energetic functions within the body.

candidiasis An overgrowth of intestinal yeast.

cervical dysplasia A condition of abnormal cell division of the cervix.

cervical stenosis A narrowed or constricted cervix.

chlamydia A sexually transmitted disease, often "silent" (with no symptoms). If untreated, it can cause pelvic inflammatory disease (PID) and scarring of the reproductive organs. See *pelvic inflammatory disease*.

cleavage The process of cell division in a fertilized egg.

Clomid challenge test Used to determine ovarian function.

clomiphene citrate An orally administered nonsteroidal ovulatory stimulant, one of a group of drugs categorized as selective estrogen receptor modulators (SERMs) prescribed to help correct irregular ovulation. One of the drugs given most frequently for infertility. Brand names: Clomid, Femara.

cold Abnormal cold is a TCM pattern characterized by a lack of Yang energies, which causes an organ or system to malfunction.

Conception meridian (Ren Mai) Arising from the Penetrating meridian, the Conception meridian, or vessel, is in charge of the body's Yin energy. The production of estrogen (a Yin hormone) is also connected to the Conception meridian.

corpus luteum A structure formed from the follicle after it has released its egg, this is essentially an endocrine gland, which secretes the progesterone needed to maintain a pregnancy should the egg be fertilized.

damp In TCM, one of the conditions of imbalance in the body. Dampness is an excess collection of fluid, which in severe cases becomes phlegm. See *heat*.

Dan Tien In TCM, the region two inches below the navel. A major energy spot on the body.

deficiency A TCM term used to indicate a lack of a particular energy/fluid in an Organ system or in the body overall. Also termed *vacuity*.

diindolylmethane (DIM) A component found in cruciferous vegetables, DIM stimulates more efficient use of estrogen by increasing the metabolism of estradiol.

ectopic pregnancy When a fertilized egg implants in locations outside of the uterus, usually within the fallopian tubes. The pregnancy must be terminated for the safety of the mother. Ectopic pregnancies can be caused by blockages in the fallopian tubes.

embryonic folds The fold lines that mark the separation of one group of cells from another in the developing embryo; they also mark the connection between groups of related cells. It is theorized that embryonic folds are the precursors of the meridian energy channels in the body.

endometrial glandular developmental arrest A condition in which the glands of the uterine lining fail to respond adequately to the signals of rising progesterone given by the corpus luteum.

endometriosis Abnormal growth of endometrial tissue outside the endometrium (uterine lining).

endometrium Uterine lining, which thickens and develops in response to hormones. The endometrium either receives the fertilized egg or liquefies and is shed with each monthly period.

Essence Called *Jing* in Chinese. In TCM, Essence is one of the two vital fluids of the body (the other is Moisture). Essence is stored in the Kidneys and contains the map of our genetic makeup. Essence is a key element of the body's reproductive system.

estradiol (es-tra-DIE-ol) E2 — the most prevalent form of estrogen produced by the body. Excess estradiol is associated with breast pain, weight gain, breast and uterine cancer, moodiness, and low libido.

estriol (ES-tree-ol) E3 — the weakest and friendliest (less cancer provoking) of the estrogens. It is converted from estrone and estradiol in the liver to a substance that can be excreted by the kidneys.

estrogen Estrone, estradiol, and estriol — the predominant female hormones necessary for maintaining healthy reproductive tissues, breasts, skin, and brain.

estrone (ES-trone) E1 — Intermediate in strength, estrone is the main estrogen produced following menopause.

excess A TCM term used to indicate too much of a particular energy or substance in an Organ system or in the body overall. To achieve balance, the excess condition must be resolved.

Extraordinary meridians In TCM, four deep meridians that connect several Organ systems. The Extraordinary meridians control the energies that determine growth, maturity, and aging. They also affect the hormonal aspects of reproduction and govern embryological development, genetic constitution, age, and decline. Together these meridians represent the hypothalamic–pituitary–ovarian (HPO) axis. See *Penetrating, Governing, Conception,* and *Girdle meridians.*

fibroids Uterine fibroids, or myomas, are the most common abnormal growth of the female reproductive organs. Fibroids are benign tumors that can occur on the inner or outer wall of the uterus, within the uterine muscle, or anywhere else in the pelvic cavity.

fimbriae The fingerlike ends of the fallopian tube used to "sweep" the mature egg from the ovary into the tube.

folic acid A substance extremely important in cellular division. Women who wish to become pregnant should supplement with folic acid.

follicle The structure in the ovary in which the egg develops.

follicle-stimulating hormone (FSH) Follicle-stimulating hormone is required for normal follicular growth, maturation, and ovarian steroid production. Rising FSH levels are critical for follicular development and, consequently, for the timing and number of follicles reaching maturity.

follitropins A group of drugs designed to supplement a woman's follicle-stimulating hormone (FSH). Drug brand names: Follistim, Fertinex, Bravelle, and Gonal-F.

galactorrhea Lactation not associated with childbirth or nursing.

Girdle meridian (Dai Mai) One of the Extraordinary meridians and the only meridian, or vessel, in the body that runs horizontally. The Girdle meridian "holds things in" (i.e., vaginal discharges and fetuses).

glucocorticoids Medications used by Western physicians to inhibit immunologic reactions within the body.

gonadotropin-releasing hormone (GnRH) agonists Used before IVF to suppress the normal production of FSH, LH, and estrogens so that control of these hormones may be maintained without the patient's own hormones interfering with the medically controlled hormonal stimulation.

gonadotropin-releasing hormone (GnRH) agonists Ovary-stimulating medications. See *human chorionic gonadotropin (hCG)* and *human menopausal gonadotropin (hMG).*

gonadotropin-releasing hormone (GnRH) antagonists Used during a hormonally stimulated cycle to block GnRH from reaching the pituitary, suppressing ovulation. Drug name: Antagon.

gonadotropins Naturally occurring hormones that stimulate the ovaries.

gossypol A chemical that inhibits sperm formation and is found in cottonseed oil.

Governing meridian (Du Mai) Arising from the Penetrating meridian, the Governing meridian, or vessel, controls the body's Yang energy and oversees the production of testosterone and progesterone, two Yang hormones.

guaifenesin An expectorant that can be helpful in reducing the surface tension and viscocity of both cervical mucus and sperm ejaculate.

Heart In TCM, the Organ that governs mind and spirit, controls Blood and circulatory system, and provides Blood for the Uterus.

heat Abnormal heat in the body is seen, in TCM, as a state of imbalance. Often associated with other conditions such as dampness, Kidney deficiency (**Ki–**), or Liver Qi stagnation (**Lv Q X**).

human chorionic gonadotropin (hCG) A naturally occurring hormone in pregnant and postmenopausal urine, hCG is used to induce ovulation and pregnancy in anovulatory women. Also used to stimulate increased production of follicles and eggs in women undergoing IUI or ART. Drug brand names: Pregnyl, Profasi, Novarel.

human menopausal gonadotropin (hMG) Extracted from the urine of postmenopausal women, hMG acts directly on the ovaries to stimulate follicle development. Given as part of an IVF protocol. Drug brand names: Pergonal, Repronex, Humegon.

hydrosalpinx A condition in which the fallopian tubes become filled with fluid, inhibiting fertility.

hyperprolactinemia Overproduction of the hormone prolactin, causing infertility.

hypothalamic–pituitary–ovarian (HPO) axis The system that links the brain structure (hypothalamus) with the endocrine glands (pituitary) and ovaries. Responsible for almost every aspect of hormonal regulation and ovulation.

hypothalamus Located at the base of the brain, the hypothalamus is the regulatory control center for all hormonal activity, including the production of gonadotropin-releasing hormones, which govern ovulation, menstruation, and pregnancy.

hypothyroidism A condition in which the thyroid produces too little thyroid hormone, impairing fertility and causing miscarriage or abnormal fetal development.

hysterosalpingogram (HSG) A diagnostic test during which a woman's uterus is injected with dye and then examined by X-ray to determine if the fluid spills into the pelvic cavity, assessing the patency of the fallopian tubes.

hysteroscopy A diagnostic procedure during which a small scope with a fiber-optic light is inserted through the cervix to examine the inside of the uterus.

iliac arteries Vessels that branch off the abdominal aorta, supplying blood to the pelvic organs before passing through the femoral arteries to supply blood to the legs.

immunoglobulin M (IgM) An antibody titer, found within the serum, that indicates an immune response to endometrial and other tissue. Immunologic and inflammatory conditions may produce this immune response within the body.

in vitro fertilization (IVF) A term applied to many of the ART procedures offered by Western medicine. In IVF, eggs are harvested from a woman, allowed to incubate, then mixed with sperm. Once the eggs have developed for two to five days, they are evaluated, and up to five healthy, fertilized eggs are delivered into the woman's uterus via catheter. A blood test is given ten to fourteen days later to confirm pregnancy.

indole-3-carbinol A substance produced by the body that helps the Liver rid the body of the negative (damp heat) effects of excess estrogen.

induration Hardening of surrounding tissue caused by new growth, such as fibroids.

inhibin B Inhibin B is a direct measurement of ovarian function, the ovary's capacity to produce a sufficient number of good-quality eggs capable of generating normal embryos. Granulosa cells (mostly from the dominant ovarian follicle) secrete inhibin B, which feeds back to the brain to control FSH secretion from the pituitary gland.

interleukin One of the hormonal factors in the ovaries that help determine the eventual fertility potential of the oocyte (the precursor to the egg).

intracytoplasmic sperm injection (ICSI) An assisted reproductive technique in which fertilization is forced by injecting sperm directly into the egg. Used when sperm are not healthy enough to penetrate the egg on their own.

intrauterine insemination (IUI) An assisted reproductive technique in which a washed sample of sperm is inserted directly into a woman's uterus to aid the chances of fertilization.

ischemia Decreased supply of oxygenated blood to an organ.

Jing See *Essence.*

Kegel exercise Squeezing the pelvic floor muscles that encircle the vagina.

Kidney In TCM, the Organ that contains our genetic makeup; controls the reproductive system and a woman's hormones; connects reproductive, skeletal, neurological, and endocrine systems; and stores Essence, one of the key energies of the body.

laparoscopy A surgical procedure done under general anesthetic in which the abdominal cavity is pumped full of carbon dioxide and instruments are inserted through small incisions in the abdominal wall to examine the pelvic cavity and reproductive organs.

leuprolide acetate Generic name for the drug Lupron, one of the gonadotropin-releasing hormone (GnRH) agonists.

L-glutamine L-glutamine is the most abundant amino acid in the body and is involved in many metabolic processes.

Liver In TCM, the Organ that controls smooth flow and distribution of Blood. It is responsible for all transformations in the body, including ovulation.

L-lysine An essential amino acid necessary for growth, development, and tissue maintenance and repair.

luteal phase Also known as the Yang, hyperthermal, or high-temperature phase, it lasts about fourteen days. It's called the luteal phase because the luteinized cells from the collapsed follicle undergo a structural transformation, a process known as luteinization.

luteinizing hormone (LH) A hormone produced by the pituitary gland, LH is one of the two necessary elements in preparing for fertilization and implantation of the egg.

menometrorrhagia Excessive menstruation extending beyond its normal time.

menorrhagia When menstruation is excessive.

menstruate The menstrual blood and other matter (endometrial lining) that leave the uterus during a woman's period.

meridians There are twelve major meridians, each associated to a specific Organ system. There are also four Extraordinary meridians that link the other meridians together. See *Extraordinary meridians* and *Organ systems.*

metrorrhagia A condition in which menstruation extends beyond its normal time.

moxibustion Herbal incense burned close to an acupoint during an acupuncture treatment. The heat produced by moxibustion increases the treatment's efficacy.

mucin A sticky substance produced by the endometrium. One part of mucin binds strongly to our antibodies and prevents them from harming the implanting embryo.

National Council for Certification of Acupuncture and Oriental Medicine The regulatory board responsible for ensuring national compliance with minimum educational and training requirements.

natural killer (NK) cells White blood cells that protect against foreign invaders. In women with endometriosis, thyroiditis, recurrent miscarriage, and other immune diseases, activated NK cells have been found to exist in the uterus, damaging the endometrium and any embryos that are trying to take up residence there.

network vessels Offshoots of the major meridians, like energetic capillaries.

nonsteroidal anti-inflammatories (NSAIDs) Pain relievers like ibuprofen. They block the synthesis of prostaglandins and, therefore, can inhibit ovulation.

oocyte Found in the ovary, oocytes are the precursors to a woman's eggs.

Organ/Organ system In TCM, there are twelve Organ systems consisting of six organ pairs, plus some Extraordinary organs such as the Uterus.

ovarian hyperstimulation syndrome (OHSS) In OHSS, the ovaries become enlarged and inflamed — a side effect seen with ovarian stimulation and often aggravated by hCG administration in the course of IVF treatments.

pelvic inflammatory disease (PID) Usually the result of a bacterial infection that can involve the ovaries, fallopian tubes, uterus, and cervix.

Penetrating meridian (Chong Mai) One of the Extraordinary meridians, or vessels, it communicates with the other meridians. In women, the Penetrating meridian originates in the Uterus and presides over menstruation, hormones, and our psychoneuro-endocrinological systems.

perfusion Passage of a fluid (like blood) through a specific organ or part of the body.

Pericardium The fibrous sac that encloses the heart. In TCM, the Pericardium protects the Heart from emotional stress and strain.

perineal muscles Muscles in the pelvic floor that support a woman's reproductive organs.

phytoestrogens Estrogenic compounds found in plants. Chemically similar to estrogen, phytoestrogens (like soy and Angelica) produce mild estrogenic characteristics in the body.

polycystic ovarian syndrome (PCOS) In PCOS, multiple small cysts, which are actually tiny follicles, develop inside the ovary, impairing fertility.

premature ovarian failure (POF) A condition affecting a woman's fertility in which her ovaries cease to function long before the average age for menopause.

progesterone A hormone secreted by the corpus luteum of the ovary after ovulation. Necessary for the development of the uterine lining so a fertilized egg can implant.

prolactin A lactation hormone released by the pituitary gland that is often elevated in women during times of stress.

prostaglandin(s) Hormonelike substances that act as chemical messengers and have a function in cellular regulation.

pyosalpinx A condition in which the fallopian tubes become filled with pus. Can inhibit fertility.

Qi In TCM, the universal energy contained in all things. A bioelectrical force that flows throughout the body and is carried by the meridians.

Qi Gong Ancient Taoist practices that involve certain exercises focusing on the basic life force — the breath.

rectify In TCM, the term used for correcting the energy in a particular Organ system.

RESOLVE A national support organization for women with fertility issues.

retrograde ejaculation A weakening of the muscles surrounding the bladder and the urethra, causing the ejaculate to flow backward into the bladder.

retrograde menstruation A condition in which menstrual blood is not discharged through the cervix but seeps back up through the fallopian tubes and flows into the abdominal cavity.

salpingitis Inflammation of the inside of the fallopian tubes. Can inhibit fertility.

selective estrogen receptor modulators (SERMs) See *clomiphene citrate.*

shen In TCM, a form of energy translated as Kidney and Spirit, which governs the reproductive system.

sonohysterography An ultrasound examination during which saline is injected into a woman's uterus.

spermatorrhea Seminal emission without intercourse, through nocturnal emission or masturbation.

Spleen In TCM, the Organ that governs energy production, metabolism, digestion, and elimination. A healthy Spleen is essential for a healthy menstrual cycle.

stagnation A term used to describe energies that are not circulating properly throughout the body.

stasis A term used to describe Blood that is not circulating properly. Blood stasis is analogous to silt.

Stein-Leventhal syndrome see *polycystic ovarian syndrome (PCOS).*

systemic lupus erythematosus An autoimmune disease affecting many systems of the body.

Tai Chi Traditional form of exercise and movement practiced by the Chinese.

traditional Chinese medicine (TCM) A system of medicine that originated in China thousands of years ago.

trans fatty acids Toxic form of fatty acids, which can impair the proper functioning of the immune and reproductive systems.

Trichomonas vaginitis A common yeast infection in the vaginal area.

trilaminar Used to describe the development of the three-layered endometrium prior to embryo implantation.

Triple Warmer (San Jiao) An Organ with no physical counterpart in Western medicine. In TCM, the Triple Warmer is the pathway that connects the Organs in the body that deal with water: Lungs, Spleen, Kidneys, Small Intestine, and Urinary Bladder.

Uterus In TCM, one of the Extraordinary Organs. Called the "palace of the child," the Uterus is the source of the Conception and Penetrating meridians.

varicocele A varicose vein in the blood vessels serving the testicles, sometimes causing scrotal swelling and /or a rise in scrotal temperature.

vas deferens The passage from the scrotum to the ejaculatory duct.

vascular endothelial growth factor A chemical found in a damaged heart, it is also seen in a woman's ovaries as she ages. It is a signal to the body that the follicular tissue is being starved of blood flow.

Yang In TCM, one of two opposites that create the universe and are present in everything, the other being Yin. Yang energy is hot, quick, burning, bright, light, and aggressive. Yang is also one of the four vital substances in the body.

Yin In TCM, one of two opposites that create the universe and are present in everything, the other being Yang. Yin energy is yielding, receiving, cold, slow, dim, passive, and heavy. Yin is also one of the four vital substances in the body.

zygote The term for a fertilized egg between the time when egg and sperm unite until first cleavage.

Acknowledgments

Thank you to Victoria St. George of Just Write Literary & Editorial Services for turning my professional work into poetry. I would like to thank my literary agent, Carol Susan Roth, for her expert guidance along this pathway; Brian Carli for his beautiful illustrations; and Little, Brown and Company for their careful editing and guidance.

Thanks to all the reproductive physicians who have opened themselves to incorporating this work into their practice, to my colleagues at Eastern Harmony, and to RESOLVE for offering refuge for so many women facing fertility issues. Throughout the years, I have learned a great deal from my teachers in Eastern and Western medicine, both in the United States and in China. Finally, I am very grateful to my husband, Ed, for his endless patience in this process, and to my children, Theresa, Kyra, and Lars, who are the gifts that make everything worthwhile.

My deepest gratitude goes out to my patients, who are also my teachers and whose stories make this work possible. They bring me their broken dreams and allow me to accompany them on their journey toward becoming whole. I honor their journey, and I hope their stories will inspire newfound hope and healing in others.

Index

nosis, 43; and diet, 81, 93; and exercise, 81, 93; and herbal therapies, 139–40; and luteal phase defect, 170; and male–factor infertility, 254, 257, 259; and miscarriage, 212; and premature ovarian failure, 238, 239; and Yang phase of menstrual cycle, 73; and Yin phase of menstrual cycle, 60, 61, 70, 71

Lao Tsu, 21, 25
L–arginine, 85, 184, 254
L-carnitine, 85, 254
LI 4 (Joining Valley), 114–15, 119, 121, *128*
LI 11 (Bent Pond), 117, *128*
lifestyle changes: and advanced maternal age, 180; and assisted reproductive technology, 265–66; and autoimmune infertility, 206; and balance, 55, 56; and conception, 78–79; and endometriosis, 225–26; and fallopian tube obstruction, 247; and fertility issues, 85–87; and male-factor infertility, 255–57; and sperm production, 253. *See also* exercise; meditation; relaxation techniques
light therapy, 106–7, 249
listening, and diagnosis, 40–41
Liu Wan Su, 29
liver, and Western medicine, 32
Liver/Gallbladder system: and meridians, 27; and pulses, 42; and stress, 32–33
Liver Qi: and diagnosis, 41; and estrogen, 32; and ovulation, 32, 61; and premenstrual phase, 65–66
Liver Qi stagnation: and acupuncture points, 114; and assisted reproductive technology, 267, 269, 270; and autoimmune infertility, 203, 205; and basal body temperature, 59; and Blood phase of menstrual cycle, 68; and diagnosis, 46; and diet, 97; and endometriosis, 220, 221; and fibroids, 224; and herbal therapies, 135–36, 148–49; and luteal phase defect, 168, 170; and male-factor infertility, 259; and ovulation, 72; and pelvic inflammatory disease, 243; and premenstrual phase, 74–75; and Spleen Qi deficiency, 48; and stress, 87; and unexplained infertility, 193, 194; and Yang phase of menstrual cycle, 63, 64, 65, 73, 74
Liver system: and Blood, 24; and fertility issues, 42; functions of, 35; and Kidney system, 48; and menstruation, 29; and ovulation, 61
longevity, 173
looking, and diagnosis, 37, 40
LPD. *See* luteal phase defect (LPD)
Lu 7 (Broken Sequence), 111, 121, *128*
Lung/Large Intestine system: and meridians, 27; and reproductive system, 29
Lung Qi, and meridians, 24

luteal phase, of menstrual cycle, 60, 62–65, 72–74, 137, 163–64
luteal phase defect (LPD): case study on, 170–72; causes of, 14, 62, 161; and cold Uterus, 167; diagnosis of, 162–63; and endometriosis, 217; and herbal therapies, 165, 167, 170; and Kidney Yang deficiency, 165–67, 168; and Kidney Yin deficiency, 170; and Liver Qi stagnation, 168, 170; and progesterone, 22–23; and Spleen Qi deficiency, 165, 166, 168; and Spleen system, 31; and Western medicine, 162–63
luteinizing hormone (LH): and herbal therapies, 133; and luteal phase defect, 162; and polycystic ovarian syndrome, 228; and sperm production, 253; and Yin phase of menstrual cycle, 61
Lv 2 (Moving Between), 114, 117, 121, *128*
Lv 3 (Great Rushing), 114, 115, 119, 121, *128*
Lv 8 (Curved Spring), 113–14, *126*
Lv 14 (Cycle Gate), 114, *123*
lymphatic massage, 90

magnetic stimulation, 106
male-factor infertility: case study of, 260–61; and traditional Chinese medicine, 254–61; and Western medicine, 251–53. *See also* sperm production
massage: and advanced maternal age, 184; and endometriosis, 225; and fallopian tube obstruction, 247; femoral massage, 88–89, 265; lymphatic massage, 90; ovarian massage, 249; and reproductive system, 88–90; uterine massage, 248–49, 266
maternal age: and fertility, 4, 5. *See also* advanced maternal age
mechanical infertility: and assisted reproductive technology, 263; case study on, 249–50; causes of, 242; fallopian tube obstruction, 245–46; pelvic adhesions, 247–48; pelvic inflammatory disease and, 243–45; and traditional Chinese medicine, 248–50
medications, 84, 85, 131–32, 175, 206–7
meditation: and assisted reproductive technology, 265, 267; and Heart deficiency, 97; and Spleen Qi deficiency, 95; and stress, 87; and unexplained infertility, 194. *See also* Qi Gong breathing
men: and acupuncture, 103; and diet, 85; and infertility treatment, 11. *See also* male-factor infertility; sperm production
menometrorrhagia, 67
menopause: advancing onset of, 183; and estrogen, 22; and Kidney system, 30; and premature ovarian failure, 236; and traditional Chinese medicine, 180, 282
menorrhagia, 67
menstrual cramps, 119
menstrual flow irregularities, 191–92

About the Author

Randine Lewis, Ph.D., M.S.O.M., is a licensed acupuncturist and herbalist who studied both Eastern and Western medicine. After attending medical school, she earned her graduate and postgraduate degrees in acupuncture, Oriental medicine, and alternative medicine, focusing on fertility.

Dr. Lewis directs Fertile Soul Retreats and speaks nationally on behalf of professional groups, acupuncturists, and infertility organizations. She is a professional member of RESOLVE, the American Infertility Association, and the American Society for Reproductive Medicine, and is a medical expert on the International Council on Infertility Information Dissemination. Dr. Lewis's intensive fertility retreats have been featured on many national and local television and radio talk shows that have spotlighted her successes treating infertility with traditional Chinese medicine. For more information on *The Infertility Cure,* Dr. Lewis, treatments, and infertility retreats, go to www.theinfertilitycure.com.

Look for these other books
on pregnancy, birth, and childcare

The Pregnancy Book

A Month-by-Month Guide
by William Sears, M.D., Martha Sears, R.N.,
and Linda Hughey, M.D., F.A.G.O.G

America's foremost baby and childcare experts tell you what to expect, month by month, from conception through birth.

Your Newborn: Head to Toe

Everything You Want to Know About Your Baby's Health
Through the First Year
by Cara Familian Natterson, M.D.

Unlike virtually any other book that covers childbirth, this guide focuses not on the mother's experiences but on the child's. Read it before delivery, take it along to the hospital, and consult it throughout your baby's first year.

The Birth Book

Everything You Need to Know to Have a Safe
and Satisfying Birth
by William Sears, M.D., and Martha Sears, R.N.

Straightforward, reliable answers to questions about every aspect of birthing, from selecting the right environment to decreasing the chances for a Cesarean birth.

The Baby Book

Everything You Need to Know About Your Baby
from Birth to Age Two
by William Sears, M.D., Martha Sears, R.N.,
Robert Sears, M.D., and James Sears, M.D.

The "baby bible" of the post–Dr. Spock generation — newly revised, expanded, and brought thoroughly up to date with the latest information on everything from diapering to daycare.

Little, Brown and Company
Available in paperback wherever books are sold